Introduction to Recreation Services for People with Disabilities: A Person-Centered Approach

Second Edition

Charles C. Bullock
University of Nevada, Reno

Michael J. Mahon
The University of Manitoba

SAGAMORE PUBLISHING
Champaign, IL

Interior Design: James Wilkerson, Michelle A. Summers, and Janet Wahlfeldt
Cover Design: Chuck Peters
Production Manager: Michelle A. Summers

ISBN: 1-57167-381-4
Library of Congress Card Number: 99-69187
Printed in the United States

This book is dedicated with love to our wives and best friends, Kay Holjes and Maureen Mahon, without whose constant support and encouragement this project would not have been completed.

Contents

SECTION III

APPENDICES

Acknowledgments

No book is ever written by a single author or, in this case, two authors. This book is no different. This book represents the culmination of years of reading, teaching, thinking, and talking with students, friends, colleagues, and libraries. There is no way to thank everyone who has been a part of this book. For those unnamed, however, know that your contribution was significant in the development of this book.

We want to thank our students at the University of North Carolina and the University of Manitoba who have helped us in ways that we never imagined. You are graduate and undergraduate students who span nearly thirty years collectively. We appreciate your insights and challenges. We appreciate your willingness to listen and learn from us and for our opportunity to listen and learn from you. Your patience as well as your insights have truly enriched this book.

We also acknowledge and thank our colleagues and staff at the Universities of Nevada, Manitoba, and North Carolina for countless hours of research, typing, proofing, editing, and encouraging. We are particularly indebted to Julie Baird, Hollie Johnson, Michelle Seibert, and Julie Schell from the University of Nevada at Reno, and Erika Bockstael, Heather Adams-Sdrolias, and Sandra Goatcher at the University of Manitoba, and Tammy Spurgin, Jeanette Rozier, and Mary Beth Rubano at the University of North Carolina at Chapel Hill.

Supportive colleagues in the Center for Recreation and Disability Studies at the University of North Carolina at Chapel Hill, the Recreation Studies Degree Programme at the University of Manitoba, and the Health, Leisure, and Human Performance Research Institute at the University of Manitoba deserve more thanks than we can possibly offer. Carrie, Jack, Leigh, Maureen, Kelly, Karen, Jennifer, Betsy, Zana, Dan, Laurel, Candy, Hal, and Charlsena, you provided us with a rich environment in which to work and play. Your constant support and queries helped us to continue to move forward even at times when progress seemed stalled.

You were colleagues who helped us grow and helped us continue to learn and contributed in so many ways to the realization of this book. A particular and heartfelt thanks for the contributions of Carrie McCann, who was the first member of what would become the Center for Recreation and Disability Studies. Carrie, your friendship, insights, and assistance have made a lasting impression on both of us and your contributions are sprinkled throughout this entire book. Your work with the LIFE (Leisure Is For Everyone) project is at the heart of the entire second section as well as Chapter 13. Thank you for your major contribution. We also sincerely appreciate the work of Karen Luken, also at the Center for Recreation and Disability Studies. Karen, your assistance in Chapter 12 expanded an area that would have been weak otherwise. We appreciate your assistance in the development of that chapter. We also acknowledge the contributions of Laurie Selz, a doctoral student in Special Education at the University of North Carolina at Chapel Hill. Laurie, your work on Chapter 14 made "An Introduction to Therapeutic Recreation" a chapter that we feel will give students a strong overview to this dynamic field. We acknowledge the expertise of Frank Brasile of the University of Nebraska-Omaha and Jennifer Mactavish of the University of Manitoba. Your work in the second edition revisions of Chapter 15, "Sport and People with Disabilities," has strengthened that chapter.

To Charlsena Stone, you were an untiring graduate assistant and colleague. Your assistance in finding references and graphs, typing, and editing is greatly appreciated. Your hard work and attention to detail in the development of the Instructor's Guide for this book will be a real help to instructors who use this text. And to Dr. Lee Meyer, who was both doctoral committee member for Mike and colleague and friend of both Mike and Charlie for so many years, we thank you for being our mentor and friend. Your insights too are sprinkled throughout much of this book.

We would like to thank our families, without whose love this book would not have been completed. To Katie, Brennan, and Seann, we both have felt your love and support in so many ways. To Maureen and Kay, who probably should be listed as co-authors, we thank you for helping us to achieve our goal.

Finally, the writing of this book would not have been possible were it not for the insights of the countless people with disabilities with whom we have spent time during the past few decades. Hopefully, you can hear your voices, thoughts, admonitions, and encouragement throughout this book.

Together, we have completed a text that we hope will be useful to students in a variety of fields.

Charles C. Bullock, Ph. D. - University of Nevada, Reno
Michael J. Mahon, Ph. D. - University of Manitoba
March 1999

INTRODUCTION

The second edition of this book represents a significant revision to our first edition. The fields of disability studies and recreation are rapidly changing. It is important to us that our book reflects the most current research and thinking about these interdisciplinary fields. For example, in the field of disability studies, the World Health Organization is in the final stages of approving a new definition of disability, to more aptly reflect the perspectives of the disability community. We have included this new definition in our revisions. The field of recreation and leisure studies has also made significant advances. This past year, in 1998, *Therapeutic Recreation Journal* published a series on the key practice models in therapeutic recreation, which included critical responses by practitioners and academics. This too is included in this second edition. There are many other updates and revisions we have made. One significant addition to this edition which we think will really help students as you more fully explore the issues presented is the inclusion of a related websites section at the end of every chapter. The changes are highlighted throughout this introduction.

The first edition of this book was "in the works" for many years. It was written and rewritten in our heads many times. As we worked, taught, studied, and wrote in the area of recreation and disability, we constantly thought about the full array of recreation services for people with disabilities. We devoted much of ourselves to this enterprise and we loved it. As such, we tried to add substance to the second edition to keep the information current.

It is important to us that we are on the same wavelength with you, the reader. That's why we have written this introduction to tell you our perspective. To us, recreation is very important. This book is about recreation and therapeutic recreation services for people with disabilities. There are similarities, but there are major differences in recreation and therapeutic recreation. For example, recreation services are purely enjoyable, while therapeutic recreation services are enjoyable but intentionally more goal directed and treatment oriented. In this book we will describe the full range of recreation services for persons with disabilities.

Another important part of our perspective is that recreation services must be centered within the person who is being served. That is, whether treatment-oriented recreation therapy, goal-oriented special recreation, or activity-oriented inclusive recreation, it is the person and not the professional or even the activity that must be at the center of service delivery. This is not a new concept; however, it is one that has not been adequately emphasized within the recreation and therapeutic recreation literature. If there is one central theme in this book, it is that people with disabilities are people who have the same needs and wants as anyone else and deserve the right to be at the center of recreation and therapeutic recreation services that are ostensibly "for" them.

About the Book

This book represents our personal learnings and beliefs that have come from many sources, particularly from people with disabilities with whom we have worked, our students through more than twenty-five years of collective teaching experience, and our colleagues. We both have extensive experience working with people with disabilities. As we have worked with people with disabilities, we have learned about them and learned from them. Probably the deepest learning from them, however, is that each person with a disability is a person, not a disability. For example, as a recreation leader in a special recreation program, Mike once worked with John and Sarah, who were blind. He worked with them and got to know them over a period of several months. Mike had not spent much time around people who were blind, so he did not know much about blindness. Mike assumed that by working with John and Sarah, he had learned about blindness and about people with blindness. In fact, however, Mike had learned more about John and Sarah than he had about blindness. Mike realized that even though they both were blind, they had very different needs and wants, let alone skills and capabilities. Mike had learned a lot about two people and a little about blindness!

There are countless stories from both of us that reiterate the importance of centering the services within the person. Some of these stories are from treatment settings and others are from inclusive recreation settings. The examples span the full range of recreation services. Yet, the message is always the same: "Treat me as a person first. Let me be involved in decisions that involve me. Do not stereotype me because of my disability." We heard them then and we have tried to write this book from that perspective.

Manifestations of disabling conditions differ from person to person. There are indeed some generalities about blindness or mental retardation or mental illness, but people with disabilities expect to be treated as people not prejudged because of their disability. Throughout this book, as we give examples and explanations, we will always discuss the importance of centering recreation services within the person.

In addition to the insights we have gained from people with disabilities, as we have taught students in recreation and therapeutic recreation curricula, we have learned from them as well. As professors, we always try to challenge our students and ask that we be challenged as well. We want our students to think critically and to go beyond mere memorization of information. We want the same of you, our readers. We want you to read for concepts and to think critically about these concepts. That is why there are suggested "Learning Activities" at the end of each chapter. You will see that the learning activities are practical and pragmatic and require you to go beyond the text as you think critically about your response. Through the years, our students have taught us that they are more interested and more motivated to learn when they are involved in their learning in a meaningful way. We have attempted to write this text to facilitate interest and motivation.

We have always told our students that we expect to learn from them. They often patronizingly nod affirmatively, never really believing that they have anything to "*teach*" us. Nothing could be further from the truth. We have learned countless things from students. Our students have challenged long-held beliefs and concepts and have insisted that we rethink and sometimes modify our positions. Students assume that their professors have read all of the relevant literature. Professors have not and can not read all of the relevant literature. In fact, there is often "relevant" literature in places professors may not routinely look. However, our students' work has often uncovered new literature in journals that we had yet to discover. Their papers have often sparked alternative thinking that has allowed us to go beyond thinking about issues in the same way. In this book, we have used the collective wisdom of many of our students. This book is sounder because of the contributions to our learning from our students. We hope that you will participate in this learning and that you will teach your instructors at the same time.

Not only have we learned from people with disabilities and from our students, we have also learned from our colleagues. We are indebted to the many whose work we have read. In many cases, we have had the privilege of discussing and sometimes arguing issues and topics with the authors and researchers. We count as our colleagues not only those educators, researchers, and practitioners in recreation and therapeutic recreation, but also those in special education, rehabilitation, social work, psychology, and other related and sometimes seemingly unrelated fields. This book is strengthened by the diversity of thought from so many of our colleagues.

More about the Book

This book is intended to be an introductory text for all students in parks and recreation/leisure studies curricula. Every student, whether she intends to work in a provincial park or a state hospital, a community recreation center or a community mental health center, a public school or a cruise ship, needs a basic level of knowledge about people with disabilities. As a result of current legislation and a societal sensitivity to diversity, people with disabilities are increasingly present in all types of recreation service systems. Therefore, all recreation professionals, not just therapeutic recreators, must know something about people with disabilities. You will not learn enough to become a therapeutic recreation specialist, but you will learn enough to understand therapeutic recreation. If you are interested in pursuing a therapeutic recreation specialization, you will have a strong base from which to continue your more detailed study in that area. If, on the other hand, you are interested in tourism, recreation management, or some other specialization, you will know enough to feel comfortable including people with disabilities into your ongoing activities and programs.

Following this "Introduction," the book is divided into three sections and a "Conclusion." Section I contains six chapters that establish the philosophical, conceptual, historical, and political underpinnings of recreation and persons with disabilities. Section II includes six chapters that provide both general and specific information about people with disabilities. Section III discusses the recreation service delivery system and issues and trends related to service delivery. The concluding chapter in this text revisits the central themes of this book in an effort to address issues and trends and to challenge all students to promote person-centered and responsive services and programs.

Since the central theme of this book is that people with disabilities are people who have the same needs and wants as anyone else and deserve the right to be at the center of their services, attention is given in Chapter 1 to a person-centered understanding of disability. Initially there is a discussion of the new definition of ***disability*** put forth by the World Health Organization in order to establish a continuity of terms that will be used throughout the text. This is an important addition to the 2nd Edition. Next is an introduction to "people first" and positive language that will familiarize you with preferred terms that focus attention on the uniqueness and worth of an individual rather than emphasizing the individual's disabling conditions or perpetuating stereotyping based on negative labels and images. In Chapter 1 of this second edition, we also present data on the number of people who are considered to have a disability.

To further understand the issues presented in the text, a history of the treatment of people with disabilities is presented in Chapter 2. The harsh and seemingly inhumane treatment will be eye opening to most readers. Very little of the history we present even resembles our person-centered theme. Yet, it is important to understand "where we have been." An understanding of the past makes it clear why there is a need for ever-increasing person-centered and responsive services.

Chapter 3 provides a philosophical and conceptual basis for much of the information about people with disabilities presented in Chapter 1. The major concepts covered in detail are normalization/social role valorization, self-determination, independence/interdependence, and inclusion. These concepts are consistent with a person-centered approach to recreation services and will be referred to both implicitly and explicitly throughout the text. We have expanded and significantly updated our analysis of these concepts in the 2nd Edition. It is these concepts that will ensure that people with disabilities, whether in a recreation or a therapeutic recreation environment, will be encouraged and supported to achieve their full potential. These concepts, if learned and practiced, will place the person and not the professional at the center of service delivery.

Chapter 4 recognizes the importance of legislation in understanding past and current services to people with disabilities. The chapter begins with the earliest legislation of modern times and moves toward more current legislation. We have made certain that the 2nd Edition presents the most up-to-date legislation in both the United States and Canada. To make this section more meaningful, a brief overview of how laws and their regulations are determined is presented. Following that, five U.S. laws and their subsequent amendments that form the core of current protection against discrimination for people with disabilities are presented. Throughout this section, Canadian legislation that roughly corresponds to these five core laws also is presented. The final law that is presented is the Americans with Disabilities Act (ADA), which is the most persuasive piece of civil rights legislation that has ever been passed in North America. In many ways, the ADA is the culmination of the other *core* laws. The ADA has such an impact on all areas of life that it is covered in even more detail than the other four.

Since all of these core laws deal with protection against discrimination, Chapter 5 covers how people with disabilities are treated today. We will look theoretically at attitude formation and attitude change as we suggest that as aspiring professionals in recreation, you must become advocates for the rights of all people. This chapter also covers accessibility and the removal of barriers to ensure equal access to all people. The information presented in Chapters 4 and 5 is very detailed, yet it is information that is important for all potential recreation and therapeutic recreation professionals to understand. In fact, the basic premise (person-centeredness) of this text is supported and reinforced by recent legislation, which has grown out of several pieces of core disability rights legislation.

The final chapter in Section I (Chapter 6) begins our discussion of recreation and therapeutic recreation services. We first describe recreation and leisure as important parts of the lives of all people. We juxtapose work and leisure, as is so often, although unknowingly, done. We then begin a basic overview of therapeutic recreation, special recreation, and inclusive recreation. We describe all terms as recreation-based, but we try to make clear distinctions among the various services. We particularly explain the differences in ***services*** and ***settings*** since our extant literature is filled with inaccuracies in this area. The concept of ***mandate*** for service is presented as a way of organizing and understanding various services. Throughout this chapter, attempts have been made to relate recreation and therapeutic recreation to the information presented in this section.

Each chapter in Section I (and in each subsequent section) includes thought questions as independent and/or interactive learning activities as well as references to assist you in more detailed study of a particular topic.

Section II includes chapters that familiarize you with basic information about various disabling conditions. This section begins with Chapter 7, which is a detailed discussion of a number of issues that cut across all disabilities. Issues and topics that are covered include the individual versus categorical approach to understanding and working with people with disabilities. Other topics include information about life-span issues such as the various transitions throughout life, cultural diversity, and poverty and employment. In this chapter we acknowledge the importance of focusing on the individual, rather than on the disability, but at the same time recognize the need for you to have some information about specific disabling conditions. Many people do not neatly fall into one disability category, but in fact, have more than one disabling condition. As such, we will consider the issue of multiple disabilities within this chapter. Because the field of disability studies is changing rapidly, we have revised this section quite extensively in our 2nd Edition to capture the most recent thinking on all of these topics.

Following this introductory information in Chapter 7, information about disabling conditions is presented. This information is basic, but we feel it is essential that all future recreation professionals be informed about different disabling conditions. It includes information about broad categories of disabling conditions, such as people who have mental retardation (Chapter 8), people who have physical disabilities (Chapter 9), people who have visual impairments (Chapter 10), people who have hearing impairments (Chapter 11), and people who have mental illness (Chapter 12). We believe that this level of information, as well as the knowledge of where to find more detailed information, is sufficient for any recreation professional to be able to provide responsive, person-centered recreation services to all people. Of course, the more specialized the service, the more in-depth knowledge about disabilities is needed. Since this is a textbook for all students in recreation curricula, it is not intended to provide the level of detail needed for a person to become a therapeutic recreation specialist. Rather, it is intended to provide basic information that is needed by anyone who comes in contact with people with disabilities. The person wishing to pursue a career in therapeutic recreation will no doubt need to learn more specific information about implications of disabling conditions, as well as medical/psycho-social terminology that is pertinent to clinical practice. This, hopefully, will come from future courses, as well as from practicum and internship experiences. Whatever your career aspirations, the information presented in Section II will provide a strong and needed base.

Section III moves beyond the disability-specific information to discuss the service delivery system that includes recreation, therapeutic recreation and sport. Chapter 13 explains recreation services that are available to people with disabilities. The bulk of recreation services for people with disabilities are found within public recreation programs. This is true both in Canada and in the United States. However, in both the United States and Canada, these recreation services and programs within the public sphere have mostly been segregated — that is, programs that were only available to people with disabilities. With current federal laws it is clear that there will be more and more emphasis on integrated or inclusive recreation programs. In this chapter we explain the differences between integrated and segregated/specialized programs. We describe the special recreation service delivery model and give examples of exemplary special recreation throughout the United States and Canada. We then describe the LIFE (Leisure is for Everyone) philosophy which is a philosophy of integrated/inclusive recreation services from an individual and an organizational perspective. Following an overview of the LIFE philosophy, exemplars of integrated/inclusive recreation services throughout the United States and Canada are presented.

Chapter 14 describes the nature of therapeutic recreation. In this chapter, there is a presentation of various definitions and models as well as a discussion of the various settings in which therapeutic recreation specialists work. In this second edition we have added some discussion on the review of practice models published as a special series in the 1998 volume of *Therapeutic Recreation Journal.* The first edition included only three models. In the second edition, we have added the conceptual model presented by Dattilo, Kleiber, and Williams (Self-determination and enjoyment enhancement: A psychologically-based service delivery model for therapeutic recreation) as a fourth model. There is detailed presentation of the therapeutic recreation process, including assessment, goal setting, treatment/discharge planning, intervention, documentation, and evaluation. After reading this chapter, students should have a clear picture of what a therapeutic recreation specialist does and a solid base to build the clinical skills necessary to work as a therapeutic recreation specialist. Students not interested in pursuing therapeutic recreation specialization will understand and better appreciate therapeutic recreation and the potential interfaces with other recreation settings.

Sport and people with disabilities is explored in Chapter 15. As in public recreation, there are also issues about how participation should and can occur within sport. Within this chapter we provide an overview of the history of sport for people with disabilities. In addition, we describe the benefits of sport for people with disabilities. We then describe the delivery system for sport, using wheelchair athletics and Special Olympics as examples of different types of sport systems for people with disabilities. The final part of this chapter discusses some of the controversies/issues within sport that exist today.

Chapter 16 focuses on leisure education as a key process that can be utilized in both recreation and therapeutic recreation settings. On the one hand it can be education for leisure, while on the other it can be used as an individually conceptualized intervention. In this section we describe in detail the definition and process of leisure education. We give examples from therapeutic recreation and recreation to make the concept clear both in Canada and in the United States.

The concluding chapter of this book deals with issues and trends in the area of recreation and disability. As we continue to stress the importance of person centeredness, we suggest that our field move more toward a community membership paradigm which presupposes inclusion and move away from the current recreational paradigm which allows integration. Other issues covered in this chapter are issues that are crucial to the lives of people with disabilities and are consistent with the community membership paradigm. They include supported living, advocacy, self-advocacy, friendships/community connections, natural supports, and futures planning. The concept of supported living goes beyond the fragmented treatment of housing, vocational preparation, recreation involvement, etc. Supported living looks at the whole person and asks, "What does this person need (regardless of the severity of disability) to live within his/her community?" As such this chapter considers such issues as friendship, community connections, self advocacy, natural rather than simply paid supports, and myriad other related concepts that are necessary for person rather than professional centeredness. All of these issues involve recreation in some way. Therefore, rather than to talk narrowly about recreation and only secondarily about the larger issues, we have chosen to first look at the current issues and trends and then determine how recreation can or should be involved. This is entirely consistent with centering recreation in the person and will ensure that recreation and therapeutic services are provided on the basis of needs and strengths rather than only on professional judgment.

Summary

It is our hope that you will begin to see people with disabilities as people as you learn about recreation and therapeutic recreation services. If you emerge from this book (or your class) with this person-centered knowledge, then you will have learned a lot about how to provide recreation services to people with disabilities. Whether or not you happen to be a person with a disability, our more earnest hope is that you will emerge from this with a commitment to ensure that people with disabilities are treated as people who are at the center of their programs and services. This means that you will become an advocate, maybe even a zealot, on behalf of people with disabilities. You will encourage friends and colleagues to use "people first" language. You will refrain from jokes that perpetuate stereotypes. You will be part of a new breed of recreation and therapeutic recreation professionals who celebrate differences and strive to provide person-centered and responsive services.

Learning Activities

1. How can you teach your fellow students and your instructor? Think about your previous life experiences, including but certainly not limited to how you like to be treated, a memory of a critically ill or institutionalized relative, a movie, a television show, a conversation you have had, or something you have observed but may not have even thought about. All of these experiences, combined with many others, make you who you are. This is your stock of knowledge and gives you much to share with others. Discuss with a classmate or a friend the extent to which you believe that you have or ever will have anything to teach to others. Discuss your level of confidence about sharing/teaching. What makes you reluctant to take on this role of student as *teacher*? Next, write down two things that you can teach others. (They do not have to be original, just things from your stock of knowledge that you can teach others.)

2. What do you notice about the way the authors refer to people with disabilities? What specific phrases and concepts do the authors use? Choose a person in your class who has read the same introductory material that you have read and discuss these two questions.

SECTION I

CHAPTER 1

WHO ARE PEOPLE WITH DISABILITIES?

INTRODUCTION

Who are people with disabilities? Since people with disabilities are the major focus of this book, we need to be clear about what we mean by the use of the phrase "people with disabilities." People with disabilities are often our neighbors, our family members, our teachers, and our friends. People with disabilities are not *them*. They are *us*! As Shapiro (1993, p. 5) suggests:

> There are hundreds of different disabilities. Some are congenital; most come later in life. Some are progressive.... Others are episodic and progressive. Some conditions are static .... Still others ... can even go away... Each disability comes in differing degrees of severity.

Regardless of the specifics of a particular disabling condition, first and foremost when we talk about disability, we are talking about *people* who happen to have disabilities. Beyond that, it becomes somewhat more difficult because we are talking about a wide range of people who have a wide range of conditions that may cause functional limitations in many different areas of life. We are talking about people who are considered hearing impaired, visually impaired, or cognitively impaired. We are talking about people who have psychological or emotional difficulties. We are talking about people who have significant physical limitations. But it is not that easy. Just because a person has a diagnosed disability, he may or may not consider himself to be handicapped. What one person might describe as a limitation, another person might describe as merely an inconvenience. However, to establish some common ground, we will provide definitions of some key concepts. In Section II of this text we will give considerably more detail about different disabling conditions.

DEFINITION OF DISABILITY

There is often confusion over such terms as disability, handicap, and impairment. They are often used interchangeably, yet, can imply very different things. In 1980 the World Health Organization published a definition of disability titled the International Classification of Impairments, Disabilities, and Handicaps (ICIDH). This was a cause-and-effect model which indicated that disease/injury leads to functional and organic impairment, which leads to disability in a person's behavior and activities, that results in some level of handicap. According to ICIDH and Environmental Factors International Network (1998), the model was criticized because of its linear nature — suggesting that the disablement process occurs in a linear fashion. In 1993, the World Health Organization agreed to begin a process to revise the ICIDH. Five years later, following an exhaustive international collaboration, the Beta 1 draft of the International Classification of Impairments, Activities, and Participation (ICIDH2) was presented. This draft is undergoing one final modification process with the intention being to adopt a new definition by the World Health Assembly in 1999.

Figure 1.1
The Beta 1 draft of the International Classification of Impairments, Activities, and Participation (ICIDH2) (Adapted from ICIDH and Environmental Factors International Network (1998))

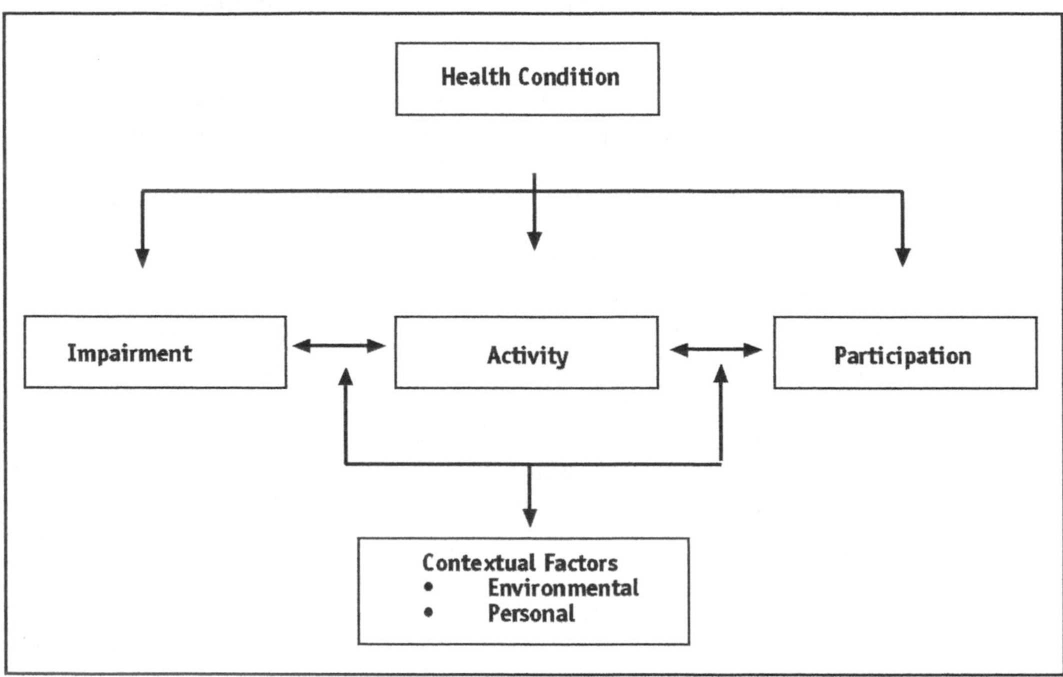

The revisions to the definition of disability have occurred within the context of a society that has developed an enhanced awareness of the functional limitations faced by many of its citizens. Such things as increased recognition of the importance of including people with disabilities in community life and a redefinition of health to move beyond the absence of illness to focus on quality of life have served as a backdrop for this new definition. The draft ICIDH2 proposes three dimensions: Impairment, Activity, and Participation. Figure 1.1 provides a graphic representation of the relationship among these dimensions.

According to this new definition, disablement is an umbrella term that includes three key dimensions — body structures or functions, personal activities, and participation in society. The Personal Activities dimension is formerly the category disability, and participation is formerly handicap. It is clear, even at this level, that the redefinition is much more focused on the abilities of the person, as compared to his disabilities, which is certainly in keeping with the philosophy of this book. Figure 1.1 also suggests that disablement is a complex relationship that includes the interaction between the disorder or disease and personal and environmental contextual factors. Personal Factors are intrinsic to the individual and include such things as gender, age, other health conditions, fitness, lifestyle, and individual psychological assets. Extrinsic to the individual are Environmental Factors such as attitudes of society, architectural structures, and legal systems.

According to ICIDH and Environmental Factors International Network (1998, p. 27), "Impairment is a loss or abnormality of body structure or of a physiological or psychological function." Rather than the underlying pathology, impairment is the manifestation of the pathology, which can be permanent or temporary. The second dimension, Activity, is the level of functioning of the person, which can be limited in the nature, duration, and quality. This dimension refers to the individual's capacity to perform things that we consider typical in our lives, such as walking, talking, driving a car, writing a letter, eating a meal, or for the Canadian reader, ice skating. The final dimension is Participation. Participation is, in a sense, the operationalisation of the disablement process, in that it refers to the person's engagement in the activities of life, as a function of his impairment(s), health conditions, and contextual factors.

What should be clear from this new definition of disability, is that the process of disablement is complex. It is a function of multiple factors that are both intrinsic and extrinsic to the individual. This book will discuss many of the factors that can contribute either positively or negatively to the disablement process. A disability is a construction of many factors, some of which we can influence. Our goal in this book is to provide you with information and ideas on how you can have a positive influence, or in a sense, work to limit the process of disablement for the people with whom you come into contact.

People-First Language

Hutchinson and McGill (1992) suggest that language tends to shape beliefs about a person's potential needs and desires. Language is very often the manner in which the subjective norm is communicated. A Parliamentary Committee on the Status of Disabled Persons in Canada concluded that:

> vocabulary can orient an entire perception in the public mind; pejorative or negative words not only bias a person's understanding, but trivialize genuine community support for people with disabilities. (Department of the Secretary of State of Canada, 1992, p. 4)

Much debate has taken place regarding the appropriate language to use in relation to individuals with disabilities. Historically, the terms disabled, handicapped, or more specific descriptors such as "blind" were most commonly preceded by the article "the." Such labels as "the disabled" or "the blind" categorize and imply that all people with disabilities are similar. Instead of making reference to the mentally retarded or the intellectually disabled, we should use the more acceptable and appropriate term: "people with mental retardation" or "people with intellectual disabilities." Referring to people with disabilities as the disabled or the mentally retarded creates an image of a group of people, all of whom have many of the same characteristics. In fact, such labels as "the blind" and "the mentally ill" often do not even include the additional word "people". A person who works in an institution for people who are mentally ill can often be heard describing her job with the phrase: "I work at Dorothea Dix State Hospital with the mentally ill." Although unintentional, such usage is dehumanizing and places more emphasis on disability than on personhood. Once such phrases become commonplace in our language, they can lead to our conscious or unconscious stereotypical attitudes that all people with disabilities are the same. Nothing could be further from the truth.

The aim of this text is to foster an individual, not a categorical, approach to understanding and working with people with disabilities. The language that we use must contribute to, rather than detract from, this goal. There is growing consensus that the use of "people first" language promotes a positive attitude toward people with disabilities and contributes to our focusing on each individual. People first means exactly what it denotes. That is, when we talk about people with disabilities, we first say "people" followed by "who are..." or "who have..." or "with..." That emphasizes personhood before acknowledging the disability. We should be careful and deliberate about the words we use and the way we refer to people with disabilities. What may seem tedious initially as we use people first language will become second nature over time. People with disabilities are individuals like any other members of society and should be referred to using people first language.

The cartoon in Figure 1.2 makes the point clearly about language and people with disabilities. It suggests that when considering the language we use, we not forget the person, whether it be Joan, Jim, or Samantha. During the past few decades, great concern has often been expressed by professionals and advocacy groups regarding the terminology we use to describe people with different types of disabilities. Nearly every professional and advocacy group in the United States and Canada have provided strong leadership in the promotion of positive language in the disability movement.

Figure 1.2

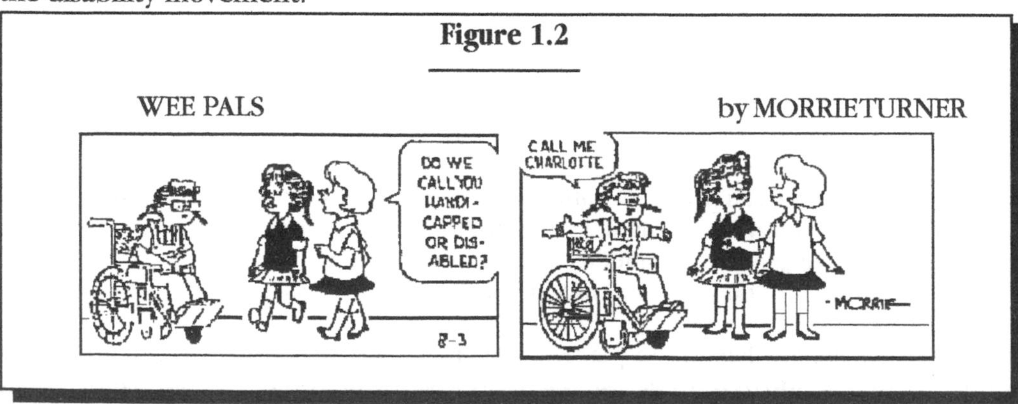
WEE PALS
by MORRIE TURNER
DO WE CALL YOU HANDI-CAPPED OR DIS-ABLED?
8-3
CALL ME CHARLOTTE
MORRIE

Create Positive Images

In addition to using "people-first" language, we should be careful not to use negative or pejorative words. Certain terms can be dehumanizing and can perpetuate negative stereotypes about people with disabilities. Terminology that emphasizes the person rather than the disability is preferred. A list of phrases in Table 1.1 gives examples of both positive, appropriate terminology as well as negative, inappropriate terminology. Many of the negative, inappropriate phrases are ones that we have heard or used throughout our lives. Many people do not even think of the negative image they present when they call a person a *cripple*. Nearly everyone has joked about *psychos* or *dummies*, thinking nothing about it. What is important, however, is to think about it, to "catch ourselves" as we unintentionally use negative or pejorative words. Others will notice our deliberateness and hopefully will model our language. Still others will not notice and we will have to explain to them why we do not say, "confined to a wheelchair." We will have to explain that we use positive, ability-oriented language rather than negative, inability-oriented language. Our persistence will be a good role model for others. Table 1. 1 provides some examples of appropriate, positive language as well as negative, less appropriate language when referring to people with disabilities.

Table 1.1

Examples of Appropriate/Inappropriate Terminology

Appropriate	Inappropriate
Person with a disability	Disabled person, the disabled, the handicapped, handicapped people
Individual with mental retardation/ intellectual disability	MRs, dummy, feebleminded, mentally retarded person, the mentally retarded
Person with a physical impairment	Disabled people, cripple, invalid
Person with Down Syndrome	Down, Mongoloid
Person who is blind	Afflicted with blindness
Person with mental illness	Lunatic, psycho, crazy, schizy
Person who is unable to hear or speak	Deaf and dumb, deaf mute
Person who uses a wheelchair	Wheelchair bound, confined to a wheelchair
Child	Special child

These preferred terms focus attention on the uniqueness and the worth of an individual rather than emphasizing the individual's disabling condition. The connotation of disability is very important to avoid. It is not uncommon to hear someone use words that are outdated or that are dehumanizing and create a negative image of the individual. Such terms contribute to negative stereotypes and should be avoided. They include such words as ***crazy, defective, deformed, retard, lame, cripple, spastic, unfortunate,*** etc. By choosing words carefully, you can convey positive images about people with disabilities. As a recreation specialist, you will be expected to model good behaviors in your communication with and about people with disabilities.

"People-first" language focuses on the sequence in which a term such as ***disability*** and words like "person" or "individual" appear in a written or spoken sentence. The sequence of the word individual before disability focuses the sender or receiver of the sentence on the reference being made to ***a person***. Reversal of this sequence, such as saying disabled people or blind people, tends to focus both the sender and receiver on the diagnostic label. It is often argued that the use of "people first" language in either written or verbal communication is awkward. Hutchison and McGill (1992, p. xvi) suggest that "Whenever we use language, we are making choices about how we want to define the situation or the person." As more people with disabilities become active participants in community life, our shared vocabulary will continue to change. When in doubt about the correct word to use, simply ask the person or his friends and family what he prefers. Remember that it is best to focus on getting to know a person, not a disability. We stress the importance of making the decision to use "people-first" and positive language as one method of fostering a person-centered approach to recreation and therapeutic recreation services.

How Many People Have Disabilities?

It is difficult to say exactly how many people there are with disabilities in the United States or Canada. A National Health Interview Survey (NHIS, 1989) estimated that there are 43 million people in the United States who have at least one disability. The estimate of Canadians with at least one disability is proportionally the same. In point of fact, however, estimating the number of people with disabilities is not that easy.

There are no simple, straightforward answers. Some people with disabilities do not admit that they have a disability, while others do not even consider themselves to have a disability (ICD survey, 1986, p. 14). Americans with disabilities are evenly divided between those who do and those who do not consider themselves disabled (handicapped) persons. About 49% of people with disabilities said they consider themselves disabled (handicapped), while 50% said they do not. However, there are dramatic differences in self-perceptions between slight or moderately disabled people and those who are severely disabled. Only 19% of people who identify themselves as slightly disabled and 32% of those who identify themselves as moderately disabled consider themselves disabled. Large majorities of those who identify themselves as severely disabled (58%) or very severely disabled (77%) consider themselves disabled (handicapped) people. People most likely to consider themselves disabled (handicapped) are those over 45 years, those disabled later in life, those most limited in their activities, and those who describe their disability as severe. But, 23% of people who identify themselves as very seriously disabled do not consider themselves disabled (handicapped). Many factors clearly influence self-perceptions about disability (handicap).

The way surveys are constructed dictates the populations that will be solicited as well as the responses that will be given by those surveyed. Already clear is that the very definition of the term disability varies depending on who asks the questions and what information is sought. As such, the statistics on the size of the population of individuals with disabilities depend on various program statistics serving selected eligible people, on information collected in surveys addressing broad social issues, or on interpretations of data designed to achieve particular programmatic purposes (*Rehab Brief*, 1993).

Indeed, there are many different answers to the question: "How many people with disabilities are there?" It is important to realize that estimates vary given the specific use for the data. For example, in pushing for legislation, advocates may adopt a larger, more general number, such as the 43 million number used in the Americans with Disabilities Act (ADA). On the other hand, a person doing a more targeted study may use a different number to refer to more specific information on particular populations or particular needs.

Clearly, there is a serious need for more and better data about people with disabilities. We need better information about the nature of disabling conditions and their social and economic consequences, both to guide policy and programmatic decisions as well as to enrich our understanding of disability. We need to know more about demographic trends, the impact of impairments on employment (recreation) and the range of life functions, the ways in which people with disabilities participate (or not) in public and private programs, and the values and attitudes of people with and without disabilities (Scotch, 1990).

The definition of disability is a critical issue. Even though we have suggested the guidelines as outlined by the World Health Organization, disability has been used to mean everything from a minor impairment that has little or no impact on activity to a condition that requires one to rely on others for assistance in one's most basic functions. When it comes to surveying for the purpose of disability statistics, no one accepted definition exists. National surveys or programs serving people with disabilities use specific stated definitions, but each program or survey uses definitions addressing its specific purposes (Scotch, 1990).

Three frequently cited surveys that measure the extent of disability in the U.S. are the Census Bureau's Survey of Income and Program Participation (SIPP) and its Current Population Survey (CPS), as well as the National Health Interview Survey it conducts for the National Center for Health Statistics.

The CPS is a more limited measure of disability, says bureau statistician Jack McNeil, because it specifically asks people only about work-inhibiting disabilities.

Respondents are asked if they have a condition that prevents them from working or limits the kind or amount of work they can do. "That could be responded to in various ways by a person with a disability," says McNeil. "If a person uses a wheelchair, but has a satisfactory job, then there wouldn't be a particular reason for that person to report that they have a disability."

The CPS question concerning work disability dates back to the 1960s when the Social Security Administration wanted to identify the number of people who might eventually apply for Social Security disability benefits. In contrast, the newer SIPP questions explore issues of functionality across the life span.

The SIPP defines functional disability as difficulty with or inability to perform age-appropriate activities due to a physical or mental condition or impairment. This includes those who have trouble seeing ordinary newsprint even with corrective lenses; those who can't hear normal conversation, or whose speech can't be understood; those who have trouble lifting ten pounds, climbing a flight of stairs, walking three city blocks, or getting around in their homes; or those who have difficulty with at least one of the five Activities of Daily Living — getting into or out of bed or a chair, bathing, dressing, eating, and using the toilet.

The SIPP also asks about people's ability to perform Instrumental Activities of Daily Living. These include: going outside the home, keeping track of money and bills, preparing meals, doing housework, and using the telephone. The survey also collects information about those who use wheelchairs, canes, crutches, or walkers, as well as those who have certain mental conditions. Finally, the SIPP asks about people's ability to work at a job.

With this set of questions, the SIPP data reveal links between disabilities and employment status. Some people who are paraplegic don't find their condition a hindrance to full-time work, while others do. With this survey, analysts can tease out the differences.

The National Health Interview Survey (NHIS) covers similar topics in the same way — i.e., self-reported. This annual nationally representative survey asks people about long-term limitations or short-term restrictions in activities due to acute or chronic conditions. Major activities for those aged 5 to 69 include going to school, working, and keeping house; non-major activities include participation in civic, recreational, and other activities. The ability to engage in normal play is the benchmark major activity for preschool children; the ability to live independently signifies the same for those aged 70 and older.

Acute conditions that could cause temporary disability include all types of illnesses and injuries. Sometimes the lasting effects of injuries become chronic impairments. Chronic conditions include the same congenital and acquired impairments tallied in the SIPP, such as visual and hearing problems, as well as paralysis and limb loss. They also include mental illness and retardation, immunity disorders, and diseases of the respiratory, circulatory, digestive, and other body systems. In other words, the NHIS allows people to indicate any kind of physical or mental condition that limits their activity in any way. Researchers in turn can define disability as they see fit, based on various combinations of responses.

The value of the SIPP and NHIS questions is that they permit customized definitions of disability. After all, the label is largely contingent on people's expectations of what they can, should, or want to do in their particular situations. If a construction worker suffers a back injury that prohibits him from doing heavy labor the rest of his life, he's permanently disabled in that line of work. An office worker with the same back problem may require ergonomic equipment and flex-time for physical therapy, but she might be otherwise unaffected as far as work goes. On the other hand, she might be unable to do certain home-maintenance tasks, like lifting children and bags of groceries (Mergenhagen and Crispell, 1997).

The choice of how to define disability is more than merely a semantic issue. In fact, the definition determines who is included and who is not. For example, for state or federal entitlement programs that commission a survey of the numbers of people with disabilities, cost containment issues limit the population count. On the other hand, larger numbers will be solicited and subsequently used by advocacy groups attempting to affect local, state, or federal policy. The definition, as a result, has a direct impact on the statistical estimates of people with disabilities. The range of estimates varies depending on the source of data and the concept to be measured. See Table 1.2 for selected disability statistics.

We must note that most national surveys cover only the noninstitutionalized population. In the United States, an additional 1.5 to 2 million individuals are unaccounted for, most of whom have disabilities and reside in institutions such as nursing homes, psychiatric hospitals, residential facilities, and facilities for people who are mentally retarded. Whatever the estimates developed as a result of survey efforts, a significant observation is that large numbers of people in North America have functional limitations. The figure in the United States that is popularly accepted is the NHIS survey that states that at least 43 million Americans have at least one impairment. Since this was the figure that was used to pass the most pervasive piece of civil rights legislation in the history of the United States, the Americans with Disabilities Act (ADA), 43 million is the figure that we will use as well.

Table 1.2
Selected Disability Statistics

Statistic	Source
54 million (20.6%) of people age 15 and over, with any disability in the U.S.	SIPP, 1994-95
15.3 million (7.6%) of people over 15 have a functional, physical limitation	SIPP, 1994-95
4.2 million (16%) of the population in Canada have some level of disability*	HALS, 1991
34.2 million (14.1 %) of U.S. residents have a limitation in activity	NHIS, 1989
43 million Americans have at least one impairment	NHIS, 1989
17.2 million (8.6%) of 16- to 64-year-olds are work disabled	CPS, 1998
2.3 million of 16- to 67-year-olds or 13% of the working age population are work disabled.*	HALS, 1991
10% of work disabled people are employed full time	CPS, 1998

People 15 years old and over were identified as having a disability if they met any of the following criteria:

- Used a wheelchair or were a long-term user of a cane, crutches, or a walker
- Had difficulty performing one or more functional activities (seeing, hearing, speaking, lifting/carrying, using stairs, or walking)
- Had difficulty with one or more activities of daily living (the ADLs included getting around inside the home, keeping track of money and bills, preparing meals, doing light housework, taking prescription medicines in the right amount at the right time, and using the telephone)
- Had one or more specified conditions (a learning disability, mental retardation or another developmental disability, Alzheimer's disease, or some other type of mental or emotional condition)
- Were limited in their ability to do housework
- Were 16 to 67 years old and limited in their ability to work at a job or business
- Were receiving federal benefits based on an inability to work

People age 15 and over were identified as having a severe disability if they were unable to perform one or more functional activities; needed personal assistance with an ADL or IADL; used a wheelchair; were a long-term user of a cane, crutches, or a walker; had a developmental disability or Alzheimer's disease; were unable to do housework; were receiving federal disability benefits; or were 16 to 67 years old and unable to work at a job or business.

Canadian information comes from the 1991 Health and Activity Limitations Survey (HALS). HALS provides information on people who have a long-term physical or mental disability (six months or more) that may or may not limit activities. Figures as provided by the complete HALS data help Statistics Canada to better understand the barriers people with disabilities face in their everyday lives.

The Social System

People with disabilities are typically a part of a number of social systems. Howe-Murphy and Charboneau (1987, p. 12), in their text *Therapeutic Recreation Intervention: An Ecological Perspective*, define a system as

> ... a complex of elements or components directly or indirectly related in a causal network, such that each component is related to at least some others in a more or less stable way within a particular period of time.

They identify six systems of which a person with a disability is often a part. The systems they identify include the following:

- the total person,
- the biological system,
- the family system,
- an agency system,
- a neighborhood system, and
- a community system.

Figure 1.3 represents graphically what is included within each of these systems. All of the systems described in Figure 1.3 compose what may be referred to as a multiple suprasystem. Every component of each system interacts with other components of other systems. For example, the spiritual component of the total person system will quite likely interact with a family component such as mother or grandfather. Howe-Murphy and Charboneau suggest that it is important to understand the boundaries of each of the systems for a particular person in order to design interventions and to determine how recreation interacts with each system. At the same time, also necessary is recognizing that within every system there is a constant flow of information, resources, and effect within and between systems that Howe-Murphy and Charboneau describe as the energy of the social system. It is particularly important to understand that each of the subsystems portrayed in Figure 1.3 may differentially interact with a person with a disability.

In considering how recreation relates to the systems described above, we must understand that each of the systems is in a constant state of flux. For ex-

Figure 1.3
Howe-Murphy and Charboneau System

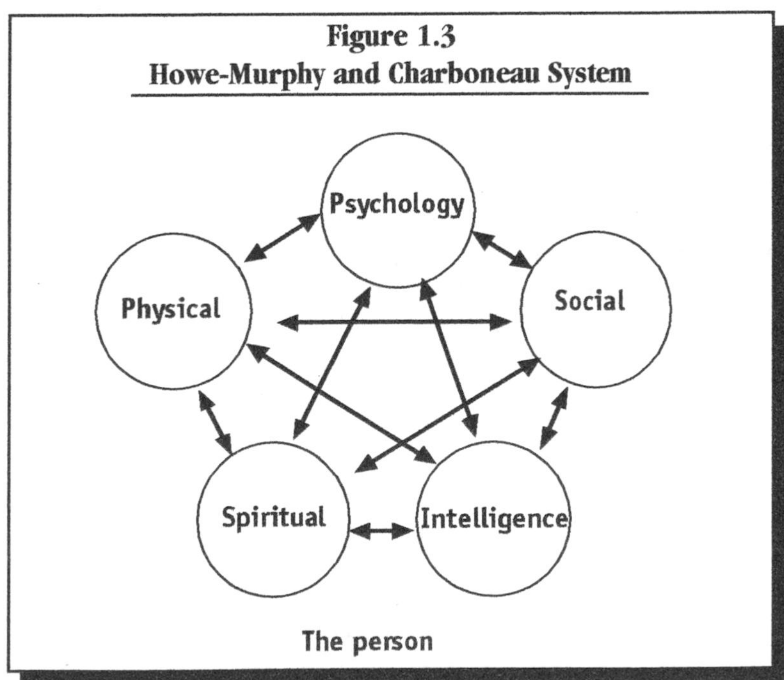

ample, the family system that includes a child with a disability will continuously undergo change. As the child moves from childhood to adolescence, she will undergo physical and social changes that will have an impact on her relationships with other family members. Sexuality will become an important consideration for both the child, her parents, and quite likely other family members. These changes may have a positive or a negative effect on the overall family system. The child's growing awareness of her sexuality may cause the parents to be uncomfortable and may introduce stress into their relationship with their daughter. In this case, the family system will be undergoing negative change. In contrast, the child and family may deal with the issue of sexuality in a positive way and their relationship may be enhanced by communicating about such life changes. This would suggest that the system would undergo a positive change.

Each of the systems will continuously undergo similar types of changes. The significance of these systems and their ongoing changes to our central focus is that the recreation delivery system must maintain itself within all of these systems and recognize the place of recreation in relation to each system and the overall suprasystem. In the case of the child experiencing sexual growth, any recreation intervention or facilitated experience must be sensitive to the child's present social system.

Beyond understanding the need for recreation services to be framed within the context of the social system of the individual with a disability, it is important to address more specifically the need for recreation services to be framed within the scope of the overall human service delivery system. This system in some ways is a combination of the agency, neighborhood, and community systems described by Howe-Murphy and Charboneau. In Figure 1.4, the most common services for people with disabilities are presented. The extent to which these services are available within a given community will vary across the United States and Canada. Existing and new recreation services must be framed within the context of these other systems. For example, a therapeutic recreation program designed to facilitate the transition of an individual from a rehabilitation setting must function in an interdependent manner with employment services, schools, and social services in order to create a transitional process that meets the overall needs of the individual. In this way, the chance of duplication or lack of services in a particular area will be diminished, and the needs of the individual will be met.

In the next chapter we will look at how people with disabilities have been treated throughout time.

Learning Activities

1. List as many words or phrases that you have heard (or said) that you would consider negative language toward people with disabilities. What makes them negative?

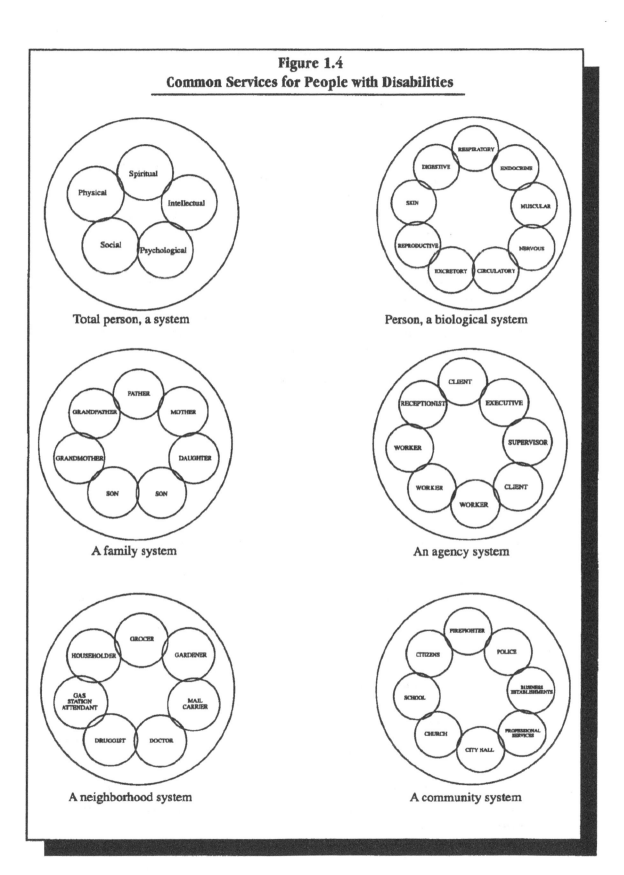

Figure 1.4
Common Services for People with Disabilities

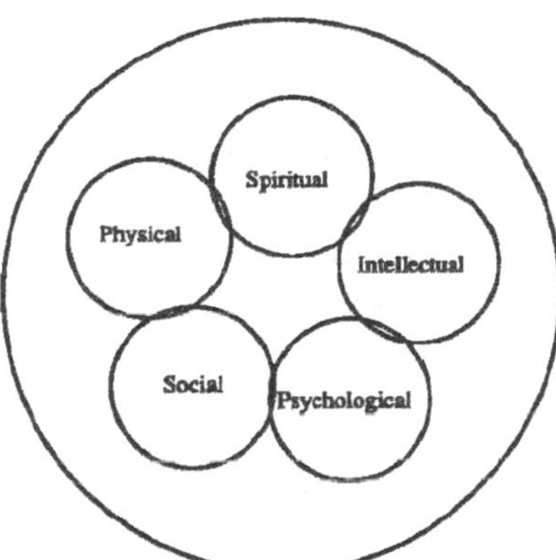

Total person, a system

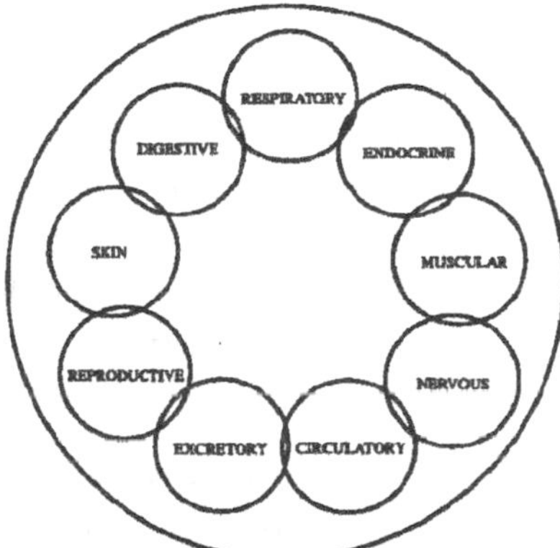

Person, a biological system

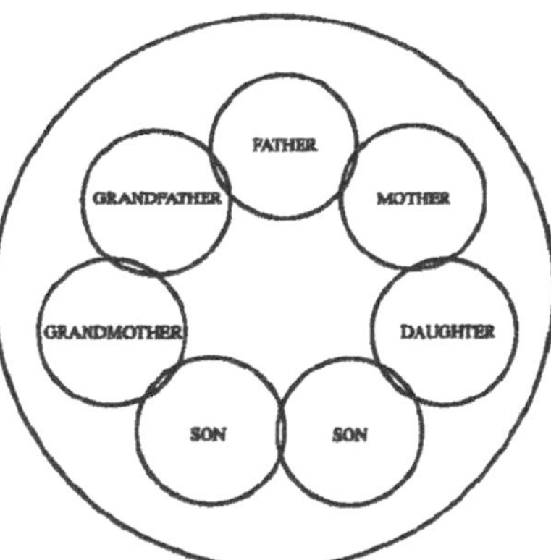

A family system

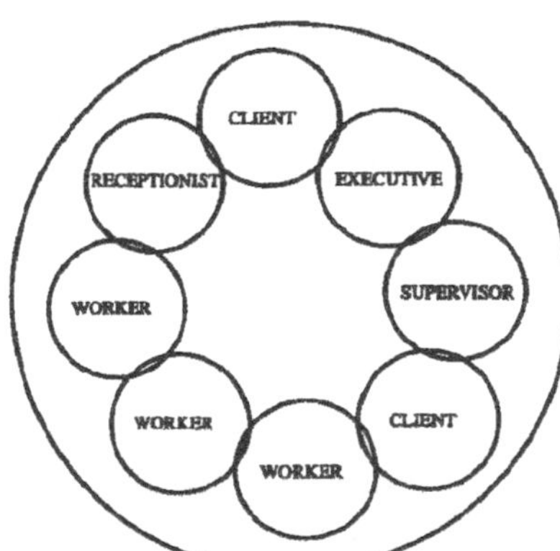

An agency system

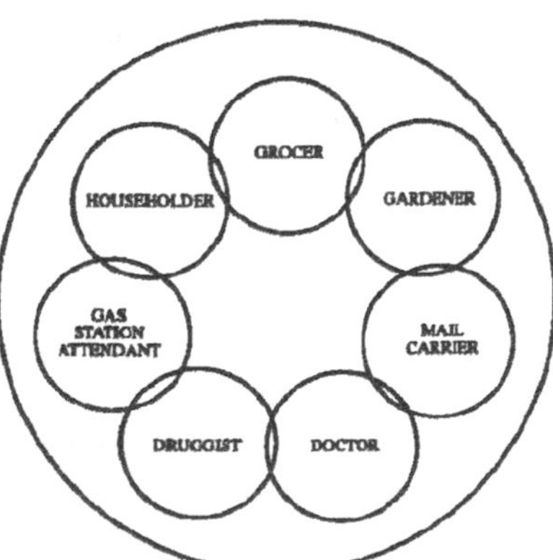

A neighborhood system

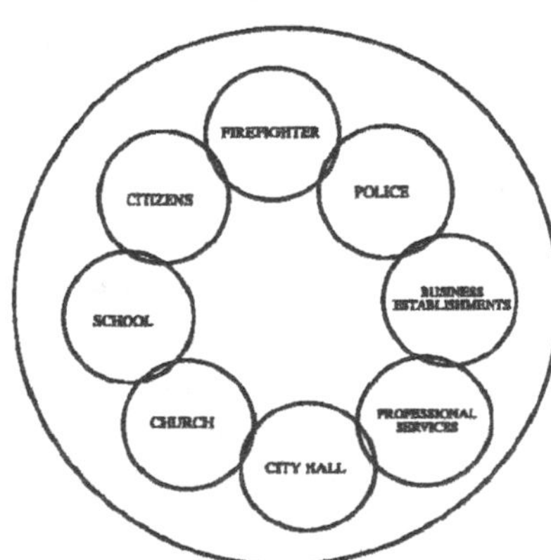

A community system

2. Using the ICIDH2 classification for a person who has become blind in her late teenage years from a degenerative eye disease, describe what might be her

    - Impairment
    - Activity
    - Participation

3. Now that you understand the distinction among terms such as impairment, activity, and participation, when you read the newspaper or when you hear people talk, pay attention to how the writers or speakers use the terms impairment and disability. How does the way the writer/speaker uses the term(s) change the meaning from your understanding of the term(s)? What term do you think should have been used and why?

4. For the next seven days, pay particular attention to the number of times that you hear or see language that is not "people first." As you listen to your friends and/or family, listen to radio and television shows, read newspapers, magazines, or books, note the "offenses." Keep a log of the number of offenses and where they occurred. Don't forget to listen to yourself!

5. Refer to Table 1. 1 and add as many additional examples of negative language as you can. After each one write a more positive and respectful alternative. Reflect on how easy it was to complete the negative list.

References

Allen, S. N. & Mor, V. (1998). ***Living in the community with disability.*** New York: Springer.

Discover together: A disability awareness resource. (1992). Ottawa: Department of the Secretary of State of Canada.

"Dispelling myths about people with disabilities." (1995). Online. Internet, retrieved 1 March 1999. Available: ***http://www.50.pccpd.gov/pcepd/pubs/fact/dispel.htm***

Helander, E., Mendis, R, & Nelson, G. (1989). ***Training disabled people in the community (RHB184).*** Geneva: World Health Organization.

Howe-Murphy, R., & Charboneau, B. (1987). ***Therapeutic recreation intervention: An ecological perspective.*** Englewood Cliffs, NJ: Prentice-Hall.

Hutchison, P, &McGill, J. (1992). ***Leisure, integration, and community.*** Concord, Ontario: Leisurability Publications, Inc.

ICIDH and Environmental Factors International Network (1998). Beta-1-draft of the ICIDH 2 (W.H.O. 1997). ***ICIDH and Environmental Factors International Network 9,*** 26-28.

"Language and disability." (1998). Online. Internet, retrieved, 28 February 1999. Available: ***http://www.austlii.edu.au/au/orgs/uts/roles/policy/aa_policy/ablist.html***

Linton, Simi. (1998). ***Claiming disability, knowledge, and identity.*** New York: New York University Press.

Lord, J. (1981). Opening doors, opening minds! ***Recreation Canada,*** Special Issue, 4-5.

Louis Harris & Associates, Inc. (1986). ***The ICD survey of disabled Americans. Bringing disabled Americans into the mainstream.*** Washington, D.C.: Author.

Mergenhagen, P. & Crispell, D. (1997). Who's disabled? American Demographics On-line. Internet, retrieved, 6 December 1998. Available: ***http://www.demographics.com/publications/ad/97_ad/9707_ad/ad970712.htm***

Rehab Brief. (1993). ***Bring research into effective focus.*** National Institute on Disability and Rehabilitation Research, Office of Special Education Research Services, U.S. Department of Education. (Vol. 14),8.

Shapiro, J.P. (1993). ***No pity: People with disabilities forging a new civil rights movement.*** New York, NY: Times Books.

Scotch, R.L. (1990, Summer). The politics of disability statistics. In I. Zola (Ed.), ***Disability Studies Quarterly, 10***(3).

Footnote

[1]In an effort to maintain the integrity of the use of the word ***disability*** in the ICD survey, the use of the parenthetical word ***handicapped*** is inserted to suggest the authors' interpretation in relation to the World Health Organization categorization previously presented.

Related Websites

http://www.isdd.indiana.edu/~cedir/languagetext.html
(The Language of Disability)

http://www.uwsp.edu/acad/educ/dupham/pplfrst.htm
(People-First Language)

http://www.libertynet.org/libres/advocacy/prefer.html
(Liberty Resources - When Referring to a Person with a Disability)

http://www.state.ct.us/ctcdd/language1.htm
(Connecticut Council on Developmental Disabilities— A Media Guide to Disability)

http://www.nc-ddc.org/people.html
(People First)

http://www.ncddr.org/icdr/isds/pages.html
(Disability Statistics Web Pages)

http://dsc.ucsf.edu/default.html
(Disability Statistics Center)

http://www.idsi.net/tri/stats.htm
(TRI Online — Statistics)

http://www.census.gov/hhes/www/disable.html
(U.S. Census Bureau)

http://www.statcan.ca:80/english/Pgdb/People/health.htm
(Statistics Canada)

http://codi.buffalo.edu/graph_based/.demographics/
(Statistics)

Chapter 2

History of Treatment of People with Disabilities

Introduction

This chapter covers more than what is generally known of the relationship of recreation and disability/illness throughout history.Whether you work in therapeutic recreation or community recreation programs, in order to be an effective professional you will need to have a comprehensive historical perspective of the treatment and services of people with disabilities.

It is hard to imagine that some of the history presented here could have happened; however, readers are cautioned to remember that what happened, occurred in an historical and cultural context. As horrific a some of it may sound, in large measure the people of the time believed that they were providing the best possible alternatives for people with disabilities in their societies. By today's standards we regard most of the ways people were treated as inadequate, if not inhumane. At the same time, some of the history—when considered in context—seems entirely adequate, if not progressive. In any case, by the standards of the day, how people were treated nearly always was considered humane—at least for the time.

Throughout human civilization, people with disabilities have been discarded and disrespected, treated like freaks, and often regarded as punishment to the parents from God. Many years were characterized by inhumane and animalistic treatment. People with disabilities were abandoned, abused, used for sport and entertainment, involuntarily sterilized, and systematically ostracized from the social mainstream. Fortunately, in recent decades an ideological shift has occurred within our collective conscious that has redefined our perception of people with disabilities. Slowly but surely, humanity has replaced inhumanity, inclusion has replaced exclusion, justice has replaced injustice, education has replaced misinformation, and consideration has replaced ignorance. But these shifts have been a long time coming. In this chapter we will look more closely at the history of treatment of people with disabilities.

Early History

Disability has existed since the beginning of time. In ancient civilizations there was public awareness of a variety of illnesses and disabilities and an organized system to treat illness. In ancient Mesopotamia, care and treatment was provided by priests because it was believed that illness and dysfunction were attributable to demons, evil spirits, and transgressions against the gods. No specific records from ancient times exist to absolutely confirm what is understood from archaeology; however, there is ample evidence to support our assertions (Avedon, 1974). There are even indications that activities were used both in ancient Mesopotamia and in ancient Greece to appease the gods and, thereby, to alleviate the illness and dysfunction that was attributable to demons, evil spirits, and transgressions against the gods.

The oldest written records of ancient Greece and Rome contain evidence that people with mental illnesses, mental retardation, and a variety of sensory and physical disabilities existed at that time. Examples of disability occur in the Bible, evidenced in the stories of people who were "crippled" and were brought for healing. There are examples during the medieval period of court jesters or people with disabilities who were used to entertain or amuse other people. Countless examples of disability occur throughout history.

Historically, determination of disability was more dependent on social factors than on a diagnosis of an illness. Whether or not a person was considered mentally ill, mentally retarded, or physically disabled depended both to the degree to which the person's behavior was different and the attitudes of members of his social group toward such deviant behavior (Rosin, 1968). "People-first" language, of course, was not even considered at the time. In fact, words like disability and the handicap have become used only in modern times. During earlier periods, people whom we today would call people with disabilities were referred to as ***dysfunctional, mad, crazy, deformed,*** or ***defective***. Many of the words and phrases that we characterized as negative in Chapter 1 have existed for many, many years. However, the definition and understanding of people as "defective" and "shameful" were overriding notions that guided the treatment and services of people with disabilities.

From the earliest times, and even through parts of this century, common wisdom among the general public was that "madness" or "defectiveness" came from demons or evil spirits and was seen as a punishment from an angry God. You may be familiar with the expression: "I'm going to beat the evil out of him." Such a colloquial comment is rooted in early treatment of people with disabilities. That is, one of the ways that people with disabilities were treated was to actually beat them in hopes of beating out the demons or evil spirits that were the reason for defectiveness. Ergo, the preceding expression.

From Roman law we see that typical members of the community were legally protected from harm from people with mental illnesses. As ***defectives***, people with mental illnesses (and indeed other disabilities) were thought to be dangerous and unpredictable. People were afraid of the members of their community who had mental illnesses. They demanded protection. As a result, specific laws were written to protect the general public. Roman law even protected the property rights of the family if the head of household had a mental disorder. An example is the story about Sophocles, who worked well into his extreme old age and often became so absorbed in his work that he neglected his business affairs. His sons believed that he was incompetent in the dealings of family property, so they took him to court to gain control of their father's property. They were successful and did in fact gain control. Roman law did not protect those with mental illness, but instead protected the right of the family and the general public from people with mental illnesses.

Two basic views in the ancient world existed regarding the etiology of disability. One attributed illness to supernatural or divine intervention, and the other view was that illness and disability were due to natural causes (Rosin, 1968). As stated above, it was not uncommon for the community to think that a "defective" child had been sent as punishment for the sins of the parents, even if those "sins" were not common knowledge to others in the community. In other cases, supernatural or divine intervention was somewhat more positive. If a person's disability was believed to be the result of or possession by a supernatural power, she was thought to have extraordinary abilities and thus considered to be "above" normal man, even sacred. Sometimes, people with mental illnesses were looked at as if they were closer to the gods than regular people. If a person was thought to be mentally ill as a result of possession, it was seen as punishment by the gods and could only be cured by forces from the heavens.

On the other hand, if a person was thought to be ill or dysfunctional as a result of natural causes, the illness or dysfunction was thought to be curable. Wide varieties of herbs, animals, and minerals were used to treat illness and dysfunction. Activity was also used. According to Avedon (1974), "...the first Greek physician, Melampus, treated the daughters of Proteus by having them play a game that involved running. This is reported to have cured them of the delusion that they were cows."

Also in the early Roman and Greek eras, music, drama, reading, and sport were used to ease dysfunction and discomfort of the mind. A number of temples were even built as curative centers. One example of such a curative center in ancient Greece that was built and continually upgraded throughout the first millennium was one that included a library, a stadium, and a theatre. Also sometimes used for treatment of mental disorders in ancient Greece was music played in conjunction with gymnastics and dancing (Avedon, 1974). In ancient Rome, as early as A.D. 124, people who were mentally ill were taken from their dark cells, brought into the sunshine, and provided music, games, poetry, and gentle exercise.

Although there are some examples of humane treatment, what is not recorded is the maltreatment of many people with serious illnesses and dysfunctions. There were few treatment facilities as we know them today. Rather, people with illnesses and dysfunctions were put in dark cells with little or no attention or were the responsibilities of families. No measures were ever taken to help most people with disabilities unless they were among the wealthy class or if they were a threat to others.

Instances of people with disabilities being "useful" exist as well. The primary mode of production throughout human existence has been foraging, and it was most likely a source of employment or even occupation for some people with less serious disabilities. As long as people were capable of "keeping up" with group movement and contributing to the gathering of necessary resources, such individuals probably survived relatively well in foraging communities (Scheerenberger, 1983). However, people with serious disabilities most likely shared the fate of people who were injured or aging: they were either euthanatized or left behind so as not to interfere with the survival of the group. As early societies moved from hunting and gathering to cultivating and harvesting, it is still likely that many people with disabilities fared well:

> In less complex, less intellectually centered societies, the mentally retarded would have no trouble obtaining and retaining a quality of realizable ambitions. Some might even be capable of gaining superiority by virtue of assets other than those measured by intelligence tests. They could make successful peasants, hunters, fishermen, and travel dancers. In other earlier societies, people with disabilities may not have fared so well. For example, in the militaristic Spartan society, infants deemed unfit for the rigors of Spartan life were thrown from cliffs to their death (Scheerenberger, 1983).

In other societies, infants believed to be defective were abandoned and left to die from exposure (Macklin & Gaylin, 1981)

Some people with disabilities who survived infancy were used to entertain. Fiedler (1978) cites exhibitions of freaks from antiquity. Welsford (1935) relates the earliest mention of the ***dwarf-fool*** with the Egyptian pharaohs who chose members of the Danga pygmy tribe as mainly a curiosity, but also for amusement. It was customary for wealthy men in the Roman Empire to keep half-witted and deformed slaves in their houses for purposes of entertainment; further, females were known to keep physically stunted and mentally deficient slaves as substitutes for "lap dogs and teddy bears" (Welsford, pp. 58-59). Throughout early history there are examples of the use of slaves for entertainment. Further examples include spectators being amused by deformed figures around A.D. 500 in the court of Attila (Wells, 1961, pp. 411-412). Bedini also mentions the ***forum morionium***, where people with disabilities were bought and sold as slaves (1991, p. 63). Such "slaves" were frequently traded or given as payments or gifts. According to Welsford (p. 107), even in death there was no peace, as people were known to break into laughter when merely looking at a ***fool's*** grave. Such abuses of people with disabilities being used for amusement robbed them of any shred of dignity and forced them into a state of dependence. At the time, the only other option appears to have been death. In the 4th century B.C., wealthy families kept people with disabilities to amuse their guests; in the 2nd century, the viewing of people with physical or developmental disabilities became a source of public entertainment (Scheerenberger, 1983; Evans, 1983).

Another era of early recorded history about which we know a considerable amount is the era in the Middle East during the early Jewish tradition. Disability was believed to be inflicted on those being punished by God. As early as the 7th century B.C., Moses told his people in the book of Deuteronomy (28:15, 28) that "if you do not obey the Lord your God and do not carefully follow all his commands and decrees...the Lord will afflict you with madness, blindness, and confusion of the mind."

As in Rome and Greece, the use of music in the Middle East was also prevalent. In biblical literature, David often played the harp in the court of Saul, King of Israel, to soothe the King's mind when the "spirit of God came upon him." From the context and everything else we know of King Saul, that phrase was a euphemism meaning when he became emotionally unstable. For example, in Samuel (16:23) is the statement:"whenever the spirit of God came upon Saul, David would take his harp and play. Then relief would come to Saul; he will feel better and the evil spirit will leave him."

Middle Ages

During the Middle Ages, people with disabilities were treated as outcasts by society. If people looked different or acted differently than normative society, they were considered outcasts. They were sent away to prisons, abandoned in the wilds, or even worse, they were killed. They were expelled from their communities where there was no one to care for them. In medieval times outcasts or people whose behavior did not fit within the norms of that particular society were often labeled as witches and were summarily persecuted and, in many cases, killed.

Also in the Middle Ages was evidence of people with disabilities being used for amusement. Billington (1984) found evidence of both English and French mobility keeping ***simpletons*** as fools throughout that time. From the 14th through the 17th centuries in France and England, people who were mentally deficient were also considered to possess supernatural powers and strengths and, as such, were an added source of "entertainment" (Welsford, 1935, pp. 78, 94). Irish court jesters were termed ***miclach, mer, and faindelach***, all denoting not only idiocy but also men who "were regarded as disreputables and in a state of semi-outlawry" (Welsford, 1935, p. 110). During the Middle Ages, a "ship of fools" sailed from port to port displaying its cargo to the curious (Foucalt, 1965). Jesters or fools were commonly attached to courts and wealthy households. In one 17th century Spanish monarchy, Philip IV was reported to have kept a sizable collection of people with disabilities (Evans, 1983). Still, however, during the Middle Ages most people with less severe disabilities were reasonably integrated into a highly stratified agrarian society. Marie Crissey (1975, p. 800) writes that "In an almost wholly illiterate population, functioning at the simplest vocational level, a group we now label ***educable retarded*** no doubt was indistinguishable."

The French Renaissance introduced the rise of humanism and the intervention of the church. By the end of the 14th century, the church had excommunicated all those who earned a living by mimicking the ***witless man*** (Billington, 1984, p. 20). In contrast to this protection by the church, any man brought before a jury in 16th century England and declared a ***purus idiota*** (simple idiot) became the property of the crown, losing all personal property (Billington).

Around the 12th or 13th centuries, some advances in the treatment of people who were different occurred. ***Defectives*** as they were often called, who had no family or nowhere to go, were put into sections of hospitals not necessarily for treatment purposes but to get them off the streets, out of the community, and out of sight. Even though we may not consider this humane treatment by today's standards, by the standards of that day this was considered extremely humane. In essence, society was taking care of those people whom they thought were completely unable to take care of themselves.

Researchers might argue that the goal was to "cast the mad out of the community and separate them from their society" (Perrucci, 1974). However, the proponents of early institutionalization felt that they were providing what was needed for the ones *defective* among them. By the 16th century an increasing tendency arose to place people with mental illnesses and other disabilities into special institutions. This was particularly influenced by policies of the religious reformers in Europe. The belief that illness and disability was caused naturally rather than supernaturally was becoming more popular, and medical treatment was beginning to be prescribed accordingly. Still, in cases where the illness seemed to be too bizarre or beyond medical explanation, supernatural explanations would be in vogue (Rosin, 1968).

Even though some people with disabilities contributed to the economy during this time, with the rise of urbanization in the 17th and 18th centuries was a need to get people "out of circulation." The removal of people with disabilities from urban areas and their incarceration along with devalued people crated new opportunities for exhibition and profit making. This occurred in one of the first ***lunatic asylums*** in Europe, the Bethlehem Royal Hospital—popularly known as Bedlam. Evans (1983, p. 37) notes that:

> In Bethlehem (Bedlam) *idiots* and *lunatics* were exhibited for a price of about a penny every Sunday. The annual revenue for these shows at Bethlehem in 1815 was 400, (which) indicated an audience of approximately 96,000 people that year. The visitors' curiosity was evoked, in part, by certain attendants who were particularly adept at getting the inmates to "perform dances and acrobatics with a few flicks of the whip."

The Enlightenment brought about some amelioration of the devaluation of people with disabilities, and its new ideas contributed to notable clinical attempts to enhance the lives of such individuals. Itard's efforts to socialize the "wild boy of Aveyron" and Johann Jacob Guggenbuhl's attempts to "cure" people with disabilities through environmental stimulation were among the first efforts to prepare people with disabilities for integration into the developing society. There were other notable exceptions. Philipe Pinel, an 18th century French physician, consciously used recreative experiences for treatment purposes. He taught that ill persons, particularly mentally ill persons, would respond and often improve (with the use of recreative activity for treatment purposes) (Albee, 1959, p. 10).

Additional evidence of the use of recreative experiences as part of the curative process is provided in an early example of self-determination and self-advocacy. An inmate of the Glasgow Royal Asylum for Lunatics tells it this way:

> For the last two years I have attended the concerts and balls given during the dark months of the year to the inmates of Gartnavel Royal Lunatic Asylum; and from what I have seen, and also what I have heard from

> the inmates themselves, I know that these meetings have soothed the excited, cheered the desponding, and turned the mind aside for the time from the corroding task of contemplating its own sorrows, and consequently ministered to the great purpose for which asylums are instituted—the cure of insanity...There are people here listening to the song and joining in the dance—enjoying the clear light, the beauty and fragrance of the fresh evergreens which festoon the hall—who under the old system would be lying in bonds and darkness, their only music the clanking of the iron bolt and the rattling (sic) of the prison keys (Anonymous, 1860).

Modern History: Early Institutional in North America

Colonial North America had no institutions because so much time was devoted to colonization. Little tolerance existed for people who were defective. A family member who was "insane" or "defective" was taken care of at home. If the family member was violent or troublesome and the family could not care for the person or was ashamed of the person, he was often locked up or chained up by his family in the cellar, a strong house, an out building, or other flimsy building with few or no amenities (Deutsch, 1967). In such cases, these ***defectives*** were given very little food and often beaten. People who were considered defective were hidden away from society and often considered a "family disgrace." During this period of pre-institutionalization, people who were "different" lived a very isolated life, if they were allowed to live at all.

In the 18th century in North America, many institutions were built. They were originally intended to house criminals, but often people with mental disorders (mental illness and mental retardation) were incarcerated and treated as if they too had committed some criminal act (Deutsch, 1967). Connecticut's first house of correction, which was opened in 1727, was mandated to include persons who "aren't fit to go at large and whose family and friends do not take care of their safe confinement" (Deutsch, 1948). Although extreme and even cruel by our standards, much of the treatment of people who were defective was more humane during this period than had been in the medieval or earlier periods. This time often saw people hanged, imprisoned, tortured, or otherwise persecuted.

In 1752, a Pennsylvania hospital was the first hospital in the country to admit mental patients for ***curative treatment***. This was the beginning of what has been called moral treatment. Treatment changed from being cruel to being kind. This was the beginning of a revolution to understand illness and disability and to treat it accordingly. Even though this was the beginning of more humane treatment for people with disabilities, treatment was still a largely custodial situation in which it was clear that the ultimate objective was to cast these people out of the community and to separate them from the rest of society. These institutions were located in the country and housed up to 250-300 patients. The asylums, as they were later called, were surrounded by a substantial wall intended to keep the patients in and away from the rest of society.

In the United States, attempts to "cure" people with disabilities through environmental stimulation began in 1848 with the opening of an experimental school in Boston. That preliminary effort was followed by state funding for the Massachusetts School for Idiotic and Feebleminded Youth, which between 1848 and 1869 was reported to have prepared 365 ***feebleminded youths*** to become self-supporting members of the community (Evans, 1983). By 1889 there were 24 state-supported institutions in the United States (Crissey & Rosen, 1986). However, support for public funding of these facilities began to erode in the late 19th century and with decreased funding, state institutions became much more custodial (Evans).

Although there had been advances in institutional care during the 17th and 18th centuries in England, many of those would not last in the new world. As institutions became more custodial, forms of recreation diminished. Populations within institutions such as these increased during the 19th century. As more and more people were placed in institutions, they quickly became overcrowded. Throughout the 19th century, asylums popped up in every state. Even as early as this period, the after-care movement began (Deutsch, 1967), during which there was the first successful attempt at assisting patients on discharge from mental hospitals.

Prior to the late 19th century, institutions and programs for "dysfunctional" people were not organized by type of disability. Rather, any person with any illness or disability was placed into an institution. Programs and services for people who were mentally ill were indistinguishable from programs for people who were mentally retarded, for people who had cerebral palsy, or for that matter, for people with any other disability. In the late 19th century and early 20th century, separate institutions began to be developed. There were institutions for people who were mentally retarded as well as special schools for people who were blind and for people who were deaf.

During the early 20th century, many scientists and professionals scapegoated ***defectives*** as the cause for increasing disorganization and crime. In 1912, Walter E. Farnald shared the following view with the Massachusetts Medical Society (Evans, 1983, p. 43):

> The social and economic burdens of uncomplicated feeblemindedness are only too well known. The feebleminded are a parasitic, predatory class, never capable of self-support or of managing their own affairs...They cause unutterable sorrow at home and are a menace and danger to the community.

> We have only begun to understand the importance of feeblemindedness as a factor in the causation of pauperism, crime, and other social problems...every feebleminded person, especially the high-grade imbecile, is a potential criminal, needing only the proper environment and opportunity for the development of his criminal tendencies.

Fearing that mental ***defectives*** were reproducing themselves in substantial numbers, many began to call for their sterilization. In 1918, Popenoe and Johnson, as cited by Evans (1983, p. 46), supported sterilization while arguing against the release of unsterilized persons. They suggested profitable use be made of the people they called ***waste humanity***:

> Feebleminded men are capable of much rough labor. Most of the cost of segregating the mentally defective can be met by properly organizing their labor, so as to make them as nearly self-supporting as possible. It has been found that they perform excellently such work as clearing forest land, or reforesting cleared land, and great gangs of them might profitably be put at such work, in most states...(Thus) these unskilled fellows find happy and useful occupation, waste humanity taking waste land and thus not only contributing to their own support but also making over land that would otherwise be useless...Nor need this be confined to the males alone. The girls-women raise poultry, small fruits, and vegetables very successfully...No manufacturer of today has let the product of his plant go to waste as society has wasted the energies of this by-product of humanity.

Many states did develop dual policies of segregation and sterilization. By 1926, 23 states had mandatory sterilization laws; in 1927, the Supreme Court upheld the constitutionality of such legislation. Justice Holmes (in *Buck v. Bell*, 1927, p. 207) wrote the following:

> It is better for all the world, if instead of waiting to execute degenerate offspring for crime, or let to them starve for their imbecility, society can prevent those who are manifestly unfit from continuing their kind...Three generations of imbeciles are enough.

Researchers have estimated that over 50,000 people with disabilities, or those who were labeled as "defective," were sterilized in the United States between 1925 and 1955 (Evans, 1983). Countless others were confined to state institutions and endured the oppressive, if not torturous, conditions documented in a variety of works (Deutsch, 1948; Blatt & Kaplan, 1966; Vail, 1966; Blatt, 1970; United States Senate, 1985).

Treatment of People with Disabilities in Nazi Germany

The oppression in the United States and Canada was bad enough, but nothing compared to what was occurring at the same time in Germany. Anyone who had a physical or mental disability was not suitable to live. The killings of people with disabilities were the Nazi's first organized mass murders and were the proving ground in which they developed their killing techniques. The murder of children with disabilities began in October of 1939. A decree ordered midwives and physicians to report all infants born with specified medical conditions such as "Down Syndrome, blindness, deafness, abnormally small head size, severe or progressive hydrocephalus, any deformities, and paralysis" (Friedlander, 1997, 48). The most common method of killing was an overdose of medication so that death was not immediately obvious as murder. Toward the end of the war, however, starvation was used often. The killings were seen as important to the advancement of science. Children with disabilities were studied before their murders and autopsies were preformed on them after their deaths. Their organs, especially their brains, were regularly removed for scientific studies. (Porter, 1-2) Many of these institutionalized children, just as many of the institutionalized children in North America, were institutionalized for less severe disabilities and sometimes because they were slow learners and/or had behavior problems. (Brack, et. al.) The project to kill children with disabilities was overshadowed by the killing of adults with disabilities (Friedlander, 1997, 66-67). The most influential criteria for deciding whether institutionalized adults were killed was ability to perform productive work. Sometimes, however, the killings were far more indiscriminate. For example, at a psychiatric hospital in Poland, members of the German security police shot 420 patients on January 12, 1940. (Friedlander, 1997, 136). The atrocities go on and on, however, the point has been made that people with disabilities at this time in Germany were seen an nonhumans. Although people with disabilities were not systematically killed in North America, the humanity of their treatment in North America as described in the previous section is suspect. Although not to the extent as in Nazi Germany, institutions in North America were on a downward spiral.

The Height of Dehumanization in Institutions

Initially, institutions were intended to serve as medical settings for people with disabilities. However, as time went on, they increasingly became places where a person was sent if he was thought to be unmanageable. Very few doctors, nurses, or psychologists worked at such institutions because they were largely custodial. Institutions were so overcrowded that eating was often done by pureeing food, and then people were given straws or allowed to drink their food. In fact, as recently as the 1950s, in a study that was conducted at an institution in New Jersey, the average feeding time at the state school for people who were mentally retarded was around three minutes (Butera, Patton, & Columbus, 1981).

During the height of institutionalization, institutions were so crowded that baths were seldom given. When they were, peoples were herded into shower stalls and hosed down in the interest of time. Because of overcrowding and understaffing, it was not uncommon in institutions for people to walk around with soiled clothes for days at a time. To deal with this problem, inmates (as they were called even though they had committed no crime) in institutions often remained unclothed. This is not surprising since leaving people unclothed was much easier than constantly cleaning clothes that had been soiled. In addition, while residents were being hosed down, floors that caught feces and urine could be hosed and disinfected as well. Needless to say, disease was high in institutions. Sanitation was not a high priority (Korbin, 1987). The workers were not intentionally trying to be inhumane, but as mentioned, many of the staff were poorly educated and often took institutional jobs as second jobs to earn money. Workers were caught in a cycle where they were overworked and underpaid in badly overcrowded institutions. Workers did the best with what they had during this period, but people in institutions lived in squalid surroundings.

Humanization of Institutions

The overcrowded and squalid conditions were ameliorated somewhat beginning in the 1950s, for several reasons. First, many citizens were repulsed by the ***eugenic solution*** practiced in Nazi Germany, where people with developmental disabilities were systematically killed along with others labeled "undesirable." Second, parents of children with disabilities began to advocate their needs. Third, the 1950s began a period of relative prosperity, and public resources again became available for services. Finally, in the early 1960s, President Kennedy—whose sister had a developmental disability—legitimized the movement by creating a Presidential Commission to recommend a national strategy to assist people with developmental disabilities. Still, despite these efforts, people with disabilities continued to suffer from stereotypes, stigma, near total economic dependency, physical and social isolation, and physical and sexual abuse. Their continued oppression is thoroughly entrenched in 20th century popular culture.

Throughout the 20th century there were a variety of attempts at improving the care and treatment of people with various disabilities. In the case of people who were mentally ill, treatment was being tested on mental disorders. An array of treatments was used, including insulin shock therapy, where a coma would be induced. By 1938, electric convulsive shock therapy was introduced and soon became a standard procedure for treating people with mental disorders. Also around this time, lobotomies were performed to treat patients (Martindale & Martindale, 1985). A lobotomy is a surgical procedure that would actually disconnect the frontal lobe of the brain, which was thought to be the area of the brain that caused mental dysfunction. In Ken Kesey's now classic book *One Flew Over the Cuckoo's Nest*, the Chief is a graphic example of the effects of a lobotomized patient who walked around zombie-like as a result of having a frontal lobotomy. In the early 1950s, drug therapy began to arise in treating a variety of disorders and is used extensively today.

In the 1950s and '60s, institutions became more humanized. Prior to that time, trained staff was uncommon, and people who staffed institutions were often the least educated and least paid members of society. During the 1950s and '60s, more trained staff were hired. Previously, people who lived in institutions were barely treated like humans. In fact, descriptions often sound like descriptions of the treatment of animals. People were "let out of their rooms" or let out of their buildings only once or twice a day and only then to walk. Inmates (as they were still called even in the 1950s and '60s, were often left unclothed and often fed and bathed in large groups.

During the 1950s and '60s, a movement occurred to improve and to further humanize institutions and to reverse the wide-scale abuses in the treatment of people in institutions. The move was toward more intervention and more habitation—where people in institutions were taught functional living skills to be able to live in society. In some states and provinces, more institutions were built to ease overcrowding. Institutions began to hire professional staff: physicians, nurses, psychologists, vocational workers, and in some cases recreational workers. Institutions also hired additional residential staff, who were still lower-educated and untrained, but were professionally functional when staff training became a priority during this period. Once staff received training on how to work with people with disabilities, they could then provide the best possible services (Biernabach, 1981).

Also during this time, populations began to be segregated by type of disability. That is, prior to this time, institutions included all types of people. For example, a person with severe cerebral palsy—yet who had relatively good cognitive functioning—might be placed with a person with severe and profound mental retardation or with a person with a serious mental illness. During this period of humanization in institutions, people were separated so that the best possible services could be provided to people according to their needs. With the addition of the professional staff, assessments and evaluations were conducted on a wide scale of determine skill level and to determine who should be institutionalized and what type of services were needed to assist the person to have an improved quality of life.

This movement to humanize institutions also included ensuring that people wore clothes—clothes that fit them rather than the old practice of no clothes or baggy or unattractive clothes. Residents were assisted in taking their own showers rather than being hosed down. Beds were provided for everyone as opposed to having beds for some and the floor for others. Residents of institutions began to have foot lockers that included their own personal things. Prior to this, residents had been stripped of everything that ever belonged to them, and everything they had was communal. For example, at the time when residents did wear clothes, after the wash was done, clothes were simply passed out with no attention to ownership. Progressively, more attention was made to choice of clothing and to personal belongings. In addition to changes such as these, there were also changes to the physical environment. In most cases residents in institutions were not "dangerous," so the fencing and walls were less necessary than they had been thought to be previously. As a result, many fences and walls came down and many doors were left unlocked. Lobotomies were performed less frequently and sterilization became a choice rather than a mandate.

During this period, there was a move toward more individuality and choices for people who resided in these institutions. Recreators were now hired; previously, if there was any recreation at all, it was conducted by staff after everything else was done. Unfortunately, when they were hired seldom were they people who were trained in recreation. Nonetheless, there was a growing awareness of the importance of quality of life, which included recreation participation.

In spite of all of the positive changes in institutions, many things were still dehumanizing about them. Institutions were started as a humane response to inhumane treatment of people with disabilities. In fact, most institutions were started to keep people out of jails or other inappropriate places where they were even more grossly ill-treated. Yet, institutions soon became ***people warehouses***. These institutions, so debased from their supposed humanitarian origins, often subjected their "inmates" to inhumane, cruel conditions more like those of a concentration camp than of a hospital. One example of such abuse was Fairview in Pennsylvania, which was referred to as "the place of no return, hell, the animal farm, Auschwitz, the last stop" (Rawls, 1980 p. 18).

Deinstitutionalization

In the late 1960s and '70s, there was a move toward deinstitutionalization. "Deinstitutionalization referred to the move away from large-scale, institution-based care to small-scale, community-based facilities" (Dear & Wolch, 1987, p. 16). People with mental or physical disabilities began moving into community facilities instead of state facilities. "Community-based care was a possible means of solving the continuing rise in mental health costs and the heavy financial burden mental illnesses posed on the states" (Halpern, Sackett, Binner, & Mohr, 1980, p. 2). Even though many people with disabilities were getting out of institutions and away from in humane treatment, funding in communities was insufficient. When 75% of the residents left the institutions to join the community, only 25% of their funding followed (Halpern et al.). At the height of the institutional period, institutions had in excess of four or five times their capacity. Today, a typical institution in the United States has only 700 or 800 people, as opposed to 2,500 or 3,500 at the height of institutionalization. Interestingly, deinstitutionalization connotes discharging people from institutions; however, reductions in admissions rather than discharges, have accounted for a large majority of the reductions.

Today's institutional population consists of those individuals who are severely disabled, are very old, have a significant disability, and have nowhere else to go. In 1964, only 27% of institutional residents had severe disabilities. In 1965, children and youth 21 years or younger made up nearly half (48.9%) of state institutional residents in comparison to the 51.1% of adults (22 years or older). By 1991, the proportion had changed to 8.7% children and youth and 92.3% adults. In 1991, 12.3% of institutional residents were reported to be functionally blind and 5.6% were reported to be functionally deaf. Also, increasing proportions of state institution residents were reported to have neurological disorders: 44.6% were reported to have seizure disorders, and 21.6% were reported to have cerebral palsy. All of the percentages are significantly higher than 15 years earlier. In addition, the proportion of residents reported to exhibit behavior disorders continued to increase, reaching almost half (47.8%) of the resident population (*Policy Research Brief*, 1993).

In other words, the decrease in total institutional population brought about a smaller but even more severely disabled population. As a results, the cost of care has dramatically increased since 1950. In 1950, the average per person annual cost of care was about $745.60 (or about $2.04 per day). By 1994 the average annual cost had risen to $75,051.30 per person (or $205.62 per day). In dollars adjusted for changes in the Consumer Price Index over this periods, cost of care in 1994 was 18 times as great as in 1950 (see Figure 2.1). Many of the statistics presented are factors that have contributed to the steady increases in the costs of state institutional care.

Today, there are moves in many states to further deinstitutionalize (see Figure 2.2) and, in fact, close state institutions for people who are mentally retarded or mentally ill. This is occurring differently in different states and different provinces. However, in some states, new institutions are being proposed and/or built.

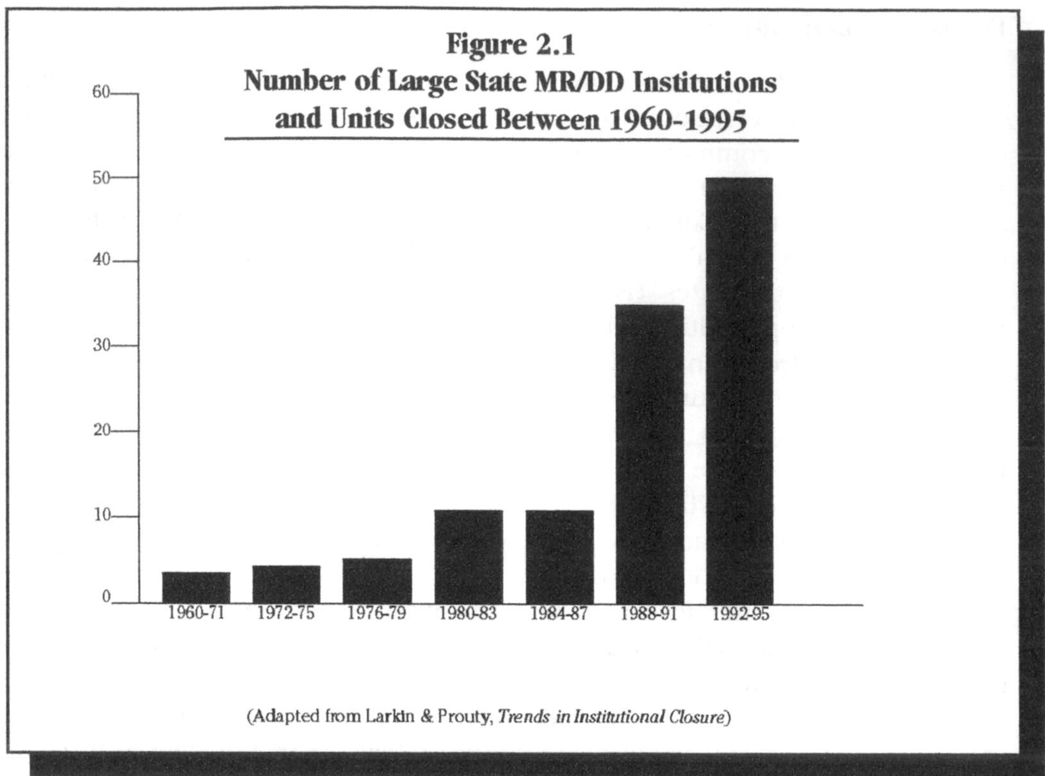

Figure 2.1
Number of Large State MR/DD Institutions and Units Closed Between 1960-1995

(Adapted from Larkin & Prouty, *Trends in Institutional Closure*)

Figure 2.2
Maryland Newspaper Article

Maryland Institution to Close in 1997

Maryland Governor William D. Schaefer announced that Great Oaks Center, a state institution housing 165 people with mental retardation, will close in 1997. Open(ed) in 1970, Great Oaks was licensed for 295 beds as an intermediate care facility for the mentally retarded (ICS/MR) but had grown to nearly 500 by 1978. Schaefer said that decision to close the facility "mirrors a national trend that people with developmental disabilities are better served in community settings." According to state officials, there will be an eighteen month "careful, deliberate, and rationale" planning process for community placements of Great Oak residents.

The United States is in the midst of a period of substantial reduction, not only of the population of state institutions but also in the number of institutions actually in operation. Even though the numbers were declining as already presented, the actual closure of institutions was relatively rare until the late 1980s (see Figure 2.3).

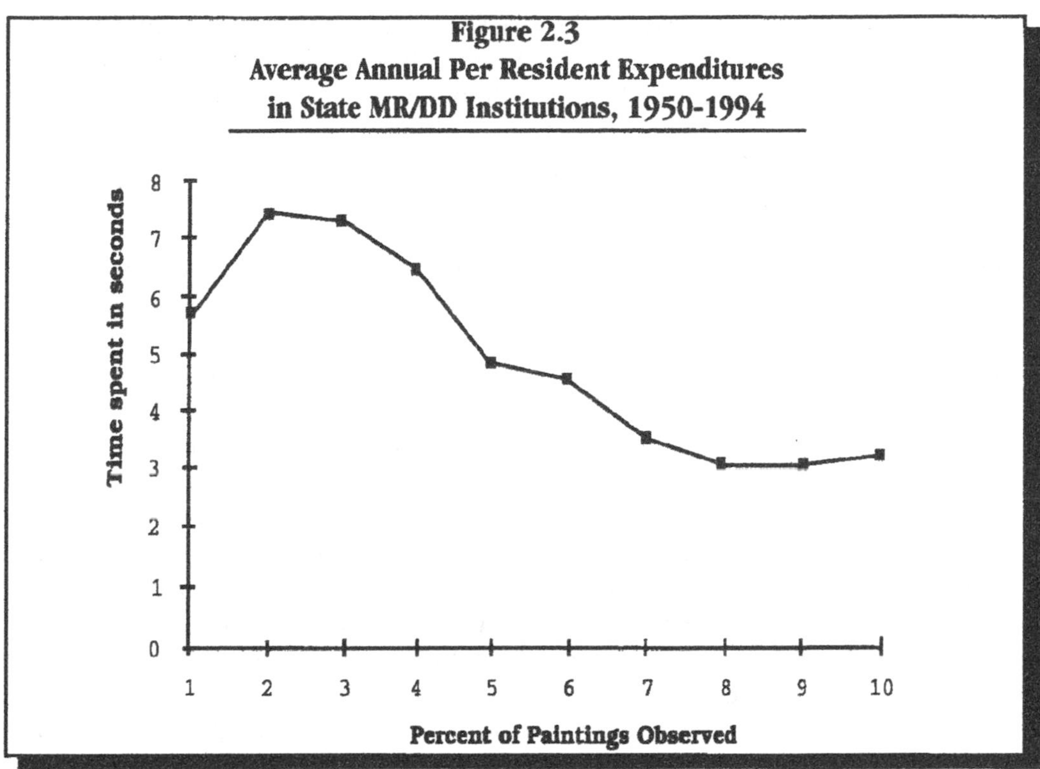

Figure 2.3
Average Annual Per Resident Expenditures in State MR/DD Institutions, 1950-1994

By the end of 1995, three states (New Hampshire, Michigan, and Vermont) had no state institutions with 15 or more residents. By the end of 1995, 32 states had closed at least one state institution. By the end of 1999, researchers project that all of Minnesota's remaining state institutions will be closed and, by the end of the year 2000, they project that all of New York's Developmental Centers will be closed. Undoubtedly, a national commitment to the depopulation and closure of state institutions is there. This trend is expected to continue.

Beyond Institutions

With the onset of deinstitutionalization, we began to see group homes, half-way houses, and other community living arrangements. The philosophy at the time was to prepare people to move *from* institutions into the community. We had come full circle. The difference is, this time people would live in homes and communities with pride rather than being hidden away. As such, prior to discharge or deinstitutionalization, people were increasingly taught to work and play. They were taught social skills so they would be able to "get along in the real world." Widely believed was that if a person who was institutionalized could be made "ready" in the institution, the institutional resident could transfer the learning and be "ready to live in the community."

This may have been logical thinking, but there were problems. Preparing people, or getting them "ready," may be a good idea, but there needs to be community support for these efforts to be continued and expanded. The problem is simple.

Initially, very little money was appropriated at state, local, or national levels to ensure effective deinstitutionalization. Essentially, no money was appropriated to follow along with people who left institutions. In most states during this period of deinstitutionalization, roughly 75% of the institutional population was discharged from institutions. However, only 25% of the money followed previously institutionalized people into the community. That left 75% of the money to the institution that housed only 25% of the former institutional residents. The fact could be argued that the residents who were left behind were more severely disabled and, in fact, that is accurate. However, the disproportionate amount of money that followed individuals from the institutions into the community made it hard for them to have appropriate habitation and treatment options available to them in the community.

Deinstitutionalization, for all of its hopes to re-humanize the treatment of people with disabilities, caused some additional problems. For example, the idea of deinstitutionalization was not to take people from the community and/or to put people with disabilities back into the community. This meant that to get back into the community, former residents had to be living in homes that were themselves in the community. Over time, however, the observation has arisen that many people without disabilities who currently reside in the community do not want groups of people with disabilities living in their neighborhoods. A number of people have even protested adamantly against that occurring. As a result, people who were once locked away in institutions were now being shunned and unwelcomed in the communities to which they were being returned. In a sense, devaluing did not end, but was renewed in new settings.

It is fair to say that even though advocates and, in most cases, previously institutionalized persons themselves were ready for deinstitutionalization, communities were not. Not only were people being discharged from institutions, but also very few people were being admitted. In other words, all of the people who had been in institutions, plus the ones that heretofore would have been sent to institutions, were now in communities throughout North America. In retrospect, deinstitutionalization happened too quickly and with too little preparation within communities. Many people with disabilities, who were no longer in institutions but were instead in local communities, had nothing to do. Few jobs, few educational or recreational opportunities, and few services were available and there was little accessibility to business and services. Inadequate transportation was the norm, as were inadequate policies and procedures. In summation, communities and their citizens were not ready for the mass of people who were turned out among them.

The biggest concern for advocates of people with disabilities who were now back in the community was that there was nothing for them to do. There were special education classes in some schools, but most of the people being deinstitutionalized were beyond school age. With so few jobs available for recently deinstitutionalized people with disabilities, a need for vocational options arose. During the period when institutions became more humanized and began preparing residents for discharge, one of the main institutional programs was vocational rehabilitation. Residents were learning work skills in institutional workshops, yet they were not skills preparing them for competitive employment. Because few options were available, one of the first services for previously institutionalized people with disabilities was increased vocational services, especially in the development of sheltered workshops. Sheltered workshops were an environment where individuals with disabilities went for work-like opportunities. They were proposed as one of the first steps to a smooth deinstitutionalization. For the most part, these were very low-skilled jobs in shelter environments (not real job sites) that provided inadequate preparation to move into competitive employment with people without disabilities. More recently, some advocates have questioned the legitimacy of sheltered workshops and have moved toward supported employment where people with disabilities are provided choices in types of work and are trained and supported in regular competitive jobs rather than the institution-like ***sheltered*** environment.

Also, no public recreation programs for people with disabilities existed. As a result of deinstitutionalization and the needs of people with disabilities for recreational services, a number of special populations' programs were started in public parks and recreation departments and YM/YWCAs, especially in larger cities. Like sheltered workshops, these programs were intended only for people with disabilities. There was no differentiation by disability. That is, whether a person had mental retardation, mental illness, cerebral palsy, blindness/visual impairment, or any other disability, he would be included within the same program or activity. Over time and as public recreators gained more training and began to provide increased specialized services, people were divided by disability groupings, which was thought to be a more appropriate way to program recreation for people with disabilities. Like sheltered workshops, special recreation programming has continued and has expanded since that time; it has filled a needed gap in the provision of services. However, today, with the passage of the Americans with Disabilities Act (ADA), as well as the legislation that will be discussed in Chapter 4, increased moves toward integrated or inclusive recreation programming is occurring. We will talk more about recreation and therapeutic recreation services in Chapter 6.

Conclusion

Although there have been periods of humanistic treatment throughout time, the bulk of history is less respectful. Since ancient times, people with disabilities have been devalued and often kept apart from the rest of society:

> By the late 19th century, people with disabilities of every kind were housed in alms houses, workhouse, penitentiaries, and hospitals of various sorts. Away from the turbulence and illicit attractions of the industrializing city, well-ordered institutions would provide *moral treatment*, and thereby instill the appropriate behavioral norms among the dependent classes (Dear & Wolch, 1987, p. 29).

Institutions moved from the ethic of moral treatment to a norm of custodial care as institutional populations steadily increase. Overcrowding and understaffing led to deplorable and squalid conditions. Blatt and Kaplan (1966) give the following description of one of the day rooms that they observed. They state:

> In each day room is an attendant or two, whose main function seems to be "stand around" and, on occasion, "hose down the floor," "Driving" excretions into a sewer conveniently located in the center of the room...In one such dormitory with an overwhelming odor, we noticed feces on the wooden ceilings and on the patients as well as the floors. (P. 22).

People with disabilities have definitely come a long way from the treatment they received only 30 or so years ago. But after the horror of institutionalization was over, the fight to provide dignity and respect for all people was not. As Blatt and Kaplan (1966, p. 1) assert, "Indeed, it appears that disabled people (sic) are some of the last people to be engaged in this historical sweep of the struggle for human rights." Even after the inhumane treatment stopped in institutions, it did not stop in the everyday world.

In the mid-1960s, in the height of the humanization of institutions, the systematic depopulation of state institutions began. Unfortunately, communities were not properly prepared to accept people who had heretofore been set apart from the mainstream of society. People with disabilities were discriminated against everywhere they went in the community because the outside world was not prepared with the facilities, let alone the attitudes needed for them.

Even now that there are fewer institutions and fewer people with disabilities who are institutionalized, there are still disturbing things that happen. Lest we are lulled into thinking that the type of dehumanization that has existed previously no longer exists, all a person needs to do is to keep up with local, regional, and/or national news. As recently as late February 1999, an article in the Reno Gazette-Journal which is an Associated Press story not only uses non- "people-first" language, but also describes treatment that reminds us of the treatment that occurred decades earlier. The opening line of the article ("Doctors charged," 1999) states, "A two year investigation of deaths at Pennsylvania's largest home for the retarded led to charges Friday against six doctors accused of such offenses as manslaughter and sewing up patients' wounds without anesthesia."

In Chapter 3 we will discuss concepts that if used in the development and implementation of recreation services will ensure respect and dignity of people with disabilities. In Chapter 4 we will discuss core legislation that has been enacted in the past quarter century that is consistent with the concepts presented in Chapter 3, which were enacted to increase the civil rights of people with disabilities.

Learning Activities

1. Pick a period in history at least 50 years ago. Do some research into that era and try to understand the widely held attitudes and values of the time. Then from the perspective of a reformer of that era, write a newspaper article about the treatment of people with disabilities. Remember not to impose your later 20th century view.
2. Contact your state/province Mental Health/Mental Retardation Division. Find out as much as you can about state/province institutions in your state/prov-

ince. How many are there now? Is the trend in your state/province to close state/provincial institutions or to build new ones? What are the timelines for closures or for opening new institutions?

3. Interview your parents about deinstitutionalization. Find out how much they know about the history of institutions and the current trends in your state. See how close their understanding is to what you find out from the state/provincial Mental Health/Mental Retardation Division.
4. Ask your parents how they would feel if a small group of people with mental illness bought a house and moved into your neighborhood? How would you feel?

References

Albee, G.W. (1959). ***Mental health manpower.*** New York: Basic Books, Inc.

Anonymous. (1860). ***The philosophy of insanity.*** Edinburgh: MacLachian and Stewart.

Avedon, F.M. (1974). ***Therapeutic recreation service: An applied behavioral science approach.*** Englewood Cliffs, NJ: Prentice Hall.

Bedini, L. (1991). Modern day "freaks?": The exploitation of people with disabilities. ***Therapeutic Recreation Journal, 25*** (4), 61-70.

Berenbaum. M. (1993). ***The world must know: The history of the Holocaust as told in the United States Holocaust Memorial Museum.*** Boston, MA. Little, Brown, and Company.

Billington, S. (1984). ***A social history of the fool.*** New York: St. Martin's Press.

Birnback, D. (1981), Backward society, 1981: Implications for residential treatment and staff training. ***Hospital and Community Psychiatry, 32*** (8), 550-555.

Blatt, B. (1970). ***Exodus from pandemonium: Human abuse and a reformation of public policy.*** Boston: Allyn & Bacon.

Blatt, B. & Kaplan, F. (1966). ***Christmas in purgatory: A photographic essay of mental retardation.*** Boston: Allyn & Bacon.

Bogdan, R. (1988). ***Freak show: Presenting human oddities for amusement and profit.*** Chicago: University of Chicago Press.

Brack, F., Halder, Hilfrich, Himmler, & Wurm. (1949-1953). Nazi extermination of people with mental disabilities. The Jewish Student Online Research Center. (JSOURCE), 15-19. Retrieved November 4, 1998 from the World Wide Web: http://www.us-isreal.org/jsource/Holocaust/mental_disabilities.html

Buck vs. Bell. (1927). ***United States Supreme Court Reports,*** 247, 200-208.

Butera, F., Patton, J., & Columbus, M. (1981). Institutions, institutional reform, and deinstitutionalization. In J. Patton (ed.), ***Mental retardation.*** Columbus, Ohio: C.E. Merrill.

Crissey, M. (1975). Mental retardation: Past, present and future. ***American Psychologist,*** 30, 800-808.

Crissey, M.S., & Rosen, M. (1986). ***Institutions for the mentally retarded: A changing role in changing times.*** Austin: Pro-Ed.

Dear, M.J., & Woch, J.R. (1987). *Landscapes of despair.* Princeton, NJ: Princeton University Press.

Deutsch, A. (1948). *The shame of the states.* New York: Harcourt Brace.

Deutsch, A. (1967). *The mentally ill in America.* New York: Columbia University Press.

"Doctors charged in abuse at retarded home." (1999, February 27). *Reno Gazette-Journal*, p. A8.

Evans, D.P. (1983). *The lives of mentally ill retarded persons.* Boulder: Westview Press.

Fiedler. L. (1978) *Freaks: Myths and images of the secret self.* New York: Simon and Schuster.

Foucalt, M. (1965). *Madness and civilizations: A history of insanity in the age of reason*. New York: New American Library.

Friedlander, H. (1997). *The origins of Nazi genocide: From euthansia to the final solution.* Chapel Hill, NC: University of North Carolina Press.

Halpern, J., Sackett, K.L., Binner, P.R., & Mohr, C.B. (Eds.).(1980). *The myths of deinstitutionalization: Policies for the mentally disabled.* Boulder: Westview Press.

Kliewer, C. & Drake, S. (1998). *Disability, eugenics, and the current ideology of segregation: A modern moral tale. Disability and Society, 13* (1), 95-111.

Korbin, J.E. (1987). Child maltreatment in cross cultural perspective: Vulnerable children and circumstances. In R. Gelles & J.B. Lancaster (eds.), *Child abuse and neglect* (pp. 31-55). New York: Aldine De Gruyter.

Larkin, K.C., & Prouty, R. (1995/96, Winter). Trends in institutional closure. In *Impact*, Vol. 9 (1).

Macklin, R., & Gaylin, W. (1981). *Mental retardation and sterilization*. New York: Plenum Press.

Martindale, D., & Martindale, E. (1985). *Mental disability in America since World War II*. New York: Philosophical Library.

Perrucci, R. (1974). *Circle of madness. On being insane and institutionalized in America.* New Jersey: Prentice Hall, Inc.

Policy Research Brief—Research and Training Center on Residential Services and Community Living. (1993), February). Institute on Community Living, College of Education, University of Minnesota, 5 (1).

Porter, John. (1997). Brains of handicapped children murdered by Nazis to be buried. *Deutsche Press-Agentur,* pp. 1-3 [Newspaper, selected stories on line]. Retrieved November 12, 1998 from internet: http://infoweb3.newbank.com/bin/gate.exe?f=doc&state=u0s0gd.3.1.

Rawls, W. (1980). *Cold storage*. New York: Simon and Schuster.

Rosin, G. (1968). *Madness in society.* Chicago: University of Chicago Press.

Scheerenberger, R.C. (1983). *A history of mental retardation.* Baltimore: Brookes Publishing.

United Sates Senate Committee on Labor and Human Resources. (1985). *Care of institutionalized mentally disabled persons, Parts 1 and 2.*

Vail, D.G. (1966), *Dehumanization and the institutional career:* Springfield, IL: Charles C. Thomas, Publisher.

Wells, H.G. (Revised, R. Postgate). (1961). ***The outline of history: Being a plain history of life and mankind.*** New York: Garden City Books.

Welsford, E. (1935). ***The fool: His social and literary history.*** London: Faber and Faber.

Related Websites

http://www.disabilityhistory.org/
(Disability Social History Project)

http://www.acf.dhhs.gov/programs/pcmr/history.htm
(President's Committee on Mental Retardation—History)

http://www.npr.org/programs/disability/
(Beyond Affliction: The Disability History Project)

http://codi.buffalo.edu/graph_based/.bibliography/woodhill/woodhill.html
(History of Disabilities and Social Problems)

http://web.syr.edu/~thechp/suprt3a.htm
(Surviving the Institution and Struggling in the Community)

Chapter 3

Conceptual Cornerstones of Service Delivery

Introduction

In Chapter 1 we discussed the importance of focusing on the individual with a disability as a person with unique talents and needs. In Chapter 2 we showed how the majority of past treatments and services for people with disabilities were not person-centered, in fact, were often not even respectful of personhood. Early moves toward institutionalization made initial attempts to recognize the need for more respectful treatment. Similarly, the later move toward deinstitutionalization was driven by advocates who demanded better treatment of people with disabilities. Today, there are federal as well as state and provincial laws that ensure humane, respectful treatment. In Chapter 4 we will highlight key-federal legislation. In this chapter we will describe theories and concepts that we believe are the cornerstones of person-centered recreation service delivery.

The people first concept of service delivery is crucial for ensuring that recreation services are responsive to individuals with disabilities. In other words, the person-centered approach is all about enhancing quality of life for persons with disabilities. Recent findings in a 1998 National Organization on Disability/Harris Survey provide critical evidence of the need to consider quality of life within the field of disability (N.O.D./Harris, 1998). The results of this survey indicated that only about one in three Americans with disabilities say that they are satisfied with their life, compared to six out of ten non-disabled Americans. This gap has widened in the last four years. In addition, fewer than half of people with disabilities believe that their quality of life will improve over the next four years. For these reasons, quality of life is a concept which has increasingly received attention by people with disabilities, families, and service providers. According to Schalock (1996, p. vii), however, it is a concept that has been around for many years, but has gained prominence as we have come to recognize the disparities regarding the quality of life of people with and without disabilities:

> . . . and what makes the concept of quality of life so important to our field is our attempt to use this concept as a process and an overriding

principle to improve the lives of persons with mental retardation and closely related disabilities.

Quality of life is foundational to the person-centered approach. In many ways, our recognition of the importance of quality of life, helps us to understand the essence of the person-centered approach. This is because, quality of life is rooted in the person. Schalock (1996) outlines some of the core principles of quality of life for people with disabilities. Those that are most germane to our discussions appear in Table 3.1.

The core principles outlined in Table 3.1 provide a useful frame of reference for later chapters in this book that address service delivery issues. In this chapter, we will discuss several other concepts, which are imbedded within the dimensions of quality of life discussed by Schalock (1996). The overarching framework of quality of life as well as the concepts of normalization, social role valorization,

Table 3.1
Principles of Quality of Life Central to the Person-Centered Approach

- Quality of life for persons with disabilities is composed of those same factors and relationships that are important to all persons.
- Quality of life is experienced when a person's basic needs are met and when he or she has the same opportunities as anyone else to pursue and achieve goals in the major life settings of home, community, school, and work.
- Quality of life is a multidimensional concept that can be consensually validated by a wide range of persons representing a variety of viewpoints of consumers and their families, advocates, professionals, and providers.
- Quality of life is enhanced by empowering persons to participate in decisions that affect their lives.
- Quality of life is enhanced by the acceptance and full integration of persons in their local communities.
- Quality of life is an organizing concept that can be used for a number of purposes including evaluating those core dimensions associated with a life of quality, providing direction and reference in approaching customer services, and assessing persons' feelings of satisfaction and well-being.

(Adapted from Schalock, 1996)

self-determination, interdependence, and social inclusion provide the conceptual cornerstones for the recreation service delivery system.

For the purposes of this text, we will consider the conceptual basis to mean the ideals that contribute to the facilitation of recreation opportunities for people with disabilities. The ideals provide something against which to measure our services. In some ways they can be utilized to ensure service quality. If these ideals are not understood and used as the basis upon which to develop and deliver recreation services, then we intend that the services rendered are not conceptually sound, and thus they do not provide a proper level of consistent, respectful, person-centered services. These ideals are the standard; they are infused both implicitly and explicitly throughout the remainder of this text. The remainder of the chapter will describe the ideals that we feel contribute to the satisfactory provision of recreation services for people with disabilities.

Normalization

The principle of normalization was first defined by Nirje in a series of papers that he presented during the late 1960s and early '70s while lecturing across Sweden, the United States, and Canada. This principle has become an internationally influential paradigm that has served as the cornerstone of service delivery for people with disabilities (Howe-Murphy & Charboneau, 1987). In a collection titled ***The Normalization Principle Papers,*** Nirje (1992, p. 16) wrote the following contemporary version of his original definition:

> The normalization principle means that you act right when making available to persons with intellectual and other impairments or disabilities patterns of life and conditions of everyday living which are as close as possible to or indeed the same as the regular circumstances and ways of life of their communities.

The attractiveness of Nirje's definition is that it is written in very basic language. His definition clearly underscores that normalization is a value that should be adopted by all, and all who do not, are not "acting right." In one of his very early works, Nirje (1969) described in great detail what he meant by patterns of life and conditions of everyday living. In this article he described ***normal patterns***. However, in a more recent article, Nirje (1985) indicated that the use of the word normal was misinterpreted overtime and should be dropped. Table 3.2 provides a summary of his description of the patterns and conditions of life that are in keeping with the principle of normalization.

When you think about your daily life, you can identify some basic areas that create a pattern: getting out of bed, going to work, eating in a family situation, and going to bed when you feel tired. Though we do not always value any one of these experiences, we do value the ability to make choices related to our daily patterns of sleeping, eating, and working. In addition, the opportunity to experience leisure during one's day is extremely important. For example, we may develop a pattern over time where we jog at noon or watch the news before we go to bed. On the other hand, we also value that we can change our patterns of the day when we

Table 3.2
Patterns of Life and Conditions of Living

1. Patterns of the day.
2. Patterns of the week.
3. Patterns of the year.
4. Developmental experiences of the life cycle.
5. Patterns of economic development.
6. Patterns of environmental conditions.
7. Sexual patterns of one's culture.
8. Respect for the integrity of the individual.

want. We may make a decision to go to a movie, which interrupts our usual pattern, yet that provide us with a different type of leisure experience. It is this type of lifestyle that Nirje suggested should exist for people with disabilities. Unfortunately, all too often these sorts of patterns are not present in the lives of people with disabilities. We have seen many instances where the daily patterns of individuals with disabilities are controlled by service providers rather than the individuals themselves. For example, consider a teenage boy who has mental retardation, who lives in a group home, and who wants to go fishing on Saturday afternoon. There is nothing out of the ordinary about a boy going fishing on a Saturday afternoon. But such an option may not be available to this teenager. State or provincial regulations may require a staff member to accompany him on the fishing trip. If the majority of other members of the group home want to go to the mall, then the staff may not be able to accommodate the fishing request. Therefore, the teenage boy may be stuck with only one option and not one that he has chosen. This is the sort of situation that goes against the ideals of normalization.

Patterns of the week and year are similar to our daily patterns. We value having set patterns, while at the same time we also value breaking such patterns. The changing nature of our world has resulted in much less "traditional" daily and weekly patterns for many people. People work at various times during the day and week. Thus, for people with disabilities, having a pattern that is "typical" is hard to achieve. However, as was mentioned earlier, one aspect that has remained over time is the opportunity to control, at least to some extent, what our daily and weekly pattern looks like. Vacations, birthdays, and holidays like Christmas or Thanksgiving are aspects of our yearly patterns that most of us dearly value. In all cases, the patterns that we see in our own lives can provide us with a yardstick by which to measure the patterns of people with disabilities. However, we may not consider our own circumstances as providing a particularly useful model against which to compare others' patterns. This being true, we need to realize that we should use patterns of days, weeks, and years that we aspire to have, if indeed we consider our own to be inadequate.

Other patterns and conditions described in Table 3.2 can be considered in much the same way as the previous three. Nirje (1969) suggests that the life cycle, sexual patterns, economic conditions, and environmental conditions in which a person lives must be comparable to those to which we all aspire, if we are to be described as adhering to the principle of normalization. The final condition, which is respect for the integrity of the individual, is in many ways the most crucial, and it underscores the humanistic and egalitarian nature of Nirje's principle.

Shortly after Nirje presented his original version of the normalization principle, Wolfensberger (1972) provided what he described as a reformulation of the principle. The principle of normalization was defined by Wolfensberger (1972, p. 28) as the "Utilization of means which are as culturally normative as possible, in order to establish and/or maintain personal behaviors and characteristics which are as culturally normative as possible."

Wolfensberger's definition has tended to receive greater attention in North America than Nirje's definition for a variety of reasons, including that he developed an evaluation system based on his definition of normalization called the Program Analysis of Service System (PASS). PASS has been used extensively throughout such countries as the United States, Canada, and Australia. However, Perrin and Nirje (1985, p. 91) argue that Wolfensberger's (1972) principle is dramatically different than Nirje's and is in fact based on a fundamentally different value base. They present the following as their argument for the differentiation:

> Normalization as originally defined is based upon a humanistic, egalitarian value base, emphasizing freedom of choice and the right to self-determination. It emphasizes clearly respect for the individual and his or her right to be different.... Wolfensberger (1972, 1980), on the contrary, interprets normalization as specifying various standards of behavior to which a mentally handicapped person must conform. He speaks openly of "normalizing" people through "eliciting, shaping, and maintaining normative skills and habits" (Wolfensberger, 1972, p. 32, 1980, p. 17) or even through the use of force: "Normalization measures can be offered in some circumstances and imposed in others" (Wolfensberger, 1982, p. 28, italics in original).

It is important to understand the distinction between these two definitions because each has quite different implications when applied to recreation service delivery. If one bases service delivery on Nirje's definition, then the rights of the individual with a disability to freely choose such things as where to participate, with whom, when, how, or whether to participate at all become central concerns.

In contrast, Wolfensberger's definition clearly suggests that services must be designed in such a way that they facilitate behaviors in individuals with disabilities that are considered normative, and also that the services themselves be normative. Choosing one or the other as a basis for service delivery is less important than ensuring that one understands the implications for each. Though Nirje's definition is in many ways more attractive, we must understand that society as a whole, and more specifically persons participating in recreation programs, often *do* have expectations about the types of behaviors that are acceptable and/or appropriate.

For example, when one attends an aerobics class, participants expect that others will do such things as follow the leader and not create unnecessary disturbances. These are culturally normative behaviors. Choosing to do otherwise is most often considered taboo. As a result, it is appropriate to consider both definitions when designing and implementing recreation services.

Beyond the fact that there has not been complete agreement on the definition of normalization, some confusion over this term has also arisen; many professionals have focused on the word "normal" in attempting to understand its application to the recreation service delivery system. It is important to understand that the intent of normalization is not to transform people with disabilities into "normal individuals." For one thing, defining what a normal individual looks or acts like is impossible. Rather, the principle should be interpreted as a process for facilitating the creation of recreation environments and experiences for people with disabilities that are typical of all people. Thus, this process has a final end goal of individuals engaging in culturally normative leisure experiences.

An additional common misconception related to the normalization principle is that special services are inconsistent with the term. According to Perrin and Nirje (1985, p. 90), however,

> The normalization principle, on the contrary, supports, indeed insists on the provision of whatever services, training, and support are required to permit living conditions and routines similar to that of others in the community.

Social Role Valorization

As a result of the misrepresentation/interpretation of the normalization principle, Wolfensberger (1983) reconceptualized the principle into that of the theory of *social role valorization*. In this reconceptualization he cited the 1977 work of Briggs' dynamic and multifaceted model of self-concept where one's perceptions of self comes from interactions with significant others. Conclusions drawn from those interactions, self-attributions, and previous life experiences are influential in his reconceptualization. With this new awareness of self-concept, Wolfensberger (1983, p. 234) said of people with disabilities:

> ...the most explicit and highest goal of normalization must be the creation, support, and defense of *valued social roles* (emphasis added) for people who are at risk of social devaluation.

Social role valorization theory advocates for each individual's right and responsibility to assume a valued social role in society and society's obligation to allow individuals to pursue that role without constraint. The overarching goal of social role valorization is according to Wolfensberger (1983), achieved via the following two sub-goals; 1) enhancement of their social image, and 2) enhancement of their competencies. Social image is influenced by such things as: 1) physical setting, 2) relationships and groups, 3) activities, programs, and other uses of time, and 4) language and other symbols and images. Similarly, personal competencies can be enhanced in relation to 1) physical setting, 2) relationships and groups and 3) activities, programs and other uses of time. Wolfensberger indicates that image and competency enhancement are generally reciprocally reinforcing. Individuals with high competency generally have a positive image, while those with low competency often are associated with negative images. The same can be said for images influencing competencies. Most importantly, those with positive images are generally afforded more opportunities and experiences to enhance their competencies.

Rancourt (1990) posed the dilemma and the challenge that social role valorization theory presents to the field of therapeutic recreation. Neither the identification with disability nor leisure are generally socially valued roles. Yet, often people with disabilities have large amounts of time free from normative constraints such as work and time, which is therefore available for leisure. Rancourt urged therapeutic recreation specialists (TRS's) to "...demonstrate the worth of that which is presently culturally deemed as worthless" (p. 52). By this she means that we must work to facilitate positive images of people with disabilities experiencing leisure. Such images will serve to create positive social roles for people with disabilities. A complementary perspective on the issues of social role valorization, leisure, and people with disabilities is that we must strive to have society value people with disabilities as people, and in so doing, we will enable people with disabilities to take on various valued social roles, including those associated with work, leisure, friendships, and other typical patterns of life.

Self-determination

Self-determination and decision making have been described as important considerations related to the facilitation of community-based recreation and leisure opportunities for people with disabilities (Brown, 1988; Dattilo & St. Peter, 1991). This is based to some extent on the contemporary definition of leisure, which suggests that choice is a critical regulator for what we do or do not define as leisure (Iso-Ahola, 1980; Neulinger, 1980). In addition, Coleman and Iso-Ahola (1993) have recently suggested that leisure-generated, self-determination dispositions may act as a buffer against stress and serve to decrease the likelihood of illness. According to these authors, people who perceive their actions as self-determined are less likely to experience illness and disease, and leisure very often provides important avenues for developing one's sense of self-determination.

Self-determination grew out of Nirje's (1972) construction of normalization. He suggested that normalization meant having (among other things he described): "Opportunities to have choices, wishes, and desires taken into consideration and respected" (Nirje, 1976). Since then, self-determination has become a well-recognized priority for people with disabilities. So much so, that in 1988 the U.S. Office of Special Education and Rehabilitative Services (OSERS) began a self-determination initiative to focus on system-wide activities that would promote greater decision-making for people with disabilities.

During these past decades a number of definitions and conceptualizations have been proposed for self-determination. Wehmeyer (1996) suggests that there have been two primary conceptualizations of self-determination, as a motivational construct, and an empowerment issue. Those that promote self-determination as an empowerment issue, portray self-determination as both a means toward empowerment and an illustration of the existence of empowerment (Kennedy, 1996; Ward, 1996). Making decisions and speaking out for oneself are examples of self-determining behaviors that lead to a greater sense of empowerment, but are at the same time illustrations of empowerment. Self-determination has also appeared in the motivation literature as an internal need that contributes to a person's performance of intrinsically motivated behaviors. In addition to these two conceptualizations, Wehmeyer argues for the appropriateness of viewing self-determination as an educational outcome, which is defined according to the characteristics of actions or events.

Wehmeyer, Agran, & Hughes (1998, p. 6) proposes that the individual actions of a self-determined person must reflect to some degree the following four essential characteristics:

1. Behavioral autonomy
2. Self-regulated behavior
3. Psychological empowerment
4. Self-realization

Behavioral autonomy refers to a person acting according to her priorities, free from any outside influences. This characteristic is extremely important, as it relates to leisure, because of the influence that personal autonomy has on our own definition of leisure. Beyond the opportunity to behave in an autonomous manner, self-determined individuals are able to regulate their own behaviors. This means that we can assess our surroundings and make decisions about how to behave in order to interact appropriately. For example, an individual who takes part in a ceramics class must be able to listen to instructions, initiate behaviors which correspond to the directions given, evaluate the extent to which his actions match the directions, possibly modify certain behaviors to match the directions, and provide personal reinforcement. The third characteristic, psychological empowerment, describes the extent to which self-determined individuals feel in control. Often described as perceived control, or self-efficacy, this characteristic refers to an individual's beliefs that they can control their environment The final characteristic, self-realization, describes the recognition of the strengths and limitations that influence our ability to behave in a self-determined manner, and the extent to which we act in a manner which capitalizes on strengths and minimizes weaknesses. This characteristic is closely connected to the notion of a self-fulfilling prophecy — the more we feel that we can control our own environment, the more likely it is that we will achieve psychological empowerment, self-regulation, and ultimately, behavioral control.

The American Institute for Research (1993) identified the process necessary for being self-determined. The process is illustrated in Table 3.3. As you can see from Table 3.3, the process of being self-determined includes the opportunity not only to make decisions about the course of one's life but also to take actions based on those decisions. Also, the opportunity to evaluate the results of actions and adjust future decisions accordingly is given as well. The last two steps in the process are particularly important. All too often we help people with disabilities to make decisions and even to carry them out. However, we will often do one of two things that disallow them from experiencing these last two steps. The first thing is not allowing people with disabilities to make *bad* decisions. This is due to the strong need we often feel to protect people with disabilities from experiencing failure. However, by not allowing a person to make a bad decision, we negate his opportunity to evaluate the outcome of the decision and decide whether he felt the decision was bad, and then possibly alter future decisions. Secondly, if we have allowed a person to make a bad decision, we are often too quick to jump in and tell her why we thought the decision was bad in the first place and how she should change it in the future so as not to experience such an outcome again. Both of these work against a person becoming truly self-determining.

Table 3.3
Process of Being Self-determined

1. Identify and express one's own needs, interests, and abilities.
2. Set expectations and goals to meet one's needs and interests.
3. Make choices and plans to meet goals and expectations.
4. Take action to complete plans.
5. Evaluate results of actions.
6. Adjust plans and actions, if necessary, to meet goals more effectively.

When we present this concept in class, our students often challenge us on this point, suggesting a need for ***guided democracy***. When this happens, Mike often tells a story about a situation he experienced in a study he conducted a few years ago. Consider Case Example 3.1.

This short story illustrates the need to let the self-determination process follow its own course, so that the individual is able to make decisions for herself. If the TRS had pushed Liz to abandon her desire to show jump, Liz may not have been satisfied and would never have felt truly self-determined.

Many people have argued that self-determination and decision making should become incorporated into as many developmental experiences as possible for people with disabilities because they have historically had little opportunity to exercise choice within their lives, and as a result of a lack of practice, have a difficult time making decisions related to the use of their leisure time (Dattilo & St. Peter, 1991).

Case Example 3.1

The leisure education study was conceptually grounded in self-determination. Liz, who was a participant in a leisure education study, expressed a desire to take up horseback riding. Liz happened to have a severe multiple disability, used an electric wheelchair, and had little motor control. When Liz first expressed this goal, the therapeutic recreation specialist talked to her about a riding program—which was specifically for people with disabilities—that was available in her community and that could well meet her needs. Liz refused to participate in this program, saying that she wanted to be a part of "show jumping". The therapeutic recreation specialist (TRS) was at a loss as to how to help Liz facilitate her goal. The TRS felt certain that Liz's level of disability would prevent her from show jumping. She did not want to disallow Liz's decision, but at the same time, she didn't want Liz to fail. The TRS decided to take Liz to a local horse club and show her the facility and then see what happened. Once Liz arrived at the facility and had watched the riders for a while, she informed the TRS that she had never been to such a facility before, and that now that she was here and had seen the riders in action, she did not want to try show jumping. Eventually, a schedule was worked out allowing Liz to visit the horse club once a week to watch and to help groom the horses, and later begin highly structured and supervised riding.

Yates (1990) has suggested that there is a three-level hierarchy within which we can place decisions. Yates' (p. 3) hierarchy is as follows:

Level 1: Choices. The task of the decision maker is to choose from a set of well-defined alternatives presented to him or her.

Level 2: Evaluations. The decision maker's task is to consider one alternative at a time and to consider the worth of that alternative. The decision maker then expresses an evaluation for each alternative. Evaluations are sometimes expressed as a rank or may be expressed in more subjective terms such as good as opposed to excellent.

Level 3: Constructions. The decision maker is presented with a set of limited resources. The task is to use the resources to construct the most satisfactory alternative. This is the most complex of decision-making tasks.

Dattilo and his colleagues (Dattilo, 1986; Dattilo & Barnett, 1985; Dattilo & Rusch, 1985) have demonstrated that people with severe mental retardation are capable of making choices regarding leisure activities, and that such choices can be assessed in a consistent fashion. Within the framework proposed by Yates (1990), these decision-making studies have focused on the first level of decision-making: choices. Research by Mahon (1994) and Mahon and Bullock (1992), which used the Decision Making in Leisure (DML) Model (Mahon, 1990), showed that by using self-control techniques, constructive decision making could be taught to people with mental retardation.

As suggested by Wehmeyer, Agran, and Hughes (1998), self-determined behavior is reflected not only in making decisions but also in carrying out such decisions. They have suggested that independent planning and initiation are important skills related to self-determination. Few studies have been conducted within the field of recreation and leisure related to independent leisure initiation by people with mental retardation. The few investigations that have appeared in the literature have tended to either prescribe to a "plan *for* the participant" approach to facilitating initiation (Pollingue & Cobb, 1986) or have used techniques within applied behavior analysis to facilitate independent initiation (Duffy & Nietupski, 1985; Wuerch & Voeltz, 1982). In contrast, Mahon (1994) found that planning and initiation skills could be facilitated through the use of self-monitoring.

As has been pointed out by Wehmeyer (1992), self-regulation, or self-control (the two terms are often used synonymously), is a construct closely related to self-determination. Wehmeyer (p. 304) indicates that

> In order to show dynamic self-regulation, individuals must make decisions as to what skills to use in what situation, examine the tasks at hand and their strategic repertoire, and formulate, enact, and evaluate a plan of action, with revisions, if necessary.

Evident from this statement is that self-control, decision making, and action planning are inextricably linked to one another.

As can be seen, self-determination and decision making are important concepts related to individuals with disabilities and recreation participation. The long-held assumption that they were not capable of making their own decisions about what to do for recreation certainly has been dispelled. This is an important implication for those responsible for designing and implementing recreation programs and services. Table 3.4 provides a list of ***keys*** for enhancing self-determination for people with disabilities within the context of leisure.

Interdependence

As we have suggested, self-determination is an important concept relative to facilitating the leisure needs of people with disabilities. Condeluci (1995) notes, however, that a state of interdependence between people with and without disabilities is most conducive to facilitating social inclusion and quality of life. Interdependence focuses on relationships that lead to a mutual acceptance and respect between people with and without disabilities. Interdependence is only achieved by those who are independent. Covey (1989) describes interdependence in this way:

Table 3.4
Keys for Enhancing Self-determination

1. Teach decision-making skills that include setting goals, weighing options, identifying resources and supports, identifying consequences, and solving problems.
2. Provide opportunities for choice making across environments—schools, homes, community.
3. Identify and establish with the individual the necessary and appropriate supports.
4. Provide opportunities for challenge and success.
5. Project belief in a person's ability to succeed as well as in the person's ability to survive failure.
6. Allow individuals the opportunity to take risks.
7. Allow individuals the opportunity to make mistakes and/or fail and to learn from those mistakes.
8. Provide specific, positive feedback to facilitate self-awareness, confidence, and self-efficacy.
9. Allow the individual to accept and take responsibility for his decisions and actions.
10. Provide environments that are accessible and promote individual's utilization of strengths and abilities.
11. Offer reinforcement and acknowledgment of efforts and process of achieving goals.

> Interdependence is a choice only independent people can make. Dependent people cannot choose to become interdependent. They don't have the character to do it; they don't own enough of themselves....As you become truly interdependent, you have the foundation for effective interdependence.

Thus, according to Covey, self-determination is a precursor to interdependence. If an individual is self-determined and independent, he is capable of being interdependent.

Why do we want people with disabilities to be interdependent? Most of what has been written in the field of disability during the past decade has emphasized the need to facilitate self-determination and *independence* in people with disabilities. Most have argued that people without disabilities (often parents, institutional staff, etc.) have had far too much control over people with disabilities, and we must work to sever such control.

Is it not dangerous to speak of interdependence, which by its nature puts some control in the hands of the people without disabilities? Schoeller (1993,94) suggests that our brain, our spirit, our emotions, our psyche, and our sexuality all function better in social interaction than in isolation. Positive interaction, facilitated through an interdependent relationship, can in fact allow people to experience more choices and opportunities, leading to a determined spirit. Nevertheless, we must ensure that the individual with a disability, who represents one person in an interdependent relationship, is a valued and contributing member of the relationship.

Condeluci's (1995) notion of interdependence is closely tied to the concept of reciprocity, which is one of the five elements of the social exchange theory. Gouldner (1960) has observed that the two central elements of reciprocity are that people should help those who help them, and that people should not injure those who have helped them. He argues that reciprocity is a universal norm. In order for interdependence to exist, then, there must be reciprocity within the relationship. In lay terms, we often describe reciprocity as the "give and take" necessary for a relationship to work. This means that interdependence can and does exist between people with and without disabilities if both contribute to the relationship by giving and receiving. Condeluci (p. 93) identifies actions of the interdependent paradigm that "are designed to promote and empower the distantiated person to take more charge of their life." These actions are depicted in Table 3.5.

Table 3.5
Actions of the Interdependent Paradigm

1. Allow the consumer to define the problem.
2. Focus on capacities.
3. Establish the importance of relationships.
4. Develop supports.
5. Recognize system change.

The first action identified by Condeluci is similar to the first component of the self-determination process (i.e., identify and express one's own needs, interests, and abilities). This is consistent given the relationship between self-determination and interdependence. Condeluci suggests that most often the first action is facilitated by people with disabilities being listened to. So, in a sense, you move beyond the paradigm of self-determination when you move from people articulating goals and making decisions based on those goals, to other people listening to the goals and making related decisions. If we think about Liz in Case Example 3.1, we notice that Liz and the TRS started to move toward an interdependent paradigm once the TRS decided to respect Liz's decision about show jumping.

Very often, even when we have honored a person's decision, we may harbor doubts about her ability to achieve her goal because of deficits we have identified. Again, in regard to Liz, although the TRS did not disallow Liz's decision to show jump, she harbored grave doubts about Liz's ability to do so. Many of us who have worked within the field of disability for a number of years were trained to identify deficits, and then we worked to alleviate them. Though in some cases it is important to work to limit the impact of deficits, it is equally or more important to identify the capacities of the individual. Mount and Zwernik (1987) call this ***capacity hunting***. Focusing on interdependence challenges us to work with people with disabilities to find capacities that they have. In the field of recreation this means that we move beyond the common model to improve such things as the skills of individuals to enable them to participate in recreation.

Relationships are the cornerstone of interdepenence. As we identified earlier, relationships need to be based on the norm of reciprocity. In addition, also important is that relationships are based on the interest of each person in each other. In the field of recreation, much interest has arisen in the facilitation of friendships between people with and without disabilities (Stainback & Stainback, 1987; Heyne, Schleien, & McAvoy, 1993; Hamre-Nietupski, Hendrickson, Nietupski, & Sasson, 1993). Much of this interest has grown from the fact that often people with disabilities have few friends and very small, social support networks. It is crucial that any focus on friendship development be framed within the interdependence paradigm and the norm of reciprocity. Condeluci (1991, p. 98) supports the following:

> To achieve interdependence mandates that we understand the reasons why friendships break up after injury, or for the person with a congenital defect rarely form in the first place. Then we need to turn out attention to the ways whereby people can have the opportunity to forge new acquaintances that can mature over time.

Closely connected to the issue of relationships is that of natural supports. There is a strong need to identify situations where it makes sense to create supports in the environment that enable people with disabilities to reach given goals. Though at first glance this may seem to be in opposition to the concept of self-determination, it is not. People with disabilities must be given the opportunity to decide when and if they would like to be supported. If a decision is made by a person that he wishes to be given support, then it is important for the community to support that decision. Within the field of recreation we have spent a great deal of time determining how we can best teach people skills they will need to achieve particular goals. In particular, the works of Stuart Schleien and John Dattilo have been exemplary in this arena. In our rush to help individuals develop leisure skills, however, we must ensure that we do not insist on individuals developing skills they may not want or be able to achieve. By this we mean that it is the values and goals of the individuals that matter, not the values and goals of the staff.

In relation to the issue of supports, we need to recognize that very often natural supports (versus paid) can be developed within the community to help individuals achieve goals. A colleague recently told us about a beautiful example of natural supports within recreation. In a retirement planning meeting with John, an older adult who has a developmental disability, John and the facilitator were exploring John's options for retirement. John lives in a rural setting and indicated that he "just wanted to go fishing." The two were having some difficulty figuring out how John could fish regularly because John could not drive and the river was two miles out of town. One evening the facilitator was talking to a friend who told him that his dad (Larry) had retired recently and had taken up fishing with a vengeance, something he had always wanted to do. The light came on for the facilitator. Today, John and Larry go fishing three or four times a week, enjoy each other's company, and are catching lots of fish. This is natural support at its best!

The final action of the interdependent paradigm is system change. This action recognizes that such systems as the traditional medical model and others within the expert paradigm have created many constraints for people with disabilities. They have led to the creation of delivery systems that are more responsive to the needs of professionals than people with disabilities. As Condeluci (1995) points out, the most dramatic example of systems change is the Americans with Disabilities Act. As we will discuss in more detail in the next chapter, this Act had legislated that our system become responsive to people with disabilities. Indeed, the ADA mandates that our system change so that people with disabilities become a part of our system, rather than innocent bystanders, or worse, victims. Within the field of recreation, we must begin to recognize that our systems of service delivery often do not facilitate interdependence. We have worked within an expert system where the professional decides what is best for individuals with disabilities and also whether and when an individual is able to or capable of controlling her leisure experiences.

We have begun to recognize the need to allow individuals to become more self-determining in leisure. However, in order that we function more within an interdependent paradigm and move away from an expert system, we must begin to listen to people with disabilities and restructure our systems so that they are indeed designed to foster the actions inherent in the interdependent paradigm and, therefore, are person-centered.

Integration, Mainstreaming, and Inclusion

Integration, mainstreaming, and inclusion have been some of the different concepts used to help people with disabilities gain access to recreation and education opportunities. Integrating people with disabilities into community life is an important issue for people with disabilities, their families, community support personnel, and policy makers. Mainstreaming and integration have been defined by a number of authors (Bullock, 1979; Hutchison & McGill, 1992; Nirje, 1985, Wolfensberger, 1972). The two terms are relatively synonymous, as they are most commonly used. Both are commonly accepted as a process that consists of both the physical presence of people with disabilities in settings where people without disabilities are typically present and participation in social interactions and relationships between people with and without disabilities in typical settings (Wolfensberger & Thomas, 1983). Mainstreaming and integration are concepts that deal with *selective placement.* Mainstreaming proponents usually argue that a participant must earn his opportunity to be placed in a regular recreation setting by keeping up with the class and showing appropriate behavior. Integration is the placement of someone who has a disability with her peers in the regular setting. This method of placement makes the participant feel as though she is different and not capable. On the other hand, inclusion is the best of both worlds. Inclusion provides opportunities for a participant to choose to be with her peers in the regular setting and also provides the supports and accommodations needed to ensure personally satisfying and valued participation.

The physical component of integration is considered a necessary precondition for social integration. However, often physical integration is used as the only indicator for integration. For example, on numerous occasions we have spoken with municipal recreation personnel who have indicated that all of their programs are *integrated.* When questioned, these personnel have told us that this means that any person with a disability who wishes to join a program is welcome to do so. Though this is an important policy, we consider it as being only halfway to creating truly inclusive services. The social component of integration is in many ways more important than the physical component. Unless a person is socially connected within the setting into which he has been physically integrated, he is not truly included.

Many years ago, Mike was involved with three adults with mental disabilities who liked to bowl. They were a part of a local Special Olympics bowling program They were all excellent bowlers and expressed an interest in trying out other bowling programs. Mike helped them to connect with a local bowling program that had never included people with disabilities. The adults became *integrated* into the program. Mike was extremely excited about this new initiative and considered it to be quite "cutting edge." A few months later, the three bowlers came back to see Mike and told him that they were quitting the new program. Aghast, Mike asked why. They told him that they were not having any fun; they were never asked to join any of the other bowlers for a beer, and no one spoke to them much. They wanted to rejoin their friends and the Special Olympics program. Mike saw his "model program" crumbling before his eyes. He tried to convince the three bowlers to keep at it and indicated that he would help them to become more connected, but sadly it was too late. Many years later when we reflect on this story we recognize that Mike had assumed that by physically integrating the bowlers into a program, that they would be welcomed by those already in that setting. He learned the hard way that this is just not the case. Social integration is the key goal that often requires intervention to be achieved.

Within the integration movement, there has been great interest in determining the factors that contribute to social integration, thereby leading to successful independent living for persons with mental disabilities (Bruininks & Lakin, 1985). Wolfensberger (1972, p. 49) described social integration as a person "not only being in, but also of, the community." However, as Lord (1991, p. 217) has suggested, "in the community does not mean of the community." The social aspect of integration, the extent to which people are included in social networks, is arguably the more significant aspect of integration. Much has been written about social integration (Wolfensberger, 1972; Nirje, 1969; Hutchison and Lord, 1979; Blatt & Kaplan; 1966). Wolfensberger and Thomas (1983) argued that when social integration is achieved, individuals with a disability assume valued social roles which further supports the development of relationships with non-devalued members of their communities.

Integral to social integration is the belief that "being of the community" positively influences the life quality of individuals with a disability. In fact, social integration is recognized as one of the core dimensions that contributes to quality of life (Schalock, 1996; Haring, 1991; Wehmeyer & Schwartz, 1998). Beyond this conceptual link, social integration and quality of life also are acknowledged as highly complex, personally variable, and socially constructed notions that defy precise definition (Taylor & Bogdan, 1990; Storey, 1997).

Many have argued that people with disabilities continue to struggle to be part of the social fabric of their communities; to be socially integrated (Anderson, Lakin, Hill, & Chen, 1992; Burchard, Hasazi, Eliason, 1998; Lord, 1991; Pedlar, 1990; Ralph & Usher, 1995). Implicit in this argument is a definition and understanding of social integration that is rooted in the knowledge and opinions of researchers, service professionals, and other individuals who work in support of people with a disability (Goode, 1988; Rosen, Simon, & McKinsey, 1995; Schalock, 1996). Consequently, a number of researchers have criticized this body of knowledge because of its failure to include the perspectives of individuals with a disability (Biklen & Moseley, 1988; Schalock, 1996; Taylor & Bogdan, 1990, 1996). For example, Biklen and Moseley (1988) argued that researchers are "outsiders" who "cannot take for granted the views or positions of insiders (people with a mental disability)...but must formulate enhanced understanding by directly studying the perspectives of "insiders" (p. 155).

One of the most recent, comprehensive investigations of the relationship between social integration and leisure was conducted by Mahon, Mactavish, and Rodrigue (1998). The purpose of this research investigation was to explore the relationship between social integration and leisure over the life span of persons with a mental disability, to enable individuals with a mental disability, their social support networks, service providers, and policy makers to foster social integration. In addition, because the vast majority of literature on social integration is reflective of the perspectives of families/social supports, service providers and policy makers, an important goal within this study was to include the perspectives of people with mental disabilities. As a result, the findings place the perspectives of people with disabilities front and centre. The perspectives of service providers, policy makers, and families/social supports are presented as points of contrast for the perspectives of people with disabilities.

The researchers used triangulation in order to develop a rich understanding of social integration. Focus groups were held with people with mental disabilities. Separate focus groups were also held with families and social supports. A total of 18 focus groups were conducted with 10 taking place in urban settings and 8 in rural settings. In the metropolitan and non-metropolitan settings one focus group consisted of parents of children with mental disabilities (ages 0-11). Then there were two groups (one for people with mental disabilities and one for social supports to people with mental disabilities) for each of the following age categories, adolescents (12-21), young adults (22-34), adults (35-59, and older adults (60 and over). Age categories were constructed to reflect a typical aging process, but in selecting participants it was understood that some individuals who were well below the age of 60 years (e.g. people with Down syndrome) would be most similar to those in the older adult category and would be grouped accordingly. In order to gain further insight into social integration and leisure for people with mental disabilities, following the focus groups, key informant interviews were conducted with 40 service providers and policy makers from communities in which the focus groups were conducted.The key informants consisted of individuals identified by the investigators and partners as being able to provide insight into the relationship between service provision, policy development, and social integration.

The themes which emerged from the series of focus groups and interviews conducted over a three-year period provided an important perspective on the relationship between leisure and social integration for people with mental disabilities. Three of the themes which emerged (personal characteristics, families, and structured activities) were consistent across the focus groups for people with mental disabilities and social supports and the interviews held with service providers and policy makers. All of the informants identified the personal characteristics of people with mental disabilities as having a great deal to do with the extent to which they are socially integrated in leisure activities within their community. This included such things as the physical appearance of the person, how outgoing they are, their social and communication skills, and the nature and severity of their disability. Speaking about her 4 year old with Down Syndrome who has diabetes, one parent said "... they have to know what to do if he goes low, they have to know what the signs are if he goes low and he doesn't know and he doesn't have the communication skills to tell you, so that (in our minds) has been an overriding issue. Yeah, I'd love to put him in some play group in the evenings."

All three groups also felt that families and social supports can be both a positive and negative force regarding social integration and leisure. Families provide opportunities and situations where social integration can occur, across the life span. As one service provider put it, "the ones that have a lot of parental support, they're in everything...most of the ones that flourish are the ones in lots of other programs." At the same time, families can also constrain social integration by being overprotective and not allowing their children to make independent decisions. As a result, people with mental disabilities are often not able to choose their preferred activities, and/or the people with whom they wish to participate.

The final theme which cut across the three groups relates to the relationship between social integration and structured activities. The structure of activities tell us about the patterns, forms, and relationships within social integration. It appears that the majority of social encounters with people with mental disabilities occur in somewhat structured environments, such as social clubs, family recreation experiences, and even Special Olympics, which is often not thought of as a forum for facilitating social integration. According to one service provider, "We meet people by taking part in activities that we enjoy.... If you do things with people who have a common interest, you' re going to form common bonds."

Beyond these themes which cut across the three groups, there were themes which emerged specific to each of the three informant groups. For people with mental disabilities, friendships are an important ingredient to consider in social integration. Friendships appear to be setting or context specific. In a sense, there appear to be what the research team came to describe as "islands of social integration," in which social contacts established in one context (e.g. recreation) were seldom extended to other settings. When asked whether he participated with friends from school or other contexts such as the neighborhood in recreation, one person with mental disabilities said, "No...just people...just a team, a regular team." Service providers felt that friendships contribute to social integration, often providing the opportunity for people to be in the community, and meet people without disabilities. The following quote nicely summarizes this theme: "The opportunity to meet other people, that's really important, and where do we do most of that? It's our leisure and recreation...so when your going to that place, you have something in common to talk about...and that's how we often start relationships."

A theme which emerged from the perspective of social supports was the issue of vulnerability. Parents are especially concerned about the vulnerability of their children of all ages, and this influences the extent to which they facilitate opportunities for social integration in the context of recreation. One parent said, "Maybe I'm too protective...she has no idea what you want her to do or what you expect of her...so there's no way I would send her there (to camp) this summer." A final theme, specific to service providers and policy makers, was staff and staff training. This group felt that staff within a setting often determine the extent to which people with disabilities are or are not socially integrated. Residential staff who encourage choice making and community connections can greatly enhance the opportunity for people with disabilities to be socially integrated. Similarly, staff in recreation settings such as community centres, physical activity centres, or structured recreation programs often "make or break" the social integration process. The essence of this theme is contained in a quote from one of the service providers: "But when it came down to it, the person supporting and helping was maybe an untrained volunteer, and then it's been a disaster, an absolute disaster." Service providers in particular felt that where staff are trained to facilitate social integration, it happens fairly consistently, where they are not, it is "hit and miss."

The literature on social integration and leisure for people with mental disabilities describes the importance of leisure in facilitating social integration (Hutchison and McGill, 1992). This widely held belief has been the basis for intervention studies designed to establish the efficacy of leisure-based interventions for fostering social integration and community participation (Mahon & Martens, 1996; Bullock & Howe, 1987). Unfortunately, as has been pointed out by Pedlar (1992), many people with mental disabilities are still not socially integrated within the context of leisure and recreation. This study was designed to explore the issue of social integration and leisure from the perspective of different informant groups. The themes that emerged in this study provide some insight into why people with mental disabilities do or do not hold such community membership. It is important to point out that the different groups involved in this study share a fairly consistent perspective on the essence of social integration and leisure. The relationship between social integration and leisure is a complex phenomenon, dependent upon the interaction between many different factors. The factors that appear to facilitate social integration in leisure relate to the individual, such as personal characteristics, parents/social supports, and the community within which they live. What seems clear from this study is that social integration can and does occur within the context of leisure, given the existence of the factors which have been identified. Integration may vary when one contrasts the data from the metropolitan versus nonmetropolitan focus groups and interviews, and relating to different points of the life span.

Integration has also been described as "based on recognition of a person's integrity, meaning to be able to be yourself among others" (Nirje, 1985). This definition, in keeping with Nirje's definition of normalization, focuses on enabling an individual to be a part of her home community, while still maintaining her sense of self. This is a unique perspective on integration that has not received much attention either in the literature or in the field of recreation and leisure. However, it provides a distinctly different orientation to the concept of integration. Rather than focusing on the manner in which people with disabilities connect with the environment and people within it, this definition underscores the need to ensure that as we work to support people with disabilities in typical settings, we ensure that we do not try to change who they are as people. Rather, we ***include*** people and not simply physically integrate them.

Recently, many people have begun using the term inclusion instead of integration. Inclusion has been defined as a process that enables an individual to be a part of his environment by making choices, being supported in what he does on a daily basis, having friends, and being valued (Dattilo, 1994; Berger, 1994). There is a vast literature discussing the differences between mainstreaming, integration, and inclusion. Like so many concepts, depending on what you read, they seem more alike than different. When one reviews some of the more contemporary descriptions of integration (e.g., Hutchison & McGill, 1992) what becomes evident is that some definitions of integration include the same key elements as the definition of inclusion that we just described. However, the concept of inclusion was introduced because of a concern with some of the failings of the process of integration. More specifically, these failings related to social integration. As we discussed earlier, many agencies have been very successful in physically integrating individuals with disabilities, but much less successful at social integration. This has led many to search for a means of achieving social integration in more meaningful ways. The introduction of the term inclusion served notice that there is dissatisfaction with the extent to which people with disabilities have become a part of their communities. Inclusion gives people equal opportunity to grow and develop to their fullest potential. The fundamental principle of inclusion is the valuing of diversity within the human community. When inclusion is fully embraced, we abandon the idea that children or adults have to become "normal" in order to contribute to the world. We begin to look beyond typical ways of becoming valued members of the community, and in so doing begin to realize the achievable goal of providing all people with an authentic sense of belonging.

Inclusion is about programs that embrace differences; where all people have their needs met; where people learn to live with one another; where basic values are important to each child, not just some of the children (Strully, 1990, p. 26). As we discussed in Chapter 1, language has tremendous impact on action. Our feeling is that the movement toward the term inclusion gives more attention to some key areas not yet dealt with successfully; those areas include the cultivation of friendships, the development of natural supports in the community, and related things that are necessary for a person to be reciprocally and mutually accepted in, and connected to, his community. Interestingly, those are the very things that people such as Nirje (1969), Wolfensberger (1972), Hutchison and Lord (1979), and others have advocated for years.

Conclusion

We have discussed what we believe to be the key cornerstones to service delivery within the fields of recreation and therapeutic recreation. We believe that the concepts of normalization, social role valorization, self-determination, interdependence, integration, and inclusion provide important ideals for recreation-based programs. Throughout this chapter we have given some examples of how these concepts specifically relate to recreation. This chapter will serve as a basis for other chapters within the book. Throughout you will read numerous examples of how adherence to these ideals serves to create programs and services responsive to the needs of people with disabilities. As we have just discussed in relation to the concepts of inclusion and integration, we should never be satisfied with our present ideals. We should always strive to create new ideals or retool existing ones so as to continue to improve the lives of people with disabilities. Chapter 4 will discuss legislation that has been introduced over the years to create opportunities for people with disabilities in keeping with the concepts discussed in this chapter.

Learning Activities

1. Think of as many words as you can that reflect the concepts of normalization, integration, self-determination, and interdependence.
2. James lives in a group home with five other adults. He has lived there since moving from a state-provincial institution. He works at a local workshop, where he is the leader of one of the work crews. In his spare time he participates in Special Olympics; he also enjoys going to movies and to a local pub at odd times. Discuss what aspects of this scenario are consistent/inconsistent with the concepts in this chapter. For those that are inconsistent, how might they be altered to become more consistent?
3. Do a time log for a few days. Record everything that you do from when you wake up until you go to bed. How much of your day is spent in activities that are dependent (you dependent upon another person), independent, or interdependent?
4. How would your life change if you lost your ability to be self-determining?

References

The American Institute for Research (1993). *Self-determination assessment.* Washington D.C.

Anderson, D. J., Lakin, K. C., Hill, B. K. & Chen, T. H. (1992). Social integration of older persons with mental retardation in residential facilities. *American Journal on Mental Retardation, 96*(5), 488-501.

Bergner, A. (1994). Inclusion: Not an ideology, but a way of life. *Newsletter: The Association for Persons with Severe Handicaps, 20* (1), 4-7.

Biklen, S. K., & Moseley, C. R. (1988). "Are you retarded?" "No, I'm Catholic" Qualitative methods in the study of people with severe handicaps. *Journal of the Association for Persons with Severe Handicaps, 13*(3), 155-162.

Blatt, B. & Kaplan, F. (1966). *Christmas in Purgatory: A Photographic Essay of Mental Retardation*. Boston: Allyn & Bacon.

Brown, P.J. (1988). *Effects of self-advocacy training in leisure on adults with severe physical disabilities.* Unpublished doctoral dissertation, Virginia Polytechnic Institute and State University, Blacksburg, Virginia.

Bruininks, R.H., & Lakin, C. (Eds.) (1985). *Strategies for achieving community integration of developmentally disabled citizens.* Baltimore: P.H. Brooks.

Bullock, C.C. (1979). Mainstreaming: In recreation too? *Therapeutic Recreation Journal*, 13 (4), 5-11.

Bullock, C. C. and C. Z. Howe (1991). "A model therapeutic recreation program for the reintegration of persons with disabilities into the community." *Therapeutic Recreation Journal 25*(1), 7-17.

Burchard, S. N., Hasazi, J. S., Gordon, L. R. & Yoe, J. (1991). An examination of lifestyle and adjustment in three community residential alternatives. *Research in Developmental Disabilities, 12*, 127-142.

Coleman, D., & Iso-Ahola, S.E. (1993). Leisure and health: The role of social support and self-determination. *Journal of Leisure Research,* 25 (2), 111-128.

Condeluci, A. (1995). *Interdependence: The route to community*. Winter Park, FL: GR Press.

Covey, S. (1989). *The 7 habits of highly effective people.* New York: Simon & Schuster.

Dattilo, J. (1986). Computerized assessment of preference for severely handicapped individuals. *Journal of Applied Behavior Analysis, 19* (4), 445-448.

Dattilo, J. (1994). *Inclusive leisure services: Responding to the rights of people with disabilities.* State College, PA: Venture Publishing.

Dattilo, J., & Barnett, L.A. (1985). Therapeutic recreation for individuals with severe handicaps: An analysis of the relationship between choice and pleasure. *Therapeutic Recreation Journal, 19,* 79-91.

Dattilo, J., & Rusch, F.R. (1985). Effects of choice on leisure participation for persons with severe handicaps. *Journal of the Association for Persons with Severe Handicaps, 10* (4), 194-199.

Dattilo, J., & St. Peter, S. (1991). A model for including leisure education in transition services for young adults with mental retardation. *Education and Training in Mental Retardation, 26* (4), 420-432.

Duffy, A.T., & Nietupski, J. (1985). Acquisition and maintenance of video game initiation, sustaining, and termination skills. ***Education and Training of the Mentally Retarded***, 157-162.

Goode, D. (1988). ***Discussing Quality of Life: The Process and Findings of the Work Group on Quality of Life for Persons with Disabilities.*** Valhalla, NY: Mental Retardation Institute, Westchester, County Medical Center.

Gouldner, A.W. (1960). The norm of reciprocity. ***American Psychological Review***, 25, 161-178.

Hamre-Nietupski, S., Hendrickson, J., Nietupski, J., & Sasson, G. (1993). Perceptions of teachers of students with moderate, severe, or profound disabilities on facilitating friendships with nondisabled peers. Education and Training in Mental Retardation, 28 (2), 111-127.

Haring, T. G. (1991). Social relationships. In L. H. Meyer and C.A. Peck (Eds.), ***Critical Issues in the Lives of People with Severe Disabilities*** (pp. 195-217). Baltimore, MD: Paul H. Brookes Publishing Co.

Heyne, L.A., Schleien, S.J., & McAvoy, L.H. (Eds.). (1993). ***Making friends: Using recreation activities to promote friendship between children with and without disabilities***. Minneapolis, MN: Institute on Community Integration (UAP).

Howe-Murphy, R. & Charboneau, B.G. (1987). ***Therapeutic recreation intervention: An ecological perspective***. Englewood Cliffs, NJ: Prenctice-Hall.

Hutchison, P. & McGill, J. (1992). ***Leisure, integration, and community.*** Concord, Ontario.: Leisurability Publications, Inc.

Hutchison, P., & Lord, J. (1979). ***Recreation integration: Issues and alternatives in leisure services and community involvement.*** Ottawa, Ontario: Leisureability Publications.

Iso-Ahola, S.E. (1980). ***Social psychological perspectives on leisure and recreation***. Springfield, IL: C.C. Thomas.

Lord, J. and A. Pedlar (1991). "Life in the community: Four years after the closure of an institution." ***Mental Retardation*** 29(4), 213-221.

Mahon, M., Mactavish, J., & Rodrigue, M. (1998). Islands of social integration. ***Abstracts from the 1998 Symposium on Leisure Research***. Arlington, VA: National Recreation and Park Association.

Mahon, M.J. (1990). ***Facilitation of independent decision making in leisure with adolescents who are mentally retarded.*** Unpublished manuscript, University of North Carolina at Chapel Hill, Division of Special Education, Chapel Hill, North Carolina.

Mahon, M.J. (1994). The use of self-control techniques to facilitate self-determination skills during leisure in adolescents with mild and moderate mental retardation. ***Therapeutic Recreation Journal, 28*** (2), 58-72.

Mahon, M.J., & Bullock, C.C. (1992). Teaching adolescents with mild mental retardation to make decisions in leisure through the use of self-control techniques. ***Therapeutic Recreation Journal, 26*** (1), 9-26.

Mahon, M.J. & Martens, C. (1996). Leisure education in supported employment: Assessing the impact on leisure satisfaction and community adjustment. ***Journal of Applied Recreation Research, 21***, 283-312.

Mount, B., & Zwernik, K. (1987). Person-centered planning. In J. O'Brien & C.L. O'Brien (eds.), ***Framework for accomplishment*** (pp. 1-4). Lithonia, GA: Responsive Systems Associations.

Neulinger (1980). Leisure counseling theory and practice: Different goals require different approaches. In F. Humphrey, J. Kelly, & E. Hamilton (eds.), *Facilitating leisure development for the disabled.* Washington, D.C.: University of Maryland.

Nirje, B. (1969). A Scandinavian visitor looks at U.S. institutions. In R. Kugel & W. Wolfensberger (eds.), *Changing patterns of residential services for the mentally retarded.* President's Committee on Mental Retardation: Washington, D.C.

Nirje, B. (1972). The right to self-determination. In W. Wolfensberger (Ed.). *Normalization: The Principles of Normalization in Human Services*. Toronto, Ontario: The National Institute on Mental Retardation.

Nirje, B. (1976). The normalization principle and its human management implications. In M. Rosen, C. R. Clark, & M. S. Kivitz (Eds.), *The History of Mental Retardation: Collected Papers* (Vol. 2, pp. 363-376). Baltimore, MD: University Park Press.

Nirje, B. (1985). Setting the record straight: A critique of some frequent misconceptions of the normalization principle. *Australian and New Zealand Journal of Developmental Disabilities, 11,* 69-74.

Nirje, B. (1992). *The normalization principle papers*. Uppsala: Centre for Handicap Research, Uppsala University.

Pedlar, A. (1990). Normalization and integration: A look at the Swedish experience. *Mental Retardation, 28*(5), 275-282.

Pedlar, A. (1992). Deinstitutionalization and normalization in Sweden and Ontario, Canada: Supporting people in leisure activities. *Therapeutic Recreation Journal.*

Perrin, B., & Nirje, B. (1985). The basis and logis of the normalization principle. *Australia and New Zealand Journal of Developmental Disabilities*, 11 (2), 65-68.

Pollingue, A.B., & Cobb, H.B. (1986). Leisure education: A model facilitating community integration for moderately/severely mentally retarded adults. *Therapeutic Recreation Journal, 20* (3), 54-62.

Ralph, A. & Usher, E. (1995). Social interactions of persons with developmental disabilities living independently in the community. *Research in Developmental Disabilities, 16*(3), 149-163.

Rancourt, A. (1990). Older adults with developmental disabilities/mental retardation: A research agenda for an emerging subpopulation. In M.E. Crawford & J.A. Card (eds.), *Annual in therapeutic recreation: Volume one* (pp. 48-55). Reston, VA: American Alliance for Health, Physical Education, Recreation and Dance.

Rosen, M., Simon, E.W. & McKinsey, L. (1995). Subjective measure of quality of life. *Mental Retardation,* 33(1), 31-34.

Schalock, R.L. (1996). *Quality of Life Volume I: Conceptualization and Measurement*. Washington, DC: American Association on Mental Retardation.

Schalock, R.L. (1996). Reconsidering the conceptualization and measurement of quality of life. In R.L. Schalock (ed.), *Quality of Life Volume I: Conceptualization and Measurement*. Washington, DC: American Association on Mental Retardation.

Schloss, P.J., Alpen, S., & Jayne, D. (1994) Self-determination for persons with disabilities: Choice, risk, and dignity. *Exceptional Children*, 60 (3), 215-225.

Schoeller, K. (1993/94). Standing together: One family's lessons in self-determination. *Newsletter: Impact, 6* (4).

Stainback, W., & Stainback, S. (1987). Facilitating friendships. ***Education and Training in Mental Retardation, 22,*** 18-25.

Storey, K. (1997). Quality of life issues in social skills assessment of person with disabilities. ***Education and Training in Mental Retardation and Developmental Disabilities, 32***(3), 197-200.

Strully, J. (1990, February). Schools as inclusive communities. ***State Government News,*** 26.

Taylor, S. J. & Bogdan, R. (1990). Quality of life and the individual's perspective. In R. L. Schalock & M. J. Begab (eds.), ***Quality of Life: Perspectives and Issues*** (pp.27 40). Washington, DC: American Association on Mental Retardation.

Taylor, S. J., & Bogdan, R. (1996). Quality of life and the individualís perspective. In R. L. Schalock (ed.), ***Quality of Life Volume I: Conceptualization and Measurement*** (pp.11-22). Washington, D.C.: American Association on Mental Retardation.

Wehmeyer, M.,Agran, M., & Hughes, C. (1998). ***Teaching self-determination to students with disabilities.*** Baltimore, MD: Paul H. Brookes.

Wehmeyer, M. & Schwartz, M. (1998). The relationship between self-determination and quality of life for adults with mental retardation. ***Education and Training in Mental Retardation and Developmental Disabilities, 33***(1), 3-12.

Wolfensberger, W. (1972). ***The Principle of Normalization in Human Services.*** Toronto, Ontario: National Institute on Mental Retardation.

Wolfensberger, W. (1983). Social role valorization: A proposed new term for the principle of normalization. ***Mental Retardation, 21*** (6), 234-239.

Wolfensberger, W., & Thomas, S. (1983). ***PASSING (Program Analysis of Service Systems' Implementation of Normalization Goals): Normalization criteria and ratings manual*** (2nd ed.). Toronto, Ontario: National Institute on Mental Retardation.

Wuerch, B.B., & Voeltz, L.M. (1982). ***Longitudinal leisure skills for severely handicapped learners: The Ho'onanea curriculum component.*** Baltimore: P.H. Brookes.

Yates, J.F. (1990). ***Judgment and decision making.*** Englewood Cliffs, NJ: Prentice Hall, Inc.

Related Websites

http://www.ohsu.edu/selfdetermination/selfdet.shtml
(Center on Self-Determination — Oregon Health Sciences University)

http://www.libertynet.org/speaking/
(Speaking for Ourselves)

http://www.independentliving.org/index.html
(Institute on Independent Living)

http://www.self-determination.org/
(National Program Office on Self-Determination)

http://web.syr.edu/~thechp/nrc.htm
(National Resource Center)

http://circleofinclusion.org/index.html
(Circle of Inclusion)

http://www.ed.psu.edu/ci/ci412/inclusion.html
(On-Line Resources for Teachers - Inclusion)

http://www.nichcy.org/pubs/newsdig/nd24txt.htm
(Planning for Inclusion)

Chapter 4

Legislation

Introduction

Relatively few federal laws related to the treatment or well-being of people with disabilities were passed prior to World War II. Those that did exist were intended to address the needs of war veterans with service-connected disabilities. This meant that for most of North America's history, schools, businesses, recreation and parks agencies, and other public entities were allowed to, and often did, exclude children and adults with disabilities.

The first federal laws in the United States designed to assist individuals with disabilities date back to 1798 when the Fifth Congress of the United States passed the first federal law concerned with the care of people with disabilities (Braddock, 1987). This first law authorized a Marine Hospital service (which became known as the United States Public Health Service in 1912) to provide medical services to sick and disabled seamen. Although some legislation already addressed the needs of people with disabilities, there was actually very little legislation passed between that time and the 1960s. Since the 1960s, however, an enormous amount of federal legislation has passed in the United States that relates directly to individuals with disabilities. As a result, today people with disabilities have accomplished more than ever dreamed possible—due to more and better programs, better trained professionals, continuous research, information dissemination, and technical assistance—much of which is the direct result of federal and state/provincial legislation.

To provide the best possible services to all people, we must understand not only what has happened to people with disabilities historically but also what has happened and is happening recently and currently. Many recreation professionals have little knowledge about these laws. Knowledge of the law can assist them in understanding the entire service delivery system, can ensure the protection of civil rights, and can improve collaboration with other agencies and families. Before presenting an overview of the most important recent laws, we will illustrate how ideas become laws and regulations.

How Laws and Regulations Are Determined

The focus in this section is on federal legislation in the U.S. A number of differences exist in federal and provincial lawmaking in the Canadian parliamentary government, however, there are a number of similarities. Basically, ideas for laws can come from anyone or from anywhere. The idea must "catch the eye" of an elected official before it can be introduced as a draft bill. In order to do that, there must be a compelling reason to draft a law to ensure the protection of citizens. Therefore, long before ideas become draft bills, a lot of behind-the-scenes work must be done by individuals and groups to convince elected officials that there is broad-based support for their idea to become a law. Once the elected official or officials are convinced that an idea has sufficient merit, it is then introduced as a draft bill that is soon debated, revised, and ultimately passed or defeated. This entire process can take years of hard work and political maneuvering. The following figure (Figure 4.1) shows how a federal bill becomes a law (The Indiana Governor's Planning Council for People with Disabilities, 1992).

When an act is passed by the United State Congress and signed into law by the President, it is given a number, such as PL (Public Law) 101-476. The first set of numbers represents the session of Congress during which the law passed. For example, the 101 means the 101st session (which, incidentally, was in 1990) of Congress. The second set of numbers represents the sequence of passage and enactment of that act during that session. Thus, 101-476 means that this was the 476th law that Congress passed and the President signed during the 101st session of Congress.

It is also important to understand that laws are reauthorized regularly. That is, they are reviewed and, if needed, changed or amended, and then repassed. Each reauthorization then becomes a new public law. For example, Public Law 94-142, the *Education for All Handicapped Children Act*, has had several reauthorizations since its passage in 1975. The 1990 reauthorization, PL 101-476, even changed the name of that statute to *Individuals with Disabilities Education Act.* Recreation professionals need to keep up-to-date on these changes because they often affect the programs and services that we provide.

Laws passed by Congress provide a general framework of policy related to a particular issue. Once a law is passed, Congress delegates to an administrative agency within the Executive Branch the task of developing detailed regulations to guide the law's implementation. In the case of the previously mentioned PL 101-476, the *Individuals with Disabilities Education Act*, it was delegated to the Department of Education to develop the regulations of the education focused law. Federal regulations are detailed in the *Code of Federal Regulations (CFR)*. The *CFR* interprets the law, discusses each point of it, and then further explains it. Copies of most federal regulations are available in your university library. The *CFR* is readable and helpful in understanding the laws. State agencies must comply with federal laws and regulations.

Figure 4.1
How a Federal Bill Becomes a Law

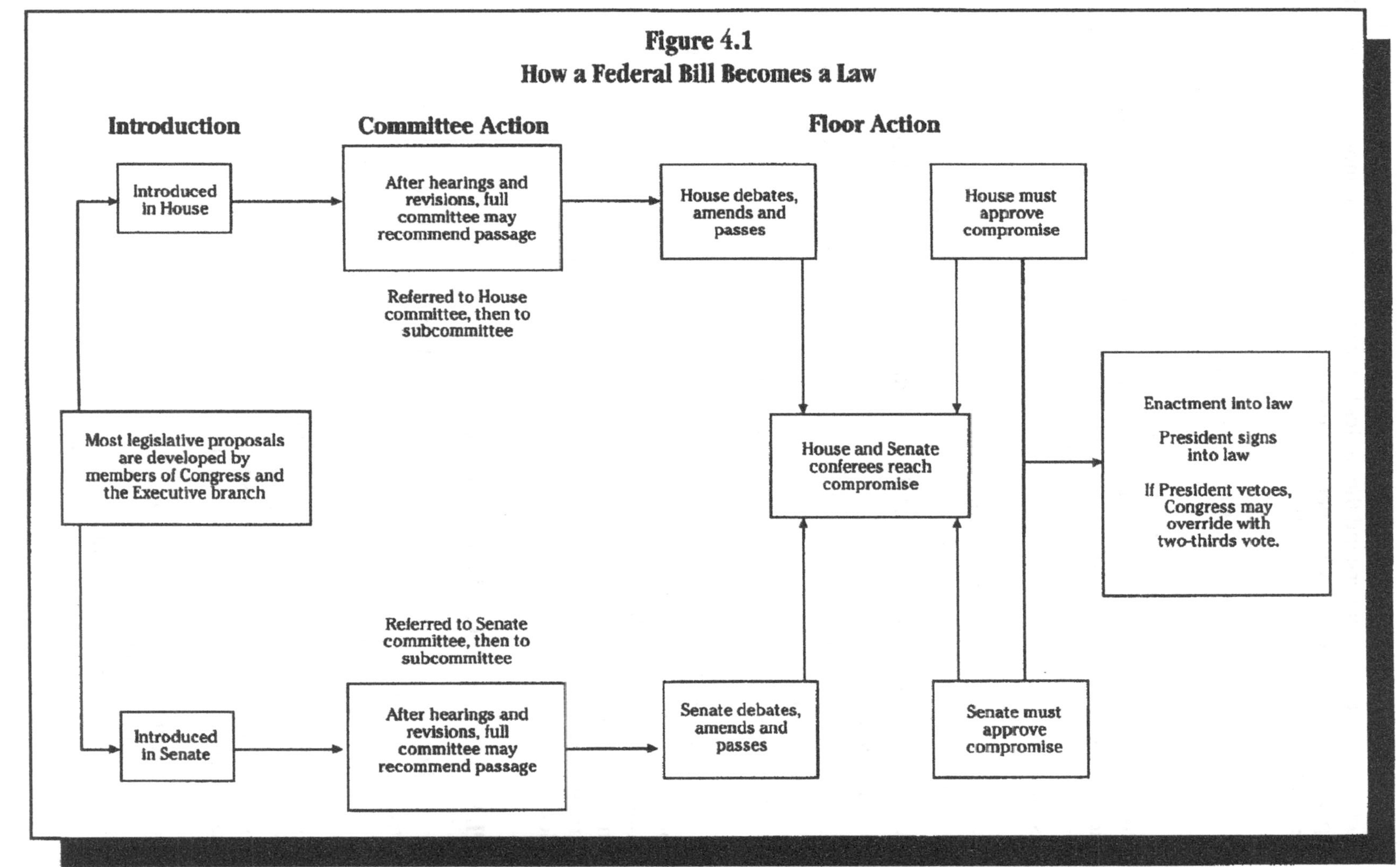
Introduction
Committee Action
Floor Action
Introduced in House
After hearings and revisions, full committee may recommend passage
House debates, amends and passes
House must approve compromise
Referred to House committee, then to subcommittee
Most legislative proposals are developed by members of Congress and the Executive branch
House and Senate conferees reach compromise
Enactment into law
President signs into law
If President vetoes, Congress may override with two-thirds vote.
Referred to Senate committee, then to subcommittee
Introduced in Senate
After hearings and revisions, full committee may recommend passage
Senate debates, amends and passes
Senate must approve compromise

This is a very basic overview of the process of law and rule-making. It is helpful, however, to understand the basics before moving on to more detail about specific laws. In the following section we will briefly explain the core of the U.S. laws affecting people with disabilities.

Current U.S. Laws Affecting People with Disabilities

Although there have been many state and federal laws that have included disability-related issues in the United States, the rights of individuals with disabilities have been most significantly strengthened by the passage of five federal laws and their subsequent periodic amendments and reauthorizations. These laws are as follows:

1. PL 93-112, the *Rehabilitation Act of 1973*.
2. PL 94-142, the *Education of All Handicapped Children Act of 1975*.
3. PL 100-146, the *Developmental Disabilities and Bill of Rights Act Amendment of 1987*.
4. PL 100-407, the *Technology-Related Assistance for Individuals for Disabilities Act of 1988*.
5. PL 101-336, the *Americans with Disabilities Act of 1990*.

These five laws, and their subsequent amendments, form the core of current protection against discrimination and current guarantees of equal opportunity that individuals with disabilities have in the United Sates. Because these laws are so important to ensuring the rights of those with disabilities, you should become familiar with both the laws and their regulations. Each law is described in some detail below.

PL 93-112, The Rehabilitation Act of 1973

There are a number of sections of the Rehab Act. This law grew out of and strengthened earlier acts, including PL 90-480, the *Architectural Barriers Act of 1968*, and the Vocational Rehabilitation Act of 1962. Among other things, the Rehab Act provides funds for vocational rehabilitation and independent living services. However, the most noteworthy part of the Rehab Act is that it addresses discrimination against people with disabilities. As such, it is the first major piece of civil rights legislation that relates specifically to people with disabilities. The law has different sections which refer to different areas of discrimination, as follows:

- Section 501: Employment;
- Section 502: Architectural and Transportation Barriers Compliance Board;
- Section 503: Employment under federal contract;
- Section 504: Nondiscrimination under federally funded programs.

The most important section was and continues to be Section 504, often called the ***nondiscrimination section.*** Even today Section 504 provides individuals with disabilities with basic civil rights protection against discrimination in *federal* programs. The law states that:

> no otherwise qualified handicapped individual in the United States shall, solely by reason of his (her) handicap, be excluded from the participation in, be denied the benefits of, or be subjected to discrimination under any program or activity receiving federal financial assistance.

To be eligible for the protection under Section 504, an individual must meet the definition of an ***handicapped person***. This definition includes any person who 1) has a physical or mental impairment that substantially limits one or more of such person's major life activities, 2) has a record of such impairment, or 3) is regarded as having such an impairment.

Major life activities include self-care, performing manual tasks, seeing, hearing, speaking, breathing, learning, and walking. Section 504 covers only those people with disabilities who would otherwise be qualified to participate and benefit from the programs or other activities receiving *federal* financial assistance.

Section 504 assures equal opportunities for people with disabilities in programs receiving federal funds—municipal and county recreation departments, YM/YWCAs, state institutions, colleges and universities, hospitals and clinics, and public and private groups of all kinds that receive any federal financial assistance. Agencies that persist in acts of discrimination face the loss of federal funds.

From 1972 (prior to the passage of the law) through 1975, the National Recreation and Park Association assigned one of its five governmental affairs specialists to solely represent the issues and concerns of its National Therapeutic Recreation Society (NTRS). This was a critical time in legislation related to people with disabilities. In part, due to the efforts of the NTRS as well as the National Consortium on Physical Education and Recreation for the Handicapped (NCPERH), the Rehab Act included recreation as an important part of the rehabilitation process and established funding for recreation research, training, and special projects (Shank, 1989; Patrick, Hillman, & Park, 1989). In fact, through funds authorized by Public Law 93-112, a number of therapeutic recreation students received funding for their graduate education. In addition, since 1979, over 200 special recreation projects supported from Section 316 funds have been initiated. The funds for these projects indicate the continued importance of recreation in the rehabilitation process. PL 93-112 has been amended several times since its inception. During each reauthoritzation, the NTRS and the NCPERH have remained as involved legislative advocates.

In 1983, PL 98-221, the ***Rehabilitation Act Amendment of 1983,*** authorized several demonstration projects regarding the transition of youth with disabilities from school to work and adult life. Through the efforts of NTRS and the NCPERH, the words recreation and therapeutic recreation were included throughout the reauthorize bill, which has allowed therapeutic recreation specialists to be involved in this transition effort. Similarly, when in 1986 PL 99-506, the ***Rehabilitation Act***

Amendments, provided for programs in supported employment services for individuals with disabilities, recreation and therapeutic recreation became ***allowable*** services in the supported employment process. In practice, few supported employment programs have actually included recreation or therapeutic services as part of supported employment services. Notable exceptions are Community Partnerships, Incorporated, an agency in Raleigh, North Carolina, and SCE Lifeworks in Winnipeg, Manitoba. Both of these agencies regularly include recreation as a part of their supported employment services. In a recent study of long-term supports of people in supported employment, the number one need as identified by parents and service providers was the need for recreation and leisure supports (Dalton, Test, Dotson, & Beroth, 1994). This suggests that recreation and leisure supports should be included in supported employment programs from the outset rather than after the bulk of employment services are completed. By having recreation and therapeutic recreation infused throughout the act, such services that have already been verified as an important part of the rehabilitation process may become even more utilized in the future. Since the mid-1980s, the American Therapeutic Recreation Association (ATRA) has joined the National Therapeutic Recreation Society (NTRS), and the National Consortium on Physical Education and Recreation of Individuals with Disabilities (NCPERID—formerly NCPERH) to continue legislative advocacy related to the Rehabilitation Act as well as several other laws discussed below.

The Rehabilitation Act still remains a core piece of civil rights legislation. In a recent reauthorization, the ***Rehabilitation Act Amendments of 1992,*** Congress took the principles and policies of the Americans with Disabilities Act (ADA) (discussed later in this chapter) and translated them into statutory language that relates specifically to rehabilitation. The reauthorized law now includes new sections that clearly tie the overall purpose of the Rehab Act to achieving the goals and objectives of the ADA. This is significant because the ADA is no doubt the most pervasive piece of civil rights legislation ever passed. By making the provision of the Rehab Act consistent with the principles and policies of the ADA, the importance and centrality of the Rehabilitation Act is confirmed. The law now is based on principles of presumed ***ability to become employed and to remain employed, to be integrated and included in all aspects of everyday life, to be provided meaningful and informed choices, and to achieve involvement of families and natural supports***.

The 1992 reauthorization includes amendments that promote streamlined access to services; it mandates strong transition requirements for students exiting the schools; and it requires provision of personal assistance services, rehabilitation technology services and devices, and supported employment, when appropriate. People with disabilities are provided significant opportunities for input into how services and supports are organized in each state through a new state rehabilitation advisory council. And, significantly, the Secretary of Education must write regulations to enable people with disabilities to secure their own goods and services following development of their IWRP (Individualized Written Rehabilitation Program). The product of over two years of advocacy, this reauthorization legislation puts a federal policy in place that empowers individuals with disabilities in the rehabilitation agencies that they must change with the times. These changes are entirely consistent with the conceptual cornerstones discussed in Chapter 3. Recreation remains specifically mentioned in the 1992 reauthorization as an important part of the rehabilitation process. Practitioners in recreation and therapeutic recreation are empowered to ensure that recreation is utilized to the fullest extent to enhance the quality of life and rehabilitation of all people. The Rehabilitation Act Amendments of 1992 (PL 102-569) and 1993 (PL 103-73) were concerned with enhancing the effectiveness of rehabilitation programs. However, the most notable addition was the change to the use of people-first language in place of demeaning language that had been used previously within the wording of the Rehab Act.

In August of 1998, President Clinton signed the Workforce Investment Act of 1998 (PL 105-220) which included amendments to the Rehabilitation Act. The bill empowers workers, not government programs, by offering training grants directly to them, so they can choose for themselves what kind of training they want and where they want to get it.

The Individualized Written Rehabilitation Program (IWRP) was changed to the Individualized Plan for Employment (IPE). The amendment adds a provision that the IPE is to be developed and implemented in a timely manner subsequent to the eligibility determination. Options for the development of the plan must be provided to the individual in writing and in appropriate modes of communication including information on the availability of assistance to be determined if needed by the individual. The continuity of services pending appeal is broadened to include assessment services prior to the development/implementation of the IPE.

To learn more about the precise nature of this act, including the sections not described here, how to file a discrimination complaint, or to obtain a copy of the Rehab Act's regulations, write to the U.S. Department of Education, Office of Civil Rights, Operations Support Service and Technical Assistance Branch, 330 C St., S.W., Room 5431, Washington, D.C. 20202.

PL 94-142, the Education for All Handicapped Children Act of 1975

Although there existed some early special education legislation, nothing before compared to the Education for All Handicapped Children Act of 1975 (EHA). This law was passed in 1975 and went into effect in October of 1977 when the regulations were finalized. This law grew out of and strengthened earlier acts of a similar name, including PL 91-230 and PL 93-380. Ballard, Ramirez, and Zantal-Weiner (1987) summarize the major purposes of PL 94-142 in the following statement:

> To guarantee that a *free appropriate education*, including special education and *related* service programming, is available to children and youth with disabilities who require it.
>
> To assure that the rights of children and youth with disabilities and their parents or guardians are protected (e.g., fairness, appropriateness, and due process in decision making about providing special education and related services to children and youth with disabilities).

> To assess and assure the effectiveness of special education at all levels of government.
>
> To financially assist the efforts of state and local governments in providing full education opportunities to all children and youth with disabilities through the use of federal funds.

Of particular importance to recreation and therapeutic recreation is the related service provision that legitimizes recreation as an important augmentation to special education services. Related services are defined in the law as:

> developmental, corrective, and other supportive services may be required to assist a child with a disability to benefit from special education, and includes the early identification and assessment of disabling conditions in children.

Bullock and Johnson (1998) list the related services specifically identified in the law:

- audiology,
- counseling services,
- medical services for diagnostic or evaluation purposes,
- occupational therapy,
- parent counseling and training,
- physical therapy,
- psychological services,
- *recreation,*
- rehabilitation counseling,
- school work services in schools,
- speech pathology, and
- transportation.

Recreation as a related service for students with disabilities must be administered in a manner consistent with other related educational services. As a related service, recreation assists, augments, and enhances the educational process. Recreation and leisure are essential parts of a total education (Bullock, Morris, Mahon & Jones, 1992). Recreation is further defined in the regulations of the law as having four components:

- assessment of recreation and leisure functioning,
- leisure education,
- therapeutic recreation, and
- recreation in school and community agencies.

Any child with a disability is entitled to a free and appropriate public education that emphasizes special education. The child *may* receive any of the additional related services, but the services must assist a child with a disability to benefit from special education and must be specifically identified and written into the child's Individual Education Program (IEP). Although parents and teachers work together on writing the child's IEP, often recreation is not included because it is not readily recognized as a related service.

As with the Rehabilitation Act, the National Therapeutic Recreation Society (NTRS) worked in cooperation with the National Consortium on Physical Education and Recreation for the Handicapped (NCPERH); they helped include recreation into this law. As a result of this inclusion, recreation has been statutorily validated as an important part of the education process. Funds authorized by this law have been used to train graduate and undergraduate students to work as related service personnel, to conduct research into the efficacy of this related services, and to conduct special projects. To date, this is still a very underutilized related service; however, as a result of much of the research that has been funded by the Office of Special Education Programs, increasing evidence points to the need for more use of this related service.

In 1983, through the ***Education for all Handicapped Children Act Amendments of 1983***, PL 98-199, Congress either amended or changed the law to expand incentives for preschool special education, early intervention, and transition programs. All programs under EHA became the responsibility of the Office of Special Education Programs (OSEP), which by this time had replaced the Bureau of Education for the Handicapped (BEH).

In 1986, ***EHA*** was again amended through PL 99-457, the ***Education of the Handicapped Act Amendments of 1986***. One of the important outcomes of these amendments was that the age of eligibility for special education and related services for all children with disabilities was lowered to age three, a change implemented during school year 1991-1992. The law also established the Handicapped Infants and Toddlers Program (Part H). As specified by law, this program is directed to the needs of children from birth to their third birthday who need early intervention services. In addition, under this program, the infant or toddler's family may receive services that are needed to help them assist the development of their child. State definitions of eligibility under this program vary, but, in order to receive federal funds, each state must have a comprehensive, statewide, interagency service delivery system.

The ***Education for all Handicapped Children Act*** makes it possible for states and localities to receive federal funds to assist in the education of infants, toddlers, preschoolers, children, and youth with disabilities. To remain eligible for federal funds under the law, states must follow certain guidelines, outlined in Table 4.1.

In October, 1990, Congress passed and then-President Bush signed into law the ***Education for all Handicapped Children Act Amendments of 1990***, PL 101-476. The new law has resulted in some significant changes. For example, the name of the law, the Education for all Handicapped Children Act (EHA), was changed to Individuals with Disabilities Education Act (IDEA). Many of the discretionary programs authorized under the law were expanded. Some new discretionary programs, including special programs on transition, a new program to improve services for children and youth with serious emotional disturbance, and a research and information dissemination program on attention deficit disorder were created. These additions represent a significant opportunity for therapeutic recreation to become more involved in a variety of discretionary programs. Services and rights were expanded to more fully include children with autism and traumatic brain injury. In addition, the law now includes both transition and assistive technology services as new elements of special education services that must be included in a student's IEP.

PL 102-119, the ***Individuals with Disabilities Education Amendments of 1991***, contains many amendments to strengthen participation of and control by families. The intent of these amendments is to ensure that "through informed decision making on what services exist and are recommended for a family, the family selects the services it desires at that time."

Additional amendments were included to recognize the importance of technology in liberating many infants and toddlers with disabilities and their families from barriers encountered in all aspects of daily living, including in recreation and leisure and in significantly enhancing learning and development. There is evidence that the provision of assistive technology has dramatically altered prospects for a child's future—where access to technology has results in labels being dropped, in the provision of opportunities in integrated environments, in increased confidence and ability of the child, and in changed perceptions of the child by the family and others.

The ***Individuals with Disabilities Education Act*** (IDEA), 1990 (PL 101-476) was reauthorized by Congress on May 14, 1997 and was signed into law by President Clinton on June 4, 1997. The new law is the Individuals with Disabilities Education Act Amendments of 1997 (PL 105-17). The 1997 IDEA, the most exhaus-

Table 4.1
State Requirements under EHA

1. All children and youth with disabilities, regardless of the severity of their disability, will receive a ***free, appropriate public education (FAPE)***—at public expense.
2. Education of children and youth with disabilities will be based upon a ***complete*** and ***individual evaluation and assessment*** of the specific, unique needs of each child.
3. An ***Individualized Education Program (IEP)***, or an ***Individualized Family Services Plan (IFSP)***, will be drawn up for every child or youth found eligible for special education or early intervention services, stating precisely what kinds of special education and related services, or the types of early intervention services each infant, toddler, preschooler, child, or youth will receive.
4. To the maximum extent appropriate, all children and youth with disabilities will be educated in the ***regular education environment***. Children and youth receiving special education have the right to receive the ***related services*** necessary to benefit from special instruction. Related services include...transportation and such developmental, corrective, and other supportive services that are required to assist a handicapped child to benefit from special education, and includes speech pathology and audiology, psychological services, physical and occupational therapy, ***recreation***, early

Table 4.1 Cont.

identification and assessment of disabilities in chidren, counseling services, and medical services for diagnostic or evaluative purposes. The term also includes school health services, school social work services, and parent counseling and training (CFR:Title 34; Education; Part 300.12, 1986).

5 ***Parents have the right to participate*** in every decision related to the identification, evaluation, and placement of their child or youth with a disability.

6 ***Parents must give consent*** for an initial evaluation, assessment, or placement; be notified of any change in placement that may occur; be included, along with teachers, in conferences and meetings held to draw up individualized programs; and must approve these plans before they go into effect for the first time. The right of parents to challenge and appeal any decision related to the identification, evaluation, and placement of their child, or any issue concerning the provision of FAPE, is fully protected by clearly spelled-out *due process procedures*.

7. Parents have the ***right to confidentiality of information***. No one may see a child's records unless the parents give their written permission. (The exception to this are school personnel with legitimate educational interests.)

tive collection of changes to be made in this law since 1991, aimed to strengthen academic expectations and accountability for the nation's 5.4 million children with disabilitics. It also aimed to bridge the gap that often exists between what children with disabilities learn and the regular, general education curriculum. Remarks by President Clinton at the signing ceremony of the IDEA on the South Lawn were:

> First, this bill makes it clear once and for all that children with disabilities have a right to be in the classroom and to be included in school activities...
>
> Second, this legislation mandates that with appropriate accommodations children with disabilities learn the same things with the same curricula and the same assessments as all the other children...
>
> Third, we know our children's success depends upon the quality of their teachers...And it will require regular education teachers to be involved in the development of individual education plans to help disabled children succeed...(Clinton, President. Speech. "Remarks from the IDEA 1997 Signing Ceremony" June 4, 1997.)

The Major foci of the IDEA Reauthorization are:

- strengthened parental participation;
- increased accountability for student success in the general curriculum including mastery of IEP goals and objectives in levels of general education performance;
- incorporation of behavior plans; and
- responsiveness to the growing needs of an increasingly more diverse society.

With this reauthorization, there is a presumption of general classroom placement for students with disabilities. Children with disabilities must have access to the regular curriculum. The Individualized Education Program (IEP) must relate more clearly to the general curriculum that children in regular classrooms receive. The IDEA states:

> The IEP includes...
>
> • a statement of measurable annual goals, including benchmarks or short-term objectives related to meeting the child's needs that result from the child's disability to enable the child to be involved in and progress in the general curriculum; and...
>
> • an explanation of the extent, if any, to which the child will not participate with nondisabled children in the regular class;

This calls for increased accountability for the success of the student with a disability in the general curriculum. General education teachers will have to do more classroom assessments for levels of performance on an annual basis. Provisions also require the general education teacher of the child, to the extent appropriate, to participate in the development of the child's IEP. The general education teacher is now a vital contributing member in establishing IEPs. Each IEP must have present levels of performance, plus goals and objectives for the general curriculum. The discussion of annual IEP goals should reflect the general education curriculum, as well as the special education curriculum as appropriate. There must be a statement of explanation of the extent, if for any reason, the child with a disability is not placed in the general education class or still requires segregated services. There must be documentation between the general education and the special education teachers to confirm the need for such services.

Behavioral plans must be established for those student with disabilities who need them. The IDEA states:

> • The IEP team shall...in the case of a child whose behavior impedes his or her learning or that of others, consider, when appropriate, strategies including positive behavioral interventions, strategies, and support to address that behavior...

Hence, behavioral plans which are typically initiated by the general education teacher need to be in place for these students. It is the general education teacher's responsibility to identify target behaviors, collect baseline data as the behavior changes, and implement strategies and methods to change the targeted behavior.

The definition of "child with a disability" allows the use of "developmental delay" to be used for children ages 3 through 9, rather than 3 through 5. Incorporated in a number of provisions are "at-risk infants or toddlers," defined as individuals under age 3 at risk of experiencing substantial developmental delay if early intervention services are not provided.

Another change expands enrollment on the state advisory panel, the purpose of which is to provide policy guidance on special education and related services. In addition to the members listed in the previous law, the panel must include representatives of IHEs preparing special education and related services personnel, among others. The majority of the panel shall be individuals with disabilities or parents of children with disabilities.

Another important provision of this bill required that transition service needs must now be included in the IEP beginning at age 14. This provision was designed to augment the previous transition service provision of the Act by focusing attention on how the child's educational program can be planned to facilitate a successful transition to his or her goals for life after high school.

In developing an IEP, the bill requires that the IEP team consider the strengths of the child and the concerns of the parents for enhancing the education of the child. In cases where the child is receiving related services, that related services personnel should be included on the IEP team to ensure the most efficient implementation of the plan. The bill also requires that the IEP team consider the need for assistive technology devices and services when developing the IEP.

IDEA 1997 aimed to improve considerably the communication among parents, general education teachers, and special education teachers. It should ensure the general education teacher's involvement in the planning and assessing of children with disabilities. And it should lead to high expectations and significantly improved student achievement for children with disabilities.

The regulations that cover the Education for all Handicapped Children Act can be found in the ***Code of Federal Regulations (CFR***: Title 34; Education; Parts 300-399). You can obtain the latest copy of the Federal regulations implementing the Education of the Handicapped Act by sending a check or money order for $12.00 (made out to the Superintendent of Documents). Mail it to the Superintendent of Documents, U.S. Government Printing Office, Washington, D.C. 20402.

PL 100-146, the Developmental Disabilities and Bill of Rights Act Amendment of 1987

The original law, the ***Mental Retardation Facilities and Community Mental Health Centers Construction Act of 1963***, PL 88-164, which includes a Bill of Rights section for people with developmental disabilities, was amended in 1987. People covered under this law now include not only those with mental retardation but also those with autism, cerebral palsy, epilepsy, and other disabling conditions as defined in the act. The term ***developmental disability***, as defined in the act, means the following:

...a severe, chronic disability of a person that

1) is attributable to a mental or physical impairment or combination of mental or physical impairments;
2) is manifested before the person attains age twenty-two;
3) is likely to continue indefinitely;
4) results in substantial functional limitations in three or more of the following areas of major life activity: a) self-care, b) receptive and expressive language, c) learning, d) mobility, e) self-direction, f) capacity for independent living, or g) economic sufficiency; and
5) reflects the person's need for a combination and sequence of special, interdisciplinary, or generic care, treatment, or other services that are of lifelong or extended duration and are individually planned and coordinated.

Each state may have a more inclusive definition of developmental disabilities, yet a definition should be at least as inclusive as the federal law. The act mandates the establishment and operation of a federal interagency committee to plan for and coordinate activities related to people with developmental disabilities. This federal agency is the Administration on Developmental Disabilities and is often referred to as ADD. This act also authorizes money to support four distinct programs:

1. ***Basic grants to states*** to support the planning, coordination, and delivery of specialized services to people with developmental disabilities. These are often referred to as state DD (Developmental Disabilities) Councils.
2. ***A formula grant program*** to support the establishment and operation of state protection and advocacy systems. These are often described as the state's P and A (Protection and Advocacy), even though each state's P and A may have a different name. For example, in North Carolina the P and A is administered under the Governor's office and is called The Governor's Advocacy Council for People with Disabilities (GACPD).
3. ***A project grant program*** to support university-affiliated programs (UAP) for people with developmental disabilities. These are often referred to as UAPs and carry out training, demonstration projects, and/or research specific to persons with developmental disabilities.
4. ***Grants*** to support nationally significant projects aimed at increasing the independence, productivity, and community integration of people with developmental disabilities.

All services provided under this law must be aimed at providing opportunities and assistance for people with developmental disabilities to enable them to "achieve their maximum potential through increased independence, productivity, and integration into the community."

Amendments to this law, the ***Developmental Disabilities Assistance and Bill of Rights Act of 1990***, PL 101-496, were passed by Congress and signed into law by President Bush in 1990. The most recent amendments, the Developmental Disabilities Act Amendments of 1994, were signed into law by President Clinton in April 1994. The new law does not make major changes to the DD Act, but rather fine tunes it. New language has been added to ensure the act's four programs address the needs of unserved and under-served populations, particularly those from racial and ethnic minority backgrounds. The new act will allow state DD Councils and state protection and advocacy systems to continue existing efforts to expand community-based services and to fully protect individuals in any residential setting.

The purpose of the Developmental Disabilities Act is to assure that individuals with developmental disabilities and their families participate in the design of and have access to culturally competent services, supports, and other assistance and opportunities that promote independence, productivity, and inclusion into the community. The most recent reauthorization of the DD Act is currently (March, 1999) underway. It is expected that the 1999 reauthorization will include significant changes that will:

- keep the Act current and on the cutting edge
- improve provisions which are currently causing problems in a significant number of States/territories
- make nationwide consensus recommendations

Specifically, the proposed changes will strengthen systems change as the major function of Developmental Disabilities (DD) Councils. As such, DD Councils will have a more explicit directive to improve the system of services, supports and other assistance for people with developmental disabilities and their families. Another proposed change is to redefine the federal priority areas to be consistent with other civil rights legislation. The federal priority areas are those areas to which states are allowed to allocate their federal money to improve services and supports for people with developmental disabilities and their families. Although there have been priority areas in previous authorizations of the DD Act, the proposal in the current reauthorization is to redefine the federal priority areas as:

- Self-Determination
- Employment
- Homes and Housing
- Health
- Education
- Child Development
- Community Inclusion and Community Education
- System Coordination

Note the new inclusion of "self-determination," one of the conceptual cornerstones of person-centered services discussed in the previous chapter. It is being proposed that this concept be infused throughout the entire reauthorization. Note also, the exclusion of recreation. It could be argued that recreation could be included under health or community inclusion, it is disturbing that overt mention of recreation is not proposed. In this chapter and in the final chapter of this book, we talk about the importance of advocacy. This is a perfect example where recreation and therapeutic recreation advocates have not been actively involved in this important piece of legislation. We challenge individuals and professional organizations to remain active in federal, state, and local legislation to ensure that the recreation needs of people with disabilities are always explicitly addressed.

The other important change being proposed in the 1999 reauthorization is to add needed definitions to the major purpose of the act. Concepts such as systems change, capacity building, advocacy, integration, and inclusion have been part of the legislation for a number of years, but not been defined. In recent reauthorizations of some of the other disability civil rights laws, these concepts have been defined. Since these concepts are central to a person-centered approach and are parts of other laws, they are listed below.

- Systems Change means the activities designed to result in laws, regulations, policies, practices, or organizational structures that are consumer and family responsive and directed so that services, supports, and other assistance are more flexible and provide enhanced opportunities for individuals with developmental disabilities to be independent, productive, integrated, and included in the community.
- Capacity building means activities designed to increase the ability of organizations, systems, and communities to serve, support, assist, and include people with developmental disabilities and their families.
- Advocacy means activities designed to inform policymakers regarding how to improve policies and practices which promote and enhance the independence, productivity, integration, and inclusion of people with developmental disabilities and their families to advocate for themselves.
- Integration means the equal right of individuals with developmental disabilities to use the same community resources that are used by and available to other citizens.
- Inclusion means the acceptance and encouragement of the presence of developmental disabilities by people without disabilities in social, educational, work, and community activities, enabling people with developmental disabilities to have:
    - friendships and relationships with individuals and families of their own;
    - live in homes close to community resources, with regular contact with citizens without disabilities in their communities;

- enjoy full and active participation in the same community activities and types of employment as citizens without disabilities; and,
- take full advantage of their integration into the same community resources as citizens without disabilities, living, learning, working, and enjoying life in regular contact with citizens without disabilities.

It is extremely important that recreation and therapeutic recreation professionals be aware of the DD Act because of the importance of recreation in enhancing the quality of life of people with developmental disabilities. Although the legislative cooperative of NTRS, NCPERID, and ATRA were not involved in the passage of the most recent reauthorizations of the DD Act, nor the 1999 deliberations, that group must monitor legislation that is related to therapeutic recreation in order to be proactive if and when specific professional advocacy is needed.

You can obtain the latest copy of the law and the federal regulations of the Developmental Disabilities Act by contacting the Superintendent of Documents, U.S. Government Printing Office, Washington, D.C. 20402.

PL 100-407, the Technology-Related Assistance for Individuals with Disabilities Act of 1988

Commonly referred to as the Tech Act and signed into law by President Reagan in August 1988, this was the first federal legislation with the sole purpose of expanding the availability of assistive technology services and devices to individuals with disabilities. The law is a systems change initiative enacted to increase access to assistive technology for individuals with disabilities, including the promotion of access to financing. Its three purposes are as follows:

1. *To provide financial assistance to the states* to help each state develop and implement a consumer-responsive statewide program of technology-related assistance for individuals of all ages with disabilities.
2. *To identify federal policies* that facilitate payment for assistive technology and those that impede such payment and to eliminate inappropriate barriers to such payment.
3. *To enhance the ability of the federal government* to provide the states with technical assistance, information, training, public awareness programs, and funding for model demonstration and innovation projects.

The legislation was enacted in recognition that for

> ...individuals with disabilities, assistive technology is a necessity that enables them to engage in or perform many tasks...(and) to have greater control over their own lives; participate in and contribute more fully to activities in their home, school, and work environments, and in their communities; interact to a greater extent with nondisabled individuals; and otherwise benefit from opportunities that are taken for granted by individuals who do not have disabilities.

The act also references underserved groups, defined as

> any group of individuals with disabilities who, because of disability, place of residence, geographic location, age, race, sex, or socioeconomic status, have not historically sought, been eligible for, or received technology-related assistance.

A comprehensive definition of assistive technology is used to include services that help individuals select, acquire, and use assistive technology devices as well as the devices themselves. *Assistive technology device* is defined by the act as:

> any item, piece of equipment, or product system—whether acquired off the shelf, modified, or customized—that is used to increase, maintain, or improve functional capabilities of individuals with disabilities.

The broad definition of devices included under the law gives states great flexibility in the programs to be developed.

Title I of the act established a program of federal grants to the states. Development grants were provided for a three-year period, with a two-year extension grant. From 1989 through 1993, all states and U.S. territories received development grants. The minimum grant award was $500,000.

Title I of PL 100-407 provided states with funds to develop a consumer-responsive state system of assistive technology services, including the following:

- model delivery systems;
- statewide needs assessment;
- support groups;
- public awareness programs;
- training and technical assistance;
- access to related information;
- interagency agreements; and/or
- other activities necessary for developing, implementing, or evaluating a statewide service delivery system.

Title II of PL 100-407 authorized the federal government to perform various activities to help states develop their service delivery systems. This included a study to be undertaken by the National Council on Disability to identify practices that facilitate or impede the financing of assistive technology devices or services and a study of the need for a National Information and Program Referral Network to assist states in responding to technology-related information needs.

The most recent reauthorization is the Assistive Technology Act of 1998 (ATA). The purposes of the Assistive Technology Act of 1998 are to:

- support States in strengthening their capacity to address the assistive technology needs of individuals with disabilities;
- across Federal agencies and departments, focus the investment in technology that could benefit individuals with disabilities; and

- support micro-loan programs to provide assistance to individuals who desire to purchase assistive technology devices or services.

The ATA reaffirms the federal role of promoting access to assistive technology devices and services for individuals with disabilities. The bill allows states flexibility in responding to the assistive technology needs of their citizens with disabilities, and does not disrupt the accomplishment of states over the last decade through the State assistive technology programs funded under the Tech Act.

Title I authorizes funding for multiple grant programs from fiscal years 1999 through 2004: continuity grants, challenge grants, millennium grants, grants to protection and advocacy systems, as well as a funding for a technical assistance program.

Title II provides for increased coordination of federal efforts related to assistive technology and universal design. Universal design means to design products, buildings, etc., so they can be used without alteration by the maximum number of people whether or not they have disabilities. It also authorizes funding for multiple grants programs from fiscal years 1999 through 2004.

Title III provides for alternative financing mechanisms for people with disabilities to purchase assistive technology devices and services from fiscal years 1999 through 2004.

Assistive technology is the key that provides access to employment, education, transportation, and other activities of daily living for many people with disabilities. As technology becomes more prevalent in our culture, there is increasingly a need for a national program with state-level flexibility to ensure that employment, education, and independent living become more accessible. The Assistive Technology Act of 1998 will meet these challenges and people with disabilities, and society as a whole, will benefit.

Technology can be a double-edged sword for people with disabilities. It can provide access to new and heretofore inaccessible activities, or it can serve as yet another barrier to access.

Although the legislative cooperative of NTRS, NCPERID, and ATRA were not involved in the passage of PL 100-407, that group monitors legislation related to therapeutic recreation in order to be proactive if and when specific professional advocacy is needed.

You can obtain the latest copy of the law and the federal regulations of the Developmental Disabilities Act by contacting the Superintendent of Documents, U.S. Government Printing Office, Washington, D.C., 20402.

PL 101-336, the Americans with Disabilities Act of 1990

The Americans with Disabilities Act (ADA) was signed into law by President Bush on July 26, 1990. The ADA has been referred to as the 20th century emancipation proclamation for individuals with disabilities. The central purpose of this act is to extend to individuals with disabilities civil rights protections similar to those provided to individuals on the basis of race, sex, national origin, and religion. Based on the concepts of the Rehabilitation Act of 1973, the ADA guarantees equal opportunity for individuals with disabilities in employment, public accommodation, transportation, state and local government services, and telecommunications. The ADA is the most significant federal law assuring the full civil rights of all individuals with disabilities.

The Americans with Disabilities Act (ADA) is a comprehensive civil rights law intended to eliminate discrimination against people with disabilities in all aspects of American life. When each of the previously discussed laws come up for reauthorization, the reauthorization process is and will continue to be influenced by ADA. The following overview will include each of the key sections and a brief description of enforcement methods.

Title I: Employment

Any employer of 25 or more people is prohibited from discriminating on the basis of disability against a "qualified individual with a disability" in any aspect of employment—advertising, recruiting, hiring, training, promoting, and discharge. Employers should develop a job analysis to determine the essential functions of each job. When an individual with a disability meets legitimate educational, skill, and experience qualifications for a position, and can perform the essential functions of a job, the employer must make a reasonable accommodation. Reasonable accommodations include, but are not limited to, reassignment of nonessential tasks, providing auxiliary aids or services, removing architectural barriers in the workplace, changing the individuals' work schedule, permitting supplemental unpaid leave, or reassignment of an employee to a vacant position. This, of course, includes employment in recreation and therapeutic recreation settings. Title I employment complaints are to be enforced by the Equal Opportunity Commission.

Title IIA: Government Services

Any unit of state or local government, or any extension or instrument thereof, is prohibited from discriminating on the basis of disability in the provision of state or local government services against an individual who, with or without a reasonable accommodation, meets essential eligibility requirements for receipt of that service. State and local government services are broadly interpreted to include every program, service, and activity of such an entity. A reasonable accommodation shall include, but is not limited to, the changing of rules, policies, and practices; the removal of architectural, transportation, and communication barriers; and the provision of auxiliary aids and services. Units of local government must conduct a self-analysis to identify discriminatory practices and barriers and shall remove all barriers as soon as possible. Title IIA is particularly important to recreation professionals who work in state, county, or municipal parks and recreation departments. Title IIA complaints against units of local government can take three routes. First, complains may be filed with the municipality or state for internal resolution. Second, complaints may be filed with the U.S. Department of Justice or a designated federal agency, e.g., parks and recreation, the Department of Interior. Or third, a lawsuit may be filed in federal court.

Title IIB: Public Transit

State and local governments that operate public transit systems may not discriminate on the basis of disability in the provision of these services. Public transit includes fixed route systems, demand responsive systems, para-transit systems, and rapid rail systems. Certain requirements are phased in over a period of time because of the anticipated difficulty in funding massive structural changes. Two of note are the requirement that one car per train must be accessible by July 26, 1995, and that key rail stations must be accessible not later than July 26, 2020. Title IIB complaints must be filed with the U.S. Department of Transportation. Or, a lawsuit may be filed in federal court.

Title III: Public Accommodations

A place of public accommodations is a private establishment (for profit or for nonprofit) that provides goods, services, or facilities; examples include hotels, restaurants, theaters, banks, stores, and health clubs. Public accommodations may not discriminate against qualified individuals with disabilities from participating in, or benefiting from, full and equal enjoyment of the services, goods, facilities, and advantages provided by that entity. Reasonable accommodations include, but are not limited to, changing rules or practices; the removal of architectural or communication barriers; and the provision of auxiliary aids or services. Where the removal of a barrier will require structural change, removal must be readily achievable. If not, alternative methods of accommodation must be considered. New construction must be readily accessible to, and, usable by, individuals with disabilities. Title III complaints may be filed with the Department of Justice, or complainants may file a lawsuit in federal court.

Title IV: Telecommunications

Telephone companies must provide telecommunications relay services for people with hearing impairments and people with speech impairments all day, every day, with no restrictions on the number and length of calls made. Title IV complaints may be filed with the Federal Communications Commission.

The implementation of the ADA through these new federal rules will produce a fundamental and dramatic shift in the way in which America perceives and values people with disabilities. Since the ADA was passed to eliminate discrimination of people with disabilities, additional information about the ADA will be presented in Chapter 5, which deals with discrimination and barriers.

There have been no significant changes to the ADA, although it has a profound influence on opportunities for people with disabilities.

For additional information and answers to questions regarding the ADA, contact the U.S. Department of Justice, Civil Rights Division, Coordination and Review Section, P.O. Box 6618, Washington, D.C. 20035-61189. Telephone: (Voice) — (202) 514-0301 and (TDD) (202) 514-0381-83, 11 a.m. to 4 p.m. Eastern time. Every state has an ADA coordinator. Additional information can be obtained from your state's ADA coordinator, usually housed in the state's capital. For a copy of the ADA regulations for the relevant title, write to the regulatory agencies to request a copy of the regulations for which they are responsible:

- **Title I, Employment Discrimination**
  Equal Employment Opportunity Commission (EEOC), 1801 L St., NW, Washington, DC 20507, (Voice) (202) 663-4264, (TDD) (202) 663-4141.
- **Title II, Public services of state and local government**
- **Title III Public accommodation by private businesses**
  U.S. Department of Justice, Civil Rights Division, Constitution Ave. & 10th St., NW, Washington, DC 20530, (Voice) (202) 514-2000, (TDD) (202) 514-0716.
- **Title IV, Telecommunications**
  Federal Communications Commission (FCC), Office of *ADA*, 1919 M St., NW, Washington, DC 20554, (Voice) (202) 632-7000, (TDD) (202) 632-6999.

Legislation in Canada

Laws in Canada are passed at three levels: federal, provincial, and local. Laws from all three levels influence the rights of people with disabilities. Federal authority is derived from the constitution provisions laid out in the 1867 British North America (BNA) Act, and in the Canadian Constitution Act of 1982.

The history of legislation in Canada related to people with disabilities is similar to that of the United States in that very little happened until the 1960s. In 1962 Parliament passed the Vocational Rehabilitation for Disabled Persons Act (VRDP). Unfortunately, the act was passed without consultation with people with disabilities. The act defined disability in the following way: "Disabled person means a person, who, because of physical or mental impairment, is incapable of pursuing regularly any substantially gainful occupation" (Enns, 1981). The act provides for equal cost sharing of vocational rehabilitation services between provinces and the federal government. More recently criticized because of its narrow definition of disability, and rehabilitation, the act was landmark lauded in its day for providing rehabilitative supports for people with disabilities.

The VRDP framework and agreements with each province were revised in the early 1990s. For example a new Canada-Manitoba agreement was signed in 1993. These agreements give more responsibility to the provinces while still containing provisions for a continuing role for the federal government. The VRDP agreement allows for a comprehensive program of vocational rehabilitation for people with disabilities to be co-funded by each Province and the Federal Government including ongoing support for provincially-based independent living resource sectors. The program consists of:

- assessment and counseling;
- follow-up goods and services for people with disabilities;
- services and processes of restoration, training, and employment placement designed to enable a person with a disability to dispense with the necessity for institutional care or the necessity for the regular home service of an attendant;

- provisions for utilizing the services of voluntary organizations that are carrying out activities in the Province in the field of vocational rehabilitation of people with disabilities;
- the training of persons as counselors or administrators to carry out programs for the vocational rehabilitation of people with disabilities, the coordination of all activities in the Province relating to vocational rehabilitation of people with disabilities; and,
- such other services and processes of restoration, training, employment placement and follow-up goods and services in respect of people with disabilities as may, by agreement between the Minister and Province, be made part of the agreement.

Both the third and six provisions have been used in recent years to enable the introduction of therapeutic recreation as a rehabilitative service.

The International Year of the Disabled Person (1981) and International Decade of the Disabled Person (1982-93) occurred during the period of time between the initial passing and revisions to the VRDP. This was a very significant period of time for the entrenchment of disability rights in Canada. During the International Year of Disabled Persons the Canadian Federal Government appointed an all-party Special Committee on the Disabled and Handicapped. This committee, which conducted hearings across Canada, undertook a comprehensive review of federal legislation that related to people with disabilities. The report, ***Obstacles***, presented 130 recommendations on all aspects of public policy including human rights, income security, assistive devices, transportation, recreation, and communication. One of the most significant accomplishments of the Committee was the inclusion of people with physical and mental disabilities in the equality rights section of the Charter of Rights and Freedoms. At least a half a dozen reports have been published since ***Obstacles*** was released that have analyzed the success of the implementation of the 130 recommendations.

In April of 1982, the Canadian Charter of Rights and Freedoms came into being. Section 15 of the Charter, which focuses on equality rights, came into full force in April of 1985. Within it, Section 15(2) provides the foundation for the assertion of rights for persons with disabilities. It states that all individuals are "equal before and under the law," and have the "right to equal protection and equal benefit of the law without discrimination and, in particular, without discrimination based on . . . mental and physical disability." Lepofsky (1997, p. 1) suggests that this section "triggered unprecedented optimism among people with disabilities.

Lepofsky (1997) conducted a thorough analysis of the impact of Section 15(2), in an article in the ***National Journal of Constitutional Law***, titled "A Report Card on the Charters Guarantee of Equality to Persons with Disabilities After Ten Years: What Progress? What Progress?" Lepofsky considered the following areas in conducting his analysis: Access to education, community living, equality in the criminal justice system, civil justice, health care, licenses, and freedom from civil detention, discrimination due to disability-based income support, coerced sterilization. This detailed, case-by-case analysis highlights the successes and failures of Section 15(2). In his conclusion, Lepofsky (p. 430) suggests that Canada's justice system deserve a "C minus on its implementation of the equality guarantee in the disability cases" tried in the past 10 years. According to Lepofsky, the most significant accomplishment was the Ontario Court of Appeal's Eaton decision on the right to equal educational opportunities for children with disabilities, that was brought down in 1995. Notwithstanding this case, Lepofsky asserts that Canada must go much further in its second decade to secure the rights of people with disabilities.

Since the introduction of Section 15(2) of the Charter, and Lepofsky's subsequent analysis of its impact, two other significant federal initiatives have taken place. In 1997, the Federal Government initiated a Federal Task Force on Disability Issues, chaired by Member of Parliament Andy Scott. The Scott Task Force traveled across Canada, and conducted 16 public consultations. The report put forth a far reaching set of recommendations, including the creation of a Canadians with Disabilities Act, a legislative review of all laws that have the potential to impact people with disabilities, the incorporation of a disability lens in the development of all laws, policies, and programs, changes to the labor market program, improved tax assistance and income programs.

The final and most recent initiative of the Governments in Canada was the release of the report ***In Unison: A Canadian Approach to Disability Issues***. The report, which was a joint effort of the Federal, Provincial, and Territorial Ministers of Social Services, sets out a blueprint for promoting the integration of people with disabilities in Canada. The key values and principles necessary to achieve the vision of full citizenship for Canadians with disabilities are very much in keeping with the philosophy of person centered recreation. Finally, the four building blocks to achieving citizenship are policies that promote access to generic services and supports, employment, and income.

In contrast to the United States, education and many other services for people with disabilities are driven by provincial rather than federal legislation. For example, provincial authority in education relies on the statutes enacted by the legislatures that provide the legal framework by which each system of education is governed. In addition, provincial schools acts provide a variety of rules and regulations set out by various departments of education. The fact that education is a provincial responsibility in Canada, has resulted in different types of legislation dealing with people with disabilities. The majority of provinces mandate special education services for persons with disabilities; however, four provinces have only permissive legislation, meaning that services are permitted but not mandated. The same can be said for other services for persons with disabilities.

Canada does not at this time have legislation that is as far-reaching as the Americans with Disabilities Act. For the time being, Canadians with disabilities must rely on Section 15(2) of the Canadian Charter of Rights and Freedoms to provide the basis for litigation and other means of asserting rights.

Conclusion

Marked by the passage of the Rehabilitation Act of 1973 and the Americans with Disabilities Act of 1990, Congress has taken measures to include people with disabilities in the American agenda. These particular pieces of legislation have been called the two most important documents ever produced in the struggle for equality by people with disabilities. These are founded on the belief that people with disabilities deserve equal protection under the law and equal access to the services provided by it. Upon this foundation are built the guidelines and parameters for inclusion by both the Rehabilitation Act and the Americans with Disabilities Act.

The Rehabilitation Act itself was not specific recreation legislation, but it contained within it the words that would service as the launch pad for policy in a varicty of areas to follow. Section 504 of the Rehabilitation Act of 1973 states that:

> no otherwise qualified handicapped individual in the United States...shall, solely by reason of his/her handicap, be excluded from the participation in, be denied the benefits of, or be subjected to discrimination under any program or activity receiving federal financial assistance.

These words, and the sentiments expressed by them, characterized the movement and functioned as a progenitor for future legislative mandates.

The Americans with Disabilities Act (ADA) is the most recent and the most comprehensive act ever to address the civil rights of people with disabilities.

Learning Activities

1. Identify state or provincial legislation that is similar to federal legislation discussed in this chapter.
2. Study the state or provincial legislation that you discover. How is it different from federal legislation? If state or provincial legislation needs to be more person-centered and consumer responsive, brainstorm ways that you can advocate for changes in your state/provincial legislation.
3. Identify your state's ADA coordinator. If you live in Canada, who is a similar governmental official in your province?
4. Consider each of the pieces of core legislation. How are they consistent with the concepts of self-determination, normalization, social role valorization, interdependence, and inclusion?
5. Find out when the next scheduled reauthorization of each of the pieces of core legislation is scheduled. Volunteer to assist an advocacy organization or your professional organization in the reauthorization process.

References

Ballard, R., Ramirez, & Zantal-Weiner. (1987). ***Public Law 94-142, Section 504, and Public Law 99-457: Understanding what they are and are not.*** Reston, VA: Council for Exceptional Children.

Braddock, D. (1987). ***Federal policy toward mental retardation and developmental disabilities.*** Baltimore, MD: Paul H. Brookes Publishing Company.

Bullock, C.C., Morris, L.H., Mahon, M.J., & Jones, B. (1992). ***School community leisure link: Leisure education curriculum guide.*** Published by the Center for Recreation and Disability Studies, Curriculum in Leisure Studies and Recreation Administration, University of North Carolina at Chapel Hill.

Bullock, C.C., & Johnson, D.E. (1998). ***Recrealional Therapy in Special Education.*** In F. Brasile, T. Skalko, & J. Burlingame (Eds.). ***Perspectives in Recreatonal Therapy: Issues of a Dynamic Profession.*** Ravensdale, WA: Idyll Arbor.

Cernosia, A. Esq. "IDEA–1997 Reauthorization. Nevada Project LEAD." September 1997.

Clinton, President. Speech. "Remarks from the IDEA 1997 Signing Ceremony." Washington, DC. June 4, 1997.

Dalton, B.A., Tet, D.W., Dotson, N., & Beroth, T. (1994). The North Carolina Long Term Support Study: Final Report. Chapel Hill, NC: The Developmental Disabilities Training Institute.

Eischeidt, S. & Bartlett, L. (1999). The IDEA admendments: A four step approach for determining supplementary aids and services. ***Exceptional Children,*** 65 (2), 163-174.

Enns, H. (1981). Canadian society and disabled people: Issues for discussion. ***Canada's Mental Health,*** December, 14-17.

Federal/Provincial/Territorial Ministers Responsible for Social Services (1998). ***In unison: A Canadian approach to disability issues.*** Ottawa, Ontario: Federal/Provincial/Territorial Ministers Responsible for Social Services.

"IDEA 1997 General Information." Office of Special Education and Rehabilitative Services. Washington, DC: U.S. Department of Education. September 30, 1997.

The Indiana Governor's Planning Council for People with Disabilities. (1992). ***The legislative process.*** Indianapolis, IN: Author.

Lepotsky, M.D. (1997). A report card of the charters guarantee of equality to persons with disabilities after ten years – What progress? What prospects? National Journal of Constitutional Law, 7, 263-431.

Patrick, G., Hillman, W., & Park, D. (1989). Public policy: The role of the federal government. In D.M. Compton (Ed.), ***Issues in therapeutic recreation: A profession in transition*** (pp. 349-371). Champaign, IL: Sagamore Publishing.

PL 93-112, the *Rehabilitation Acts of 1973.*

PL 94-142, the *Education of All Handicapped Children Act of 1975.*

PL 100-146, the *Developmental Disabilities and Bill of Rights Act Amendment of 1987.*

PL 100-407, the *Technology-Related Assistance for Individuals for Disabilities Act of 1988.*

PL 101-336, the *Americans with Disabilities Act of 1990.*

"Recommendations to the DD Task Force of the Consortium of Citizens with Disabilities on the Reauthorization of the Developmental disabilities Act." Washington, DC: The National Association of Developmental Disabilities Councils. March 4, 1999.

Shank, J.W. (1989). Legislative and regulatory imperatives for therapeutic recreation. In D.M. Compton (ed.), ***Issues in therapeutic recreation: A profession in transition*** (pp. 405-424). Champaign, IL: Sagamore Publishing.

Special Committee on the Disabled and the Handicapped (1981). ***Obstacles: Report of the Special Committee on the Disabled and the Handicapped***. Ottawa, Ontario: Minister of Supply and Social Services, Government of Canada.

"Summary of the IDEA Amendment of 1997." The Council for Exceptional Children. May 20, 1997.

Ziegler, M. "Major Changes to IDEA." Washington, DC: Federation for Children with Special Needs. May 19, 1997.

Related Websites

http://www.icdi.wvu.edu/Others.htm#g2
(Disability Legislation and Related Law)

http://TheArc.org/misc/dislnkin.html#legislation
(Information on Disability Legislation)

http://www.seals.com/html/legislation___policy.html
(Easter Seals Ñ Legislation and Policy)

http://www.ncd.gov/publications/equality.html
(Equality of Opportunity Ñ The Making of the Americans with Disabilities Act)

http://www.independentliving.org/Library/Library_Contents13.html
(Legislation and Legal Action)

http://www.independentliving.org/ Ñ (type ÒlegislationÓin the search box)
(Institute on Independent Living)

http://indie.ca/strategy/inventry.htm
(Inventory of Disability Issues)

http://www.chebucto.ns.ca/Government/Legislation.htmlÑ (click on find, type ÒdisabilityÓin the search box)
(Legislation in Nova Scotia and Canada)

CHAPTER 5

DISCRIMINATION, BARRIERS, AND ACCESSIBILITY

INTRODUCTION

As we saw in the last chapter, the Americans with Disabilities Act (ADA) is the most important piece of civil rights legislation ever written. It was written to address the pervasive discrimination that had existed for so many years against the millions of Americans who have physical or mental disabilities. The ADA was enacted for the following reasons:

1. Society tends to *isolate or segregate* people with disabilities;
2. People with disabilities experience *intentional* as well as *unintentional* (and well-meaning) *discrimination*;
3. Discrimination is *pervasive*, occurring in all levels of society;
4. Discrimination occurs in *critical areas of life*, including employment, housing, access to government services, transportation, communication, and *recreation;*
5. There is *often no satisfactory legal recourse* for people with disabilities who have experienced discrimination;
6. People with disabilities generally occupy *inferior social positions*; and
7. People with disabilities, as a group of individuals, have been *powerless to address these social inequities* (McGovern, 1992).

As important as the ADA is, it cannot put an end to discrimination. Discrimination has arisen over centuries and it will take time for lasting change to occur. Isolation and segregation have become the norm for people with and without disabilities. Isolation has even become preferable to many people with disabilities who over time have lived in an oppressive and discriminating society. Many people with disabilities have been forced into an attitude of complacency. They have felt discrimination for so long, whether intentional or unintentional, that they have chosen to isolate and segregate themselves. Some people who have disabilities may sit at home and not become involved in things they enjoy because of the potential embarrassment of subnormal performance or of performing at a level that will alienate people without disabilities. People with disabilities may choose isolation to avoid the stares of others. As a result, people without disabilities come to assume that people with disabilities want "to keep to themselves." It all becomes a cyclical and pervasive situation that is hard to change. Discrimination leads to isolation and segregation, which creates powerless and socially inferior people who feel devalued and discriminated against. As powerless people, they find advocating for changes to be hard because the majority of the population do not even realize changes are needed.

People with disabilities did not just emerge as a segment of the population. As we saw in Chapter 2, people with disabilities have always been part of society. However, to say they "have been a part of" would be inaccurate. Such a phrase implies that they have been involved and included in society, but this does not accurately reflect history. Had this been the case, there would have been little reason for federal legislation such as the core civil rights laws presented in the previous chapter.

Many reasons exist as to why people with disabilities have been less included and less involved in society. These reasons are barriers that are faced regularly by people with disabilities and are both intrinsic and extrinsic in nature. Intrinsic barriers result from a person's own physical, psychological, or cognitive limitations. These are real barriers that are usually permanent, but they may sometimes be temporary. Regardless of the duration, intrinsic barriers reduce a person's ability to be involved in a normative society. What compounds the intrinsic barriers are the countless extrinsic barriers faced by people with disabilities. Extrinsic (sometimes called environmental) barriers are things external to people with disabilities that ***impose*** limitations upon that person.

Except in the case of temporary disability, intrinsic barriers do not just go away. For example, a cognitive deficit a consequence of mental retardation and the inability to walk as a result of a spinal cord injury are permanent conditions. Of course, through education and rehabilitation, people with various disabilities often improve physical, psychological, or cognitive functioning and therefore reduce the effects of intrinsic barriers. For people with disabilities, intrinsic barriers will likely always exist. The onus is on the person to do whatever is possible to reduce the inconvenience caused by them.

On the other hand, extrinsic barriers, while real, are changeable. They include inconveniences that are imposed on people with disabilities, such as inaccessible architecture, rules and regulations that inhibit or discourage access, and negative attitude. Many such extrinsic barriers make it difficult for people with disabilities to be included and involved in normative society. The two extrinsic barriers that have the greatest negative impact are attitudinal barriers and physical barriers.

Now, we will take a closer look at attitudinal and physical barriers and discuss ways to eliminate them. We will also address programmatic accessibility, the lack of which is perhaps the most subtle and least understood type of barrier/discrimination.

Attitudinal Barriers and Attitude Change

One of the easiest extrinsic barriers to detect is a negative attitude, but it is also a difficult one to change. There are often predetermined perceptions of people with disabilities, and when these are negative attitudes, they become extrinsic barriers. Negative attitudes create major obstacles to the free movement of individuals within society. Often, attitudes toward people with disabilities are a convenient excuse to avoid contact with them. Unfortunately, this avoidance is often motivated by fear, discomfort, and an inability to see people with disabilities as people first. Negative attitudes *impose* limitations on people with disabilities and are a form of discrimination.

Negative attitudes are not always extrinsic barriers, however. In fact, negative attitudes can be intrinsic barriers as well. A person with a disability may have a negative attitude about himself or his disability or may have a "chip on his shoulder," which may create a bad attitude from people without disabilities. In these cases, the person has created an intrinsic barrier for himself. Albeit hard, these intrinsic attitudinal barriers are changeable.

Attitude Theory

Attitude theory has important implications for our understanding of the issues surrounding recreation and individuals with disabilities. It is often suggested that the attitudes of society toward individuals with disabilities have a significant impact on their ability to be active participants in various aspects of their communities, including recreation and leisure pursuits. It is a commonly held belief that we must change the attitudes of society (and sometimes of people with disabilities themselves) to create greater acceptance of people with disabilities in our communities. However, just what do we mean by the term attitude?

An *attitude* is an idea charged with emotion that predisposes a class of actions to a particular class of social situations (Triandis, 1977). Attitudes help us to adjust to our environment by providing a certain amount of predictability. We have an established repertoire of reactions to given categories of people or objects. For example, if we see a person dressed in a clown outfit and adorned with clown makeup, we assume this person will be funny and will make people laugh. That is, once a social object (in this case a person) has been classified into a particular category (in this case a clown), we usually employ our existing set of reactions (in this case a funny person/situation). This saves us from deciding each time what reaction we should have to a particular recognizable object.

Attitudes also help us to adjust to our environment and enable us to get along with people who have similar attitudes. Behavior is a function of attitudes, norms, habits, and expectancies. Habits are established through learning processes and norms of social behavior and depend on messages that we receive from others. The majority of attitudes and consequent behaviors held by a person are acquired from talking with his family and friends (Allport, 1954).

Fishbein and Ajzen (1975) indicate that attitude can be described as "a learned predisposition to respond in a consistently favorable or unfavorable manner with respect to a given object."This definition suggests that attitudes are learned rather than innate traits, and that they are, most importantly, latent or underlying tendencies rather than observable behaviors. Attitudes are not necessarily identical with observable response consistency. While attitudes influence behavior, they deal more with how an individual feels about an object, rather than how they necessarily act toward that object.

Ajzen and Fishbein (1980), in their Theory of Reasoned Action (see Figure 5.1), indicate that subjective norms combine with the specific attitude of the individual toward a given behavior to determine a person's" behavioral intention, which then influences actual behavior. Subjective norms are the influences of significant others and the corresponding motivation of the individual to comply with these norms.

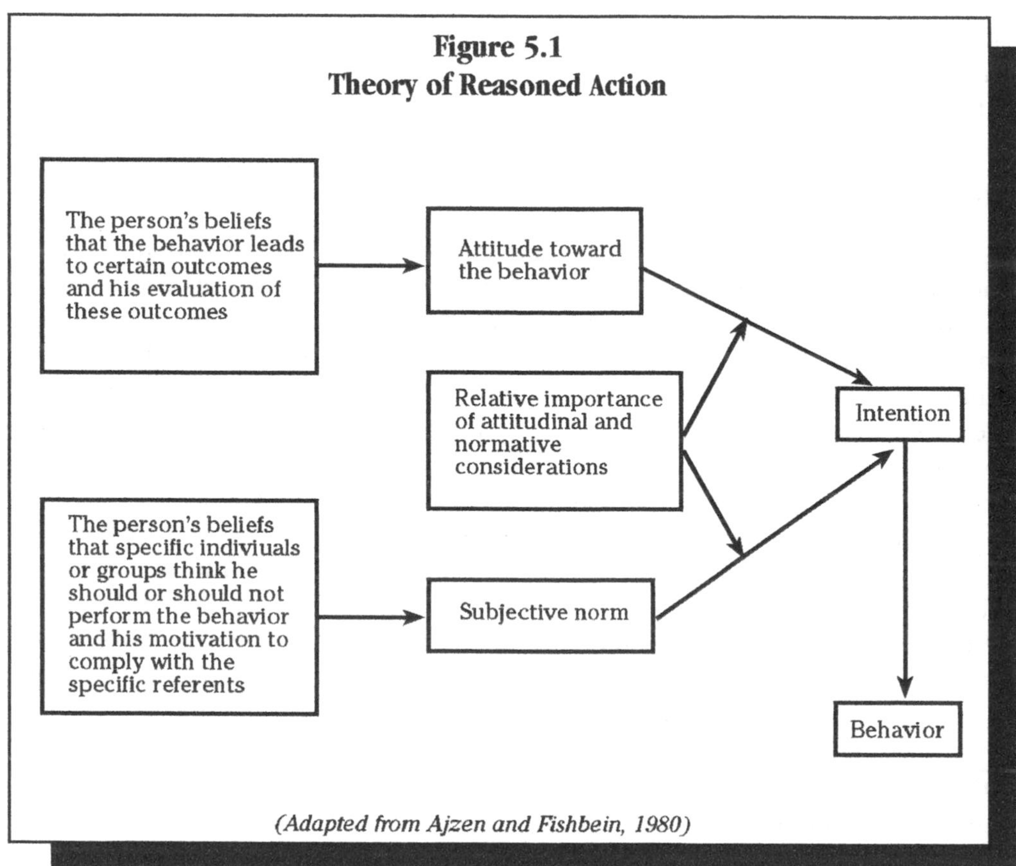

Figure 5.1
Theory of Reasoned Action

(Adapted from Ajzen and Fishbein, 1980)

Accepting the position of Ajzen and Fishbein's model relative to the influence of attitude and subjective norms on intention and behavior, we must try to understand how to create accepting behaviors of people with disabilities by society. Fishbein and Manfredo (1992) suggest that:

> ...if one wants to change or reinforce a given intention, one must change or strengthen the attitude toward performing that behavior and/or

> change or strengthen the subjective norm with respect to that behavior. Whether one should change the attitude or the subjective norm depends upon the relative importance of these two components as determinants of specific intention in the population. If the behavior is primarily under attitudinal control, attempts to change that behavior through the use of normative pressure will not be very successful. Similarly, if the members of some group perform a given behavior because their significant others think they should perform the behavior, little will be accomplished by trying to change members' attitudes toward performing that behavior (p. 37).

Attitudes and Disability

Though an understanding of the attitudes of individuals and the subjective norms that may influence them provide us with some indication of the behaviors and actions they may initiate with individuals with disabilities, a number of other factors can have an impact on behavior as well. Kennedy, Smith, and Austin (1991) point out that we must know an individual's specific attitude to understand what that person's specific behavior may be. For example, an individual may have a different attitude toward a person with mental retardation than his general attitude toward people with disabilities. This differential specific attitude is based on the amount of exposure to the person with mental retardation (attitude object), the person's personality traits, and/or the perceived consequences of the person's behavior. What this suggests is that we cannot assume that a generally positive predisposition to individuals with disabilities will necessarily result in the specific behaviors we would describe as positive and nondiscriminatory. Specific strategies must be identified to facilitate behavioral change—through changes in attitudes and subjective norms.

Prejudice and discrimination against people with disabilities remains very much a part of contemporary culture. For example, prejudice against people with disabilities may be reflected in the form of insults. One of the most pervasive ways of insulting someone is to suggest that she is somehow ***slow***. The lexicon of such terms is vast: ***stupid, dumb, nitwit, half-wit, dimwit, blockhead, bonehead, numbskull, lame brain, pea brain, fool, dopey, retard,*** etc. For the entertainment of viewers, characters in popular television programs are frequently called ***idiots, morons***, and ***imbeciles***—formerly ***scientific*** and legal classifications for levels of retardation. Equating disability with undesirability in this way stigmatizes people with disabilities. The negative value we assign to people with different levels of abilities becomes all-encompassing; it becomes their master status. People may not even realize or be willing to admit that they have negative attitudes. Nonetheless, negative attitudes get in the way of responsive, person-centered services.

Poor attitudes concerning people with disabilities are all too common among all kinds of people in all kinds of situations. Stereotyping is generally the rule and not the exception, and stereotypes typically are not positive. Stereotypes of people with disabilities as dangerous and dysfunctional have saturated the culture. For example, one of America's foremost writers, John Steinbeck, wrote a popular novel that reflected these stereotypes and has helped to perpetuate them even today. *Of*

Mice and Men describes Lenny, a large and powerful man with a disability who unintentionally kills a young woman. Lenny's character and the bare outline of the plot have been copied innumerable times in television programs, movies and even cartoons, and the novel itself has been made into a movie several times (Korbin, 1987). The most recent version, released in 1992, emphasized Lenny's dangerousness by opening with an image of a terror-stricken woman in torn clothing, running from an encounter with Lenny, even though the novel does not begin this way. The screenwriter, who is otherwise quite faithful to the original work, apparently liked the dramatic effect of such an image, demonstration that the cultural prejudice against people with disabilities that allows and accepts these stereotypes is still strong.

Frequently, villains and monsters in stories and films are characterized by some form of physical and mental disability (Korbin, 1987). Repeated exposures to such negative images cannot help but generate fear and distrust of people with disabilities.

While our society frightens itself at the expense of people with disabilities, it continues to amuse itself as well. The Three Stooges, Laurel and Hardy, Step 'n Fetchit, Jerry Lewis, and numerous other comedians have made careers out of portraying characters that have an apparent intellectual deficiency. Similarly, physical abuse of someone who does something "dumb" is seen as a normal response. Audiences laugh as Oliver Hardy hits a ***dim-witted*** Stan Laurel for doing something "stupid," as Moe hits Curly, and as Bud Abbott hits Lou Costello; on ***Cheers***, Woody Boyd is called an idiot and is sometimes struck by Sam Malone; in Disney's ***Beauty and the Beast,*** the character Gaston repeatedly punches his ***dim-witted*** sidekick, and on and on. This form of entertainment can be seen as a contemporary version of the ancient practice of "displaying" people with disabilities. Authors, screenwriters, directors, and producers typically do not intend to create and expand attitudinal barriers, but without a doubt, negative attitudes are the result.

Although attitudes are changing, attitude change is slow. For many years people with disabilities have been devalued. They have been seen as "less than" because of their differences. Condeluci (1995) recounts story after story of devaluation and oppression felt by people with disabilities. Not only have people with disabilities felt the negative attitudes toward them, but in many cases, they have come to internalize and believe them.

As a result, we could say that people with disabilities are often scripted into preconceived roles. This scripting, labeling, or stereotyping has not been malicious; however, it has had negative effects. The process works like this. We see someone who is different and we do not understand. We call on our past experiences with television shows and advertisements or comments from parents, neighbors, and friends. We use anything that we recall to help us to understand this "difference." Unfortunately, much of what we recall is negative, although almost always unintentionally so.

Wolfensberger (1972) describes various deviance roles that are often attributed to people with disabilities. He suggests that people with disabilities are often seen as menaces, objects of pity, sick, burdens of charity, objects of ridicule, eternal children, and holy innocents. These learned preconceptions create and sustain negative attitudes:

1. **Menaces**. In this situation, people with disabilities are seen as annoyances at least, and even as a threat to themselves or to the community. In the early days of institutionalization and even to some extent today, strong resistance continues against group homes being places in established residential developments. Although the objection has often been out of ignorance and lack of information, typical residents often make comments such as "I don't want to subject my children to that kind of potential danger." Another example of the annoyance or menace of people with disabilities is a comment that is often heard from parents when discussing inclusion of kids with disabilities into regular programs: "I want them to have all the opportunities they can, just not at the expense of my kids."
2. **Objects of Pity**. It is very common that people with disabilities are pitied. As we strive to elevate people with disabilities into areas of dignity and respect, the presence of pity is counterproductive. In fact, pity and respect are at opposite ends of the same perspective. A person who is pitied can never really be respected. The most obvious example of pity is telethons. For many years, telethons have been used by charitable organizations to raise funds. They are promoted as educational opportunities to help the community understand ramifications of disability by using stories or interviews about their sad lives and ways in which they have overcome great difficulty. Stories like these undoubtedly pull at heart strings of givers and as such the pity angle raises enormous amounts of money. The entire scene is very emotional and one that is intended to say "aren't we fortunate that that's not us." Pity raises funds but discourages self-determined action. [1]
3. **Sickness**. Sickness or illness is often synonymous with disability. People are often labeled as patients and less seldom as people. Although people with disabilities may indeed have some illnesses, they are far from perpetual patients and this association continues to devalue differences.
4. **Burdens of Charity**. People with disabilities are often seen as not able to take care of themselves and, therefore, must be taken care of by society. In other words, charity is the only option for people with disabilities. Charity is also associated with worthlessness. People with disabilities are perceived to not have much contribution to make; others must step in to help them. People with disabilities are a burden and need society's collective handouts.
5. **Objects of Ridicule**. Often, people with disabilities are made fun of and ridiculed. This has been a carryover from much earlier times. You will remember in the discussion of history that people with disabilities were often used in the courts of kings as jesters and fools. In fact, this period of history records time and the role of the imbecile or fool. Although not quite so ruthless today, numerous examples of people with disabilities being the brunt of jokes still exist, as discussed previously in this chapter.
6. **Eternal Children**. Regardless of age, people with disabilities are often referred to as kids. People with disabilities find themselves in the role of eternal or permanent child. This is deep-seated and insulting. Regardless of ability level or type

of disability, people with disabilities are often talked down to and attempts are made to simplify things for them. Particularly degrading and insulting is this situation for a person who has severe physical disabilities, for example, severe cerebral palsy. Although unable to speak or to move fluidity, he is often cognitively very capable. To be relegated to this eternal child is degrading.

7. **Holy Innocents**. Even today, people understand the birth of a person with a disability, the sudden onset of a debilitating disease, or an accident causing a disability to be a punishment or sometimes a gift from God. People believe that as parents or as individuals they are being tested or punished for some religious reasons. The belief is deep-seated, and as we have seen in Chapter 2, imposition of disability has for centuries been associated with deity. People who have a child born with a disability often try to understand why this "bad thing" has happened to them. They often think that they have done something "wrong" and that God is punishing them.

Although the social roles help us to understand many of the attitudes about and of people with disabilities, we need to understand the ways these roles can be adjusted to enable people who have been disenfranchised to have full access to community life.

Attitude Change

Changing negative attitudes to positive ones or even to neutral ones is a complex task that no one seems to know for sure how to accomplish. The generally accepted approach is to refute information that was acquired in the development of the negative stereotype while at the same time providing positive information and experience that supports the development of a positive stereotype, or at least a resistance to ongoing stereotyping. There are at least three ways to enhance the possibility of changing attitudes toward people with disabilities:

1. ***Personal contact and interaction*** with people who have disabilities seems to be the most effective way to change attitudes. To be in the presence of and to interact with anyone is the best way to get to know and understand him. Yet there must be more than just contact or exposure to change attitudes. There must be positive interaction that is mutual and reciprocal. As Donaldson (1980) suggests, negative attitudes may result if people without disabilities experience tension or anxiety or perceive information that reinforces existing stereotypes. Therefore, there needs to be a positive experience during personal contact with people with disabilities. Positive personal contact cannot be engineered; it must occur naturally in situations.
2. ***Persuasive communication*** is another way to change attitudes about people with disabilities. To hear someone talking about people with disabilities, trying to convince you—to persuade you that you should have positive attitudes is effective. Persuasive communication might include such phrases as "People with disabilities have the same wants and desire as anyone else" or "People with disabilities are people just like anyone else...." This book, especially cer-

tain chapters, could be called persuasive communication. Hopefully, it is effective, but is not nearly as effective as it would be for you to spend time interacting with real people with real disabilities.

3. ***Assumption of disability*** involves giving students a taste of the experience of disability. Role playing and assuming a disability for a few minutes, an hour, or a day have all been tried. Assumption of disabilities includes such things as using a wheelchair around campus for an hour, guiding a person who has been blindfolded around so she can "feel" what it is like to be blind, putting cotton in a person's ears to simulate hearing impairment, and other such role-playing exercises. All of these efforts are well intentioned, and there is research that supports assumption of disability as an appropriate method of attitude change. However, it must be remembered that this is not the best way to change attitudes and should be a last resort. There is no way a person who does not have a disability can "assume" one because at the end of the "exercise," he no longer has the disability. Such exercises give the inaccurate perception that he now knows what it is like to be blind or to use a wheelchair. Nothing could be further from the truth. After such an exercise, he knows what it is like to "not see" for a time, but there is no way that he can understand what it is like to be blind. Although one way of changing attitudes, assumption of disability should be used carefully and an extensive discussion of the experience should follow the experience itself.

As we said earlier in this chapter, the ADA was enacted to combat pervasive discrimination and to eliminate barriers. It is naïve to think, however, that by merely enacting a law we would eliminate discrimination. It is not naïve to think that the very existence of a law such as the ADA could both reduce discrimination and provide recourse to people with disabilities who have been discriminated against.

In this section we have described the pervasive and often unintentional negative attitudes. We ended the section with three suggestions of ways to be agents of attitude change. Using any of these three ways represents a proactive way to change attitudes. Sometimes, however, negative attitudes cause barriers that deny people with disabilities the very rights that the ADA is suppose to protect. Sometimes it is necessary to be reactive in an effort to "right a wrong" and to use the force of the law to remove barriers caused by negative attitudes. Consider the following excerpt from a Wyoming newspaper that serves as an example of negative attitudes and the ADA antidiscrimination guarantees.

Wyoming Complaint Cites Big Brothers/Big Sisters

The U.S. Department of Justice has agreed to investigate a complaint by the ARC of Natrona County in Wyoming that a local chapter of Big Brothers/Big Sisters excludes children with mental retardation and other disabilities from its programs.

The complaint that the organization is in violation of Title III of the Americans with Disabilities Act stems from the experience of a Casper, Wyoming, family a year ago. Sandra Petty tried to enroll her son Sean, fourteen, in the program that

> pairs children missing a parent with an adult role model for friendship. Petty was quickly advised by Big Brothers/Big Sisters of Wyoming that criteria for acceptance requires that the child not be "mentally handicapped beyond educable mental retardation…Big Brothers like to hunt and fish and be outdoors—children with mental retardation can't do those things," and it is difficult enough to find big brothers for normal kids, much less finding them for retarded children."

This is a perfect example of an extrinsic barrier on negative attitudes and stereotypes. Not surprisingly, the judge ruled in favor of the Pettys, allowed the child to be enrolled, and required the Big Brothers/Big Sisters of Wyoming to make the necessary accommodations to allow meaningful participation.

Physical Barriers and Barrier Removal

Barriers that are attitudinal are hard to deal with because they are not always easily observable, they are not always clear and obvious, and they are ever changing. Physical barriers, on the other hand, are much easier to understand. There is nothing unclear about a door that is not wide enough to allow a person who uses a wheelchair to enter. There is nothing unclear about an audible warning device that cannot be "heard" because a person cannot hear. Physical barriers are more obvious and, therefore, are easier to change.

A physical barrier is a condition of the physical environment that restricts or complicates access, movement, or participation by individuals attempting to use recreation facilities or areas. Physical barriers include more than just architectural barriers, like stairs, or curbs, or narrow hallways, or doors that are hard to open. Natural, physical barriers also abound, such as steep hills, thick tree growth, and other frustrating obstacles for many people who have mobility or visual impairments.

Here is where the ADA can help and can help quickly. As you learned in Chapter 4, public entities are required by the ADA to remove architectural barriers—those elements of facility that impede access by people with disabilities—to ensure access for customers, clients, or patrons where it is possible to do so in a readily achievable manner. Examples of barriers are curbs and steps, narrow exterior and interior doorways and aisles, rest room doorways and stalls that are too narrow for use by a person who uses a wheelchair, inaccessible drinking fountains and telephones, and many other obstacles/barriers that inhibit access.

Because of the ADA, many public and private agencies are required to ensure that they provide accessibility for all people. To do this, especially in the case of existing buildings and areas, a lot of money will be spent. The ADA recognized this and specifically provided language in the statute to prevent bankrupting businesses and government agencies. This recognition did not "let them off the hook," it simply provided a structure within which changes might be reasonably made.

Title III of the ADA requires that physical alterations to public accommodations undertaken after January 26, 1992, be readily accessible to and usable by people with disabilities to the maximum extent feasible. The term alterations refers to changes a business is undertaking for its own purposes, such as renovation, and does not refer to steps a business takes to comply with the ADA's requirements for barrier removal. Alterations do not include normal maintenance. Alterations that affect or could affect usability are required to be accessible.

When alterations are made to ***primary function areas***—work areas and areas used by the public—alterations must also be made to provide an accessible path of travel to the altered areas. ***Path of travel*** means access to restrooms, telephones, and drinking fountains serving the area. The cost of providing an accessible path of travel need not exceed 20% of the total cost of the original alteration.

While the cost of alterations to existing buildings and areas can be quite expensive, the additional cost to make a building physically accessible from the outset usually costs less than 3% more than it otherwise would. Therefore, "building in" accessibility from the beginning is much more economical than changing an existing structure to make it accessible. All newly constructed facilities must be readily accessible to and usable by people with disabilities if completed application for a building permit or permit extension was filed after January 25, 1992, and the facility was occupied after January 26, 1993. The technical standards for accessible new construction and for elimination of existing architectural barriers are set out in the Americans with Disabilities Act Accessibility Guidelines (ADAAG).

Accessibility Guidelines and Barrier Removal

The Americans with Disabilities Act Accessibility Guidelines (ADAAG) issued by the Architectural and Transportation Barriers Compliance Board can serve as a guide for the following:

1. identifying various kinds of barriers that exist; and
2. identifying measures that can be taken to remove barriers and how best to remove them.

A copy of a survey called the Americans with Disabilities Act Checklist for Readily Achievable Barrier Removal, developed by Adaptive Environments Center, Inc. and Barrier Free Environments, Inc. that use the ADAAG standards, can be found in Appendix A.

If steps lead to the front entrance and the front door is very narrow, businesses must provide a ramp and widen the door according to ADAAG standards if it is readily achievable to do so. If it is not readily achievable to follow the ADAAG standards for ramps and doorways, public accommodations must take other safe, readily achievable measures, such as installation of a slightly narrower door or a slightly steeper ramp than that permitted by the ADAAG. Although these barrier removal measures would not meet the ADAAG standards for alterations, they would nevertheless afford significant access for many customers or clients. In other words, they would be functionally usable even though not legally accessible.

Where some elements of a facility come very close to meeting the ADAAG standards and others fall far short, public entities are advised to put first priority on removing the barriers that most deviate from ADAAG standards. For example, if the front entrance already has a ramp that is just slightly steeper than that permitted by the ADAAG and the front door is just slightly narrower than that permitted by the ADAAG, but elements in the interior areas that serve clients or customers are wholly inaccessible, then public barriers that should draw first attention are those that offer the biggest impediments for customers or clients. Establishment owners should remove those that can be removed in a readily achievable manner before turning their attention to elements that deviate only slightly from the ADAAG standards.

The Department of Justice (DOJ) has recommended an order of priorities for barrier removal that it urges business to follow:

1. Provide access from parking areas, sidewalks, and entrances to the public accommodation so a person with a disability can "get through the door."
2. Provide access to those areas where goods and services are provided.
3. Provide access to rest room facilities when they are open to the public.
4. Take other measures to provide access to the goods, services, or facilities.

A good idea is to become familiar with the full array of access concerns that the ADAAG addresses. One of the ***must learning activities*** at the end of this chapter is to use the Americans with Disabilities Act Checklist for Readily Achievable Barrier Removal (Appendix A) to conduct an accessibility survey to identify existing architectural barriers and to suggest solutions for barrier removal. An excellent quick reference checklist for accessibility and ADA compliance is contained in Figure 5.2.

To date, some progress has been made toward providing entry into and use of buildings and facilities for people with disabilities. Conspicuous by its absence, however, are standards that relate to outdoor areas that are typical in public and private recreation. For example, many people with disabilities have seldom, if ever, sat directly on the grass or the beach to enjoy the sun, enjoyed flowers up-close in a garden, played in the sand with a child, or experienced an extended hike on a wilderness trail. Outdoor standards are the most difficult to address and, therefore, have been the last ones developed. The Architectural and Transportation Barriers Compliance Board (ATBCB) is currently developing and piloting standards for accessibility in outdoor areas such as campsites, swimming pools, lakes, trails, beaches, game and sports areas, and others.

In the meantime, Mig Communications has developed accessibility checklists and guidelines based on the ADA and other state and federal standards for similar elements. They are concerned with accessible surfaces in those areas as well as usability of the outdoors once people with disabilities are present in those areas. For example, they provide guidelines for the surface height of picnic tables, barbecue grills, outdoor sinks, and related amenities as well as the height, depth, and width of knee space to allow a person who uses a wheelchair to use these outdoor elements. They also provide guidelines to ensure access to and usability of event areas by people with disabilities. This includes ticket booths and counters as well as bleacher and benches. These guidelines ensure that there is adequate accessible seating for people with disabilities and that the seating allows the persons to be able to sit with whom they came rather than to be relegated to a *special* section.

Figure 5.2
ADA Compliance Quiz

How well does your organization comply with the ADA? To find out, answer "yes" or "no" to the following questions. If you answer "no" to any of the questions, take the appropriate steps to comply with the ADA.

Yes No

1. All positions (not just entry level) are open to qualified applicants with disabilities.
2. Interview areas are readily accessible to people with physical disabilities (e.g., wheelchair users).
3. Testing does not discriminate against employment applicants with speech, vision, and/or hearing disabilities.
4. Selection criteria are related to the job description and the needs of the business.
5. Applicants are not asked if they have a disability or the nature of extent of any disability. (Applicants may be asked about their ability to perform specific essential job functions.)
6. Medical examinations are not required unless they are required of all employees in similar positions.
7. Reasonable accommodations—including adaptive aids and assistive technology—are made for employees with disabilities unless they impose an "undue business hardship."
8. Existing facilities used by all employees are accessible to people with disabilities.
9. Jobs are redesigned to accommodate a person's disability. If necessary, tasks are reassigned to other employees with disabilities.
10. Part-time and modified work schedules are considered to accommodate employees with disabilities.
11. Qualified people with disabilities are considered for promotions.
12. Employees are notified of an employer's obligations under the Americans with Disabilities Act.
13. Customers are not denied service based on their association or relationship with a person with a disability.

Yes	No	
		14. Criteria for service does not limit the participation of a person with a disability unless it applies to everyone.
		15. Readily achievable, architectural barriers (narrow doorways, stairs without wheelchair ramps, heavy doors) are removed.

(Information provided by DATA, Inc., 1990)

For a free copy of the ADAAG contact:
Architectural and Transportation Barriers Compliance Board,
1331 F Street, NW Suite 1000, Washington, DC 20004-1111, (Voice/TDD)
(800) USA-ABLE.

They also ensure that there is appropriate audio amplification systems or other assistive listening systems. Other outdoor areas that are covered include swimming pool access to ensure pool entry and safety amenities such as ramps, transfer lifts, and grab bars. The number of outdoor areas that must be considered are many. For a detailed overview of guidelines for access in these area, reference the following excellent resource: Goltsman, S.M., Gilbert, T.A., & Wohlford, S.D. (1993). *The accessibility checklist: An evaluation system for buildings and outdoor settings.* Berkeley, CA: Mig Communications.

Programmatic Accessibility

Basic needs such as accessible parking, ramps, and rest rooms often have been addressed through improved planning and design. However, people with disabilities often find that although they may be able to enter a facility or even an outdoor area, they find themselves excluded from many basic activities that people without disabilities take for grated. Things as basic as orientation are often difficult for those with visual impairments or limited language skills due to inadequate or inappropriate signs. Title II of the ADA prohibits public entities from denying people with disabilities equal opportunity to participate in programs and activities because they are inaccessible. This does not mean that all buildings must be made fully architecturally accessible. The requirement is that a public entity operate each program so that, when viewed in its entirety, the program is readily accessible to and usable by people with disabilities. This is known as program accessibility and is one of the most important concepts in the ADA.

What does it mean to view a program in its entirety? The legal and ethical ideal is that all recreation programs should be equally accessible to all people, for the extent that an opportunity is not accessible, it is not really an opportunity. As we have discussed, the most commonly understood kind of accessibility is *physi-*

cal accessibility, which generally refers to the physical environment within which an activity or program is offered. Stairs, bathroom facilities, and elevators can all be physical barriers that can complicate or preclude the participation of people with certain disabilities. Program access includes physical access but it can also include administrative policies and procedures which can also be barriers to the participation of a person with a disability. The existence of such barriers is one major problem in fulfilling the mandate that people with disabilities receive equal opportunities for participation. The elimination of such barriers is essential if equal opportunity is to be achieved. Further, programmatic accessibility relates to designing programs and activities in ways that enable people with a variety of disabilities to participate fully and have fulfilling experiences. It means that any criteria for participation are applied to all potential participants equally, based on skill levels or realistic safety considerations and not on characteristics like "race, sex, religion, national origin, or ***handicap***."

In other words, a public entity is not allowed to apply eligibility criteria for its goods and services that tend to, or actually do, screen out people with disabilities except when the criteria are necessary to provide the goods or services that are being offered. A health spa cannot require a driver's license as a sole acceptable document for identification when paying membership fees by check. This policy would discriminate against people with disabilities such as blindness who are ineligible to obtain a driver's license. An exception to the policy must be made to permit these customers to present another form of identification.

The ADA requires that any criteria used be applied fairly and equally to all members of the public. It prohibits public entities from basing their eligibility criteria on assumptions that would unnecessarily exclude individuals with disabilities who, in fact, are eligible to participate in an activity. Sooner or later the public is going to run into some people, things, or conditions that have the potential to diminish their enjoyment of certain activities. These situations are not restricted to people with disabilities, but they probably occur more often to them. We refer to these situations as potential barriers to participation. Think of them as challenges to be overcome or with which to be coped. In Chapter 13 we will deal extensively with programmatic accessibility as we look at the accommodations needed to ensure equal opportunity and participation in recreation programs and services.

Achieving Program Accessibility

As we have suggested, Title I (Employment), Title II (Local Government), and Title III (Business) of the ADA are the provisions of the act that will have the greatest impact on public and the most insight into achieving program accessibility. As McGovern (1992, p. 9) states:

> The key to the Title II requirements is the determination of whether an individual with a disability could meet *essential eligibility* requirements for use or enjoyment of, or participation in, parks and recreation agency programs.

Essential eligibility means that a person either meets all of the typical requirements to be eligible for involvement in a particular activity or could meet the requirements with the provision of reasonable accommodations. In other words, when accommodations are made, people with disabilities become like other participants in terms of essential eligibility required for that particular activity. Such eligibility requirements must be applied consistently and cannot be used to screen out participants, especially participants with disabilities.

The next logical question is:"What is a reasonable accommodation?"Although the word reasonable is intentionally nonspecific, the law and its regulations name five types of reasonable accommodations. [2] McGovern (1992, pp. 12-14) lists five ways that a parks and recreation department can help people with disabilities to meet essential eligibility requirements by having them to do the following reasonable accommodations:

1. **Change policies, practices, or procedures.** This could include, but is not limited to, changing rules for the use of facilities (e.g., rules that prohibit animals from being in a recreation center could result in exclusion of an individual who is blind and uses a guide animal), changing registration policies (e.g., permitting an individual with a physical disability to set an appointment during a first-come, first-served registration process), or changing the playing rules in a particular sport (e.g., tennis players who play from a wheelchair are allowed two bounces before returning a ball hit into their court).
2. **Remove transportation barriers.** This could include providing door-to-door transportation for people with disabilities who cannot come to a park district service or facility because of the disability, or making home visits (if appropriate to the activity) to take a program to the person who cannot come to the parks and recreation department facility.
3. **Provide auxiliary aids or services.** This could include, but is not limited to, providing a sign language interpreter, a sound amplification system, an assistive system, or a text telephone for people with hearing impairments or deafness, raised lettering on signs large print brochures, Brailled communications, or a qualified reader for people with sight impairments or blindness.
4. **Remove architectural barriers.** This could include creating a path in a park between playground areas and picnic areas, beveling an uneven surface at the entrance to a doorway, or installing a lift in the deck of a swimming pool.
5. **Remove communication barriers that are structural in nature.** This could include the installation of visual alarms in a recreation center to allow individuals in a room away from other people to "get the message" transmitted by an aural fire alarm.

Many other acceptable ways exist to make reasonable accommodations; we will discuss some of them in Chapter 13.

As stated earlier in this chapter, the ADA intends to assist in protecting the rights of people with disabilities, yet it does not intend to impose an undue burden on an agency or business. As such, the ADA encourages changes that are readily achievable. The ADA defines readily achievable as "easily accomplishable and able to be carried out without much difficulty or expense." Examples of barrier removal possibilities include providing a ramp for one or even several steps, widening doorways, reconfiguring display shelves to increase aisle width, widening bathroom doorways, moving toilet stall partitions, and installing grab bars.

The readily achievable standard does not require barrier removal that involves extensive restructuring or burdensome expense. Required barrier removal for a particular public accommodation will depend on its financial and other resources. The readily achievable standard is intended to be a flexible one that is applied on a case-by-case basis. Readily achievable barrier removal is a continuing obligation. Barrier removal that was not readily achievable initially may later be required because the public accommodation has more resources available. Therefore, a public accommodation must continually monitor its accessibility as well as its financial and other resources and engage in barrier removal as new measures become readily achievable (Johnson, 1992).

Achieving effective communication for people with disabilities is also a continuing obligation. Auxiliary aids that were not required initially because they posed an undue burden may be required later in light of changing resources or changing technologies. Public entities may not add any surcharges on individuals with disabilities for auxiliary aids and services, barrier removal, or alternative measures taken in lieu of barrier removal.

Public entities are required to communicate effectively with customers or clients who are deaf or hard of hearing or who have speech or vision impairments by whatever means are appropriate. In the ADA, the term ***auxiliary aids and services*** refers to the means for achieving effective communication. This term includes sign language interpreters; written materials; assistive listening devices; Telecommunication Devices for the Deaf (TDDs); taped, Brailled, or large print materials; readers; and other communication tools (***Americans with Disabilities Handbook***, 1991).

The auxiliary aid requirements are flexible. The goal is to find an effective means of communication that is appropriate for the particular circumstance. For example, jotting down a fitness center's membership rates on a note pad for a customer who is deaf may suffice, but this means of communication will not be appropriate in a martial arts training class where complex concepts must be communicated clearly.

A business is not required to provide any particular auxiliary aid or service that it can demonstrate would fundamentally alter the nature of the goods or services being provided or would result in an undue burden on the business. It must, however, provide those needed auxiliary aids and services that would not result in an undue burden. ***Undue burden*** is defined as significant difficulty or expense when considered in light of a variety of factors, including the nature and cost of the auxiliary aid or service and the overall financial and other resources of the business. The undue burden standard is intended to be applied on a case-by-case basis.

If providing access by removing barriers is not readily achievable, the law requires public accommodations to provide readily achievable alternatives to barrier removal. For example, if barriers in a fitness center cannot be eliminated, the facility could move exercise classes or equipment to another accessible location. This is called ***post burden alternative*** thinking. It means that if an identified accommodation is too difficult or costly (i.e., if it causes a substantial economic or administrative burden or would result in a fundamental alteration of the nature of the service), the agency does not have to incur this ***burden***, but they ***must*** find an alternative method of accommodation that is not an ***undue burden***, and that allows participation by the person with a disability.

Where to Begin

It should be clear by now that accessibility is more than just ramps. Buildings and grounds accessibility is what most people think about when they think about accessibility, but there is so much more. You know that the definition of accessibility is more inclusive and that accessibility means not only getting in the door but also being able to participate once inside. Most people really want their facilities and their programs to be accessible, but just do not know how to proceed. They may feel that they need an expert before they can do anything. They do not need an expert if they have you! After reading the information in this text, completing many of the learning activities, and being aware of the additional resources available, you will be able to provide invaluable assistance. It is true that ensuring accessibility is a complicated process, but you can help your agency to remove extrinsic barriers and to achieve accessibility is a complicated process, but you can help your agency to remove extrinsic barriers and to achieve accessibility. Here are a few simple steps that the Department of Justice recommends for getting started, as cited by Gostic and Beyer (1993):

1. *Contact organizations* of or for people with disabilities in your community to help identify physical barriers to your facility or your goods or services and to familiarize you with various kinds of auxiliary aids and services that can help you communicate effectively with your customers or clients.
2. *Make a list* of architectural, policy, and communication barriers.
3. In consultation with organizations of or for people with disabilities, *set priorities* for removing architectural barriers, changing any discriminatory policies, and providing effective communication.
4. *Develop an implementation plan* designed to achieve compliance with the ADA. Such a plan, if appropriately designed and diligently executed, could serve as evidence of a good faith effort to comply.
5. *Avoid making judgments* based on myths, fears, or stereotypes.

Conclusion

All people have the right to choose what they would like to do for recreation and with whom and where they would like to do it. This is both a moral and a legal right for all people. Yet, people with disabilities often are denied access to the full range of recreation opportunities that constitute this right. Your responsibility as a recreation leader is to be sure that all your recreation programs are accessible to all people—whether they do or do not have a disability. Most recreators really want their programs to be accessible. The problem is that a lot of recreation professionals do not feel comfortable accommodating people with disabilities into their regular programs. They believe that they must have *a lot* of training or even a degree in therapeutic recreation to provide recreation programs for people with disabilities. That is just not true.

What is true is that you need to feel comfortable when working with people with disabilities, just as you would with anything that you do. In many ways, working with people with disabilities is no different than working with anyone else. People with disabilities have the same variety of needs, wants, desire, expectations, and abilities as other people. However, making programs accessible to people with disabilities may require some kind of adaptation, either by the specific participant to compensate for a skill or capability deficit or to the activity itself in a way that does not significantly affect the enjoyment and satisfaction of other participants. However, the primary reason for making programs accessible is the basic right of all people to be judged according to their capabilities, not their disabilities; their right to be included in all aspects of public life; and their right to have fun like everybody else.

People with disabilities are entitled to the full benefits of citizenship, including all of its rights, privileges, opportunities, and responsibilities. As such, the general public should support people with disabilities in the following areas:

1. Encourage and support them to achieve their full potential;
2. Grant them dignity of risk;
3. Help them to live, learn, work, play, and retire in environments of their choice; and
4. Encourage them to be primary participants in all aspects of the planning, implementation, monitoring, and evaluation of services and supports.

We believe that it is important to know about discrimination and barriers and their removal as you begin to understand more about recreation and therapeutic recreation.

Learning Activities

1. List as many extrinsic barriers to recreation participation as you can. Which barriers on your list are easiest and which are hardest to change? Why?
2. Think of popular books, television shows, or movies that include people with disabilities. How are people with disabilities portrayed? How does the portrayal affect attitude formation and/or change?

3. What is one specific action that you can do to change someone's negative attitude toward people with disabilities? Do it!
4. Conduct an accessibility survey using the ADAAG in Appendix A. What did you find? What was most surprising? What was most pleasing?
5. Plan an attitude change exercise that could be used in your class. Provide rationales to explain why you have planned the exercise in the particular way that you did. You may use the awareness exercise in Appendix B as an example.
6. As you walk around campus, try to find subtle examples of physical barriers that are often overlooked but are nonetheless problematic. Share your examples with fellow classmates and/or roommates.
7. Write to the ATBCB and/or ask your local or state ADA coordinator or similar official in your province to obtain a copy of the outdoor accessibility standards. When they arrive, use them like the ADAAG in Appendix A to conduct an accessibility survey of an outdoor recreation area.
8. Visit a YM/YWCA or other recreation agency and observe what is going on for an hour or so. What aspects could be programmatic barriers for a person who has mental retardation?

References

ADA Title II. (1992). ***Action guide for state and local governments***. Horsham, PA: LRP Publications.

Ajzen & Fishbein. (1980). ***Understanding attitudes and predicting social behavior***. Englewood Cliffs, NJ: Prentice-Hall, Inc.

Allport. (1954). ***Americans with disabilities handbook*** (1991). Washington, D.C.: Equal Opportunities Commission.

Berbe, M. (1997). The cultural representation of people with disabilities affects all of us. ***The Chronical of Higher Education***. May 30, v43 n38 p84.

Condeluci (1995). ***Interdependence: The route to community***. Winter Park, FL: GR Press, Inc.

Donaldson, J. (1980). Changing attitudes toward handicapped persons: A review and analysis of research. ***Exceptional Children*** 46(7), 504-514.

Fishbein, M., & Azjen, I. (1975). ***Belief, attitude, intention and behavior: An introduction to theory and research.*** Reading, MA: Addison Wesley.

Fishbein, M., & Manfredo, M.J. (1992). A theory of behavior change. In M.J. Manfredo (Ed.), ***Influencing human behavior*** (pp., 29-50), Champaign, IL: Sagamore Publishing.

Goltsman, S.M., Gilbert, T.A., & Wohlford, S.D. (1993) ***The accessibility checklist: An evaluation system for buildings and outdoor settings***. Berkeley, CA: Mig Communications.

Gostic, L.O., & Beyer, H.A. (1993). ***Implementing the Americans with Disabilities Act: Rights and responsibilities of all Americans***. Baltimore, MD: Paul H. Brooks.

Johnson, M. (Ed.). (1992). *People with disabilities explain it all for you:Your guide to the public accommodations requirement of the Americans with Disabilities Act*. Louisville, KY:Advocate Press.

Kennedy, D.W., Smith, R.W., & Austin, D.R. (1991). *Special recreation: Opportunities for persons with disabilities.* Dubuque, IA.:Wm. C. Brown, Publishers.

Korbin, J.E. (1987). Child maltreatment in cross-cultural perspective:Vulnerable children and circumstances. In R. Gelles & J.B. Lancater (eds.), *Child abuse and neglect* (pp. 31-55). New York, NY:Aldine De Gruyter.

Li, L., & Moore, D. (1998) Acceptance of disability and its correlates. *The Journal of Social Psychology*. 138(1). pp. 13-25.

McGovern, J. (1992). *The ADA self-evaluation:A handbook for compliance with the Americans with Disabilities Act by parks and recreation agencies*. Arlington, VA: National Recreation and Park Association.

Noe, S.R. (1997). Discrimination against individuals with mental illness. *The Journal of Rehabilitation*. V63 n1 pp. 2-3.

Triandis, H.C. (1977). *Interpersonal Behavior*. Monterrey, CA: Brooks/Cole.

Wolfensberger. (1972). *The principle of normalization in human services.* Toronto, Ontario: National Institute on Mental Retardation.

Related Websites

http://www.nrpa.org/
(National Recreation and Park Association)

http://www.ncd.gov/
(National Council on Disability)

http://asia.yahoo.com/Society_and_Culture/Disabilities/Legal_Issues/
(Society and Culture: Disabilities: Legal Issues)

http://www.indiana.edu/~nca/index.html
(National Center on Accessibility)

http://www.cais.com/naric/access.html
(The National Rehabilitation Information Center — Designing Accessible Web Pages)

http://janweb.icdi.wvu.edu/english/pcepd.htm
(PresidentÕs Committee on Employment of People with Disabilities)

http://www.yuri.org/webable/
(WebABLE!)

http://www.indiana.edu/~nca
(National Centre on Accessibility)

Footnotes

[1] In the January 1996, United Cerebral Palsy telethon, fewer instances of pity and more instances of individuals as valued, self-determined people were used throughout the fundraising campaign.

[2] Not all people with disabilities will need accommodations or assistance. Therefore, accommodation should not be provided just because a person may be blind but because a specific individual needs a specific accommodation to render him essentially eligible. When assistance is needed because of a disability, the ADA requires an agency to make reasonable accommodations for people with disabilities.

Other Sources of Information

Americans with Disabilities Act Resources

ADA Information Line, Department of Justice (DOJ), Civil Rights Division, Public Access Section, P.O. Box 66738, Washington, DC 20035-9998, (Voice) (202) 514-0301, (TDD) (202) 514-0383.

Responsible for developing and enforcing the ADA state and local government (Title II) and public accommodation (Title III) regulations; it also coordinates technical assistance programs for federal agencies.

An automated information system offers the following information 24 hours per day, 7 days per week:

1. Overview of the act and effective dates;
2. List of federal government agencies that provide assistance and information;
3. Agencies that operate information lines to assist in compliance with the act and grants from the Department of Justice;
4. Title II—Overview of major requirements;
5. Title III—Overview of major requirements;
6. How to file a complaint under Title II or III;
7. Order information—free of charge, including:
    a. the ADA information packet and accessibility guidelines,
    b. Technical Assistance Manual—Title II and III; and,
    c. ADA Handbook that includes regulations, public law, and other resource information; and
8. Staffed operator lines. Questions can be asked from 1:00 PM - 5 PM. ET. Monday through Friday.

Disability and Business Technical Assistance Centers

The National Institute on Disability and Rehabilitation Research (NIDRR) operates a network of ten regional Disability and Business Technical Assistance Centers (DBTACs).These centers provide information, training, and technical assistance to businesses and agencies covered by the Americans with Disabilities Act and to people with disabilities who have rights under the ADA.

You can contact the center in your region by calling (Voice/TDD) 1-800-949-4ADA.

Disability Rights Education and Defense Fund, 2212 Sixth St., Berkeley, CA 94710, (Voice/TDD) (510) 644-2555.

Specializes in training and technical assistance for people with disabilities and their representatives, state and local government units, businesses and trade associations; it also provides public policy advocacy and litigation.

Easter Seal Society, 70 East Lake St., Chicago, IL 60601, (Voice) (312) 726-6200, (TDD) (312) 726-4258.

Offers a catalog of books, brochures, and video cassettes that can help state and local governmental agencies and businesses to implement the Americans with Disabilities Act.

National Center on Accessibility, 5040 State Rd. 67 North, Martinsville, IN 46151 Operates a toll free number (1-800-424-1877) to offer assistance in making programs and facilities accessible to all people.

National Recreation and Park Association (NRPA), 2775 South Quincy St., Suite 300, Arlington, VA 22206, (703) 820-4940.

Has available the ADA self-evaluation: A handbook for compliance with the Americans with Disabilities Act, author John McGovern, and the ADA Resource Guide.

The ARC, formerly Association for Retarded Citizens of the U.S., 1522 K St., NW, Washington, DC 20005, (800) 433-5255.

Over 1,300 state and local chapters represent 140,000 individuals with mental retardation and their families; it also offers technical assistance and a fact sheet on the ADA.

The following is a list of sources of information and assistance available to help state and local governments understand and respond to Title II of the ADA. Many of the listed organizations and agencies produce or distribute publications relating to the ADA.

Barrier Free Environments, P.O. Box 30634, Raleigh, NC 27622, (Voice/TDD) (919) 782-7823.

Founded in 1975 by Ron Mace, AIA. It provides consulting and design services, produces accessibility guidelines, and presents educational seminars. A publications' list is available.

President's Committee on Employment of People with Disabilities, 1331 F St., NW, 3rd floor, (Voice) (202) 376-6200, (TDD) (202) 376-6205.

Organization of 600 volunteer members nationwide works to build and maintain a climate of acceptance of people with disabilities in the workforce. It produces technical assistance materials, including videotapes, public service announcements, and fact sheets. Information on job accommodation, assistive technology, tax incentives, and other topics (call for list of publications) is also provided.

RESNA Technical Assistance Project, 1101 Connecticut Ave., NW, Suite 700, Washington, DC 20036, (Voice/TDD) (202) 857-1140.

Provides information and professional consultation related to assistive technology services for states that have assistive technology grants from NIDRR. Contact RESNA to learn whether your state has a technology project.

Chapter 6

Recreation, Special Recreation, and Therapeutic Recreation Programs for People with Disabilities: An Overview

Introduction

In 1932, a recreation leader from the Los Angeles Playground and Recreation Department boldly described her desire to make possible for crippled children a "childhood as rich and diverse in its play experiences as that of any normal child" (Williams, 1932, p. 139). After describing her "Experiment" to build "figuratively a bridge for the crippled child to walk over into the natural recreation center of his community," she concluded by saying to her colleagues:

> If play is a necessity for the normal child's development, how much more is it needed for the handicapped child who is forced to make far greater adjustments to life? The recreation movement has a great responsibility and opportunity in helping the handicapped child to become a socially adjusted adult well able to use his leisure wisely" (Williams, 1932, p. 162).

Very few advocates and even fewer recreation opportunities for people with disabilities were around in 1932 when Williams made her plea. Today the context has changed somewhat. We have federal legislation to facilitate this "bridge...to walk over into the natural recreation center of his community" (Williams, 1932, p. 139). We have (and have had) specialized sections of municipal and county recreation and park agencies specifically committed to providing recreation services to people with disabilities. Yet, we still make similar pleas to the recreation profession today, albeit, using 1990s concepts and jargon. Today, we expand Ms. Williams' depression era message to say that the recreation profession has an obligation to provide inclusive and not just specialized and desperate recreation opportunities and choices to all people.

In this chapter we will introduce you to concepts of recreation, special recreation, and therapeutic recreation and will attempt to tie them into the historical and conceptual information presented earlier in Section I. A more detailed and programmatically-oriented discussion of these concepts will be presented in the third section of this book.

Work and Leisure

North America is a very work-oriented society.The ideals of the pioneers and pilgrims are still very much present. Hard work is revered. Children are taught to work hard and then play. At an early age we are told not to be lazy and all too often understand *lazy* to mean ***not working***. Adults are identified by what they do for employment and where they work. No one ever says, "What do you like to do (meaning what do you do for fun or relaxation?" Rather, they ask, "What do you do (meaning what type of work do you do)?" Jokes are sometimes made if someone "enjoys" work too much. Many people are applauded for working long hours; they are seen as being ***hard workers***, which is often interpreted and internalized as ***good, commendable***, and something of worth. Work is emphasized and assumed to be unquestionably valued by most people.

The issue is not that recreation and leisure are unimportant. It is just that with such a strong emphasis on work. Leisure is usually secondary. Leisure can never replace work as work, leisure is usually secondary. Leisure can never replace work as work so often does with leisure. Yet leisure is vehemently upheld by blue collar workers and top executives alike as a necessary part of life and that which rejuvenates them after a hard day/week of work. It makes them feel good, relaxes them, and gives them an opportunity to meet new people and to maintain existing relationships. When asked, "Where would you like to be now, if you could be anywhere in the world?" almost no one would say "at work" or "working." Nearly always, the answer involves recreation or leisure. Nonetheless, work seems to be more valued and evokes more pride among peers. It is an apparent contradiction, but one that is a systemic part of our society and an important point to make in this text.

Almost anyone would agree that leisure and recreation have myriad intrinsic and extrinsic benefits. They make people feel good about themselves and help people stay socially connected to other people. Leisure and recreation are revitalizing and rejuvenating—an important part of life. A substantial portion of a person's life requires the performance of constructive and personally significant recreation. Yet people with disabilities are often limited in their capacity to perform ordinary functions and to fulfill expected work, social, and leisure roles. Even though higher levels of involvement in leisure activities are associated with increased ratings of well-being and life satisfaction, prescribing activities for people with disabilities would not likely produce the same results because self-determination would be neglected. The role of choice that leads to personal enjoyment and meaningful involvement is crucial to feelings of life satisfaction.

A widely held belief is that social isolation or lack of social relationships can pose a major risk factor for an individual's health. In fact, there is a growing body of literature and research that suggests social supports can improve an individual's chance of recovery and sense of well-being (Coleman & Iso-Ahola, 1993). Social support can be defined in a variety of ways but needs to be individualized and contextualized so that it is personally relevant. Supports can be defined as the quantity and quality of one's friendships, the relationships that usually occur during recreation that offer connectedness, support, advice, encouragement, assistance, and material resources.

In addition to generally enhancing self-esteem and the quality of a person's life, the ability to occupy one's free time in a socially valued and acceptable manner will have a significant impact on where a person is able to live, whether he functions successfully in the community, and the quality of relationships that a person develops. Social and recreation experiences have the power to generate skills that can be transferred to work, housing, family relationships, etc. Thus, recreation experiences can facilitate an individual's successful integration into other life spheres.

Recreation in naturally occurring environments rather than in special, segregated settings can offer flexibility, choice, self-determination, individuality, and decision making. The value and benefit of recreation should be clear to professionals in recreation and therapeutic recreation although probably not as clear or at least as conscious to people with disabilities, their parents and families, advocates, or health care and rehabilitation professionals. Therefore, the value of leisure and recreation need to be consistently and eloquently reinforced in an effort to modify traditional and customary views of recreation as a secondary goal and means of intervention, a diversionary tactic, or due only as a reward for other achievements.

Most people acknowledge the importance of leisure in their lives even though they seldom elevate it to a coequal status with work or education. Leisure scholars and practitioners have debated the nature of leisure and recreation for centuries. Though various definitions of leisure have been proposed, authors have most commonly described the concept of perceived freedom and intrinsic motivation as being central to the notion of leisure (Austin & Crawford, 1996). The reader is directed to Godbey (1989), Kelly (1996), Murphy (1975), and Sessoms and Henderson (1994) for discussions on the concepts of recreation and leisure.

In this text we will help you to understand ways to ensure that recreation and leisure are an important part of the lives of people with disabilities. For now, we will talk about both recreation and therapeutic recreation for people with disabilities.

Recreation and Therapeutic Recreation in North America

Everyone agrees that recreation is important and that it is therapeutic, yet there have been differential understandings among recreation professionals about the meaning of recreation, special recreation, and therapeutic recreation. In fact, depending on which texts and authors you read, you will see the terms used differently and sometimes even interchangeably. Some argue that all recreation is therapeutic and that any recreation with people with disabilities is, therefore recreation. Others make a clear distinction between special or adapted recreation services and recreation as part of treatment or rehabilitation. Still others feel that therapeutic recreation has become too *medicalized* and is more akin to allied health professions like occupational therapy than to the field of recreation. Many others welcome the closer link with allied health and argue that therapeutic recreation is primarily concerned with treatment and is secondarily concerned with recreation.

In the midst of these differing understandings is confusion over the terms *setting* versus *service*. That is, many professionals argue that special recreation occurs in community settings and therapeutic recreation occurs in clinical settings. They are trying to label a type of service by the location in which it occurs. The confusion continues because community and clinical settings are not consistently understood. That is, clinical is a process not a place. As such, a process can occur anywhere, irrespective of place. Community is often used to mean a public parks and recreation agency, yet in today's cost-conscious medical system, clinical or treatment services increasingly occur in places other than traditional hospital or medical settings. This is all very confusing, but it is important for students to understand—whether they plan to work in recreation, special recreation, or therapeutic recreation.

In Chapters 1 through 5 we presented an in-depth look at people with disabilities from philosophical, conceptual, and historical perspectives. We have also discussed discrimination and barriers that are routinely faced by people with disabilities as well as ways to create accessible programs and environments. We barely mentioned recreation or therapeutic recreation in the previous chapters because we wanted you to have a broader context within which to understand recreation and therapeutic recreation services. In this chapter you need to understand the basics of recreation and therapeutic recreation services. This basic understanding will help in Section II of this text when you learn specific information about disabling conditions. After you have learned this specific disability information, read Chapters 13 and 14 for a detailed discussion of recreation, special recreation, and therapeutic recreation. For now, let us get back to a basic understanding of concepts.

We will start by tracing recreation, special recreation, and therapeutic recreation from an historical perspective—since you already know something of the history of treatment and services for people with disabilities. We will then define and explain what we mean by the concepts.

In the Beginning...

In the beginning there were recreation services as well as therapeutic recreation services for people with disabilities; they just were not called recreation and therapeutic recreation services. Although we think of therapeutic recreation as being relatively new, as we mentioned in Chapter 4, many examples are seen throughout history where activities were used as a form of treatment. Recently, the medical and rehabilitation literature has been filled with references to prevention of disease and disability. Although we think of those references as being new and innovative, as long ago as 3,000 B.C. (and probably much earlier if we had more detailed recorded history from earlier times), many forms of activity and exercise were used as part of the healing process. While bodily inactivity was thought to lead to disease, these activities were also thought to prolong life. As such, the basis for promoting and using recreation has a very early and rich history. Both the ancient Greeks and Romans revered recreation, leisure, and exercise as essential to good and healthy lives. In fact, there are examples in Greece and Rome of using these activities both to prevent disease as well as to assist in the healing process.

As far as we can tell, however, the deliberate *use* of recreation both as prevention and treatment of illness, disease, and disability ended for a time after the fall of the Roman Empire. Treatment of people with illnesses and disabilities was considerably less humane; in fact, it became quite cruel and punitive. Patients were often chained and tied and kept in dark, dingy dungeons. Some were also tortured and others were exhibited to the public. This was indeed a time when there were no services that would suggest the use of recreation as a part of the treatment or to improve the lives of people with disabilities. This was the norm for many centuries.

Progress was made during the 18th and 19th centuries when more humane treatment ensued. By the early 1800s there is evidence of the use of recreation as part of treatment programs, especially in psychiatric hospitals. Even as early as this time there is evidence that recreation was used both as a means to an end and as an end in itself. By far, however, most of the involvement of recreation in the lives of people with disabilities was more an end in itself. That is, literature reports many more instances of people being allowed to take walks, to listen to music, to dance and to play games, etc., rather than instances of systematic, structured, prescribed approaches that used recreation as a way to help people improve their physical, emotional, and cognitive functioning. In the mid- to late- 1800s, evidence exists of the use of big and small pets to "cheer up" patients. This approach was also used in military hospitals of the day to brighten the spirits of injured soldiers. Although in the 19th century it was not an identified profession or even a widely understood ancillary treatment service, by the early 20th century what we know today as therapeutic recreation was becoming better known. Avedon (1974, p. 12) cites an article from the ***American Journal of Insanity*** that describes how one hospital chartered a train and took 500 patients on a picnic for curative and restorative benefits.

After World War I, in the early 20th century, many soldiers who had returned from war were injured both physically and psychologically. During this time, the American Red Cross began to provide diversional recreation programs in hospital wards and convalescent centers; Red Cross recreation leaders began to be employed there in increasing numbers.

By 1919, the American Red Cross had organized a division of recreation in hospitals, and by 1930 there were 117 full-time Red Cross hospital recreation workers (Navar, 1979). In 1931, the United States Veterans Bureau (today called the Veterans Administration), recruited Red Cross workers who had previously worked in military and public health service hospitals for work in Veterans Administration Hospitals.

Interestingly, according to Shivers and Fait (1985), the first apparent use of the term ***therapeutic recreation*** appeared in federal legislation in 1938 in the act creating the Works Progress Administration (WPA). "The act used the term to describe all recreational activities intended to serve disabled, maladjusted, and other institutionalized persons" (Shivers & Fait, p. 16).

Also during the late 19th and early 20th centuries in North America, initial special recreation services for people with disabilities were more evident. In 1893, the Industrial Home for the Blind in New York City was established (Avedon, 1974), to provide recreation experiences for its clients, as well as for other reasons. In 1905, another agency devoted to the needs of people who were blind—the Lighthouse for the Blind—added donations of theater tickets to its array of available services (Avedon). These and other services for people with disabilities are not surprising since social reform was the impetus for the development of organized recreation in both America and Canada.

In North America, concern arose for the welfare of people who were trying to cope with the rapidly changing world created by the Industrial Revolution. Factory workers worked long hours for little pay and worked in squalid settings. Immigrants continued to flood onto the continent, which burdened the availability of housing. Wealthy business men bought apartment and tenement buildings to expand their businesses. Although this created new jobs, it reduced the availability of already overcrowded housing, which just exacerbated the substandard living conditions of the industrial worker. In addition, there were few places for children to play except in streets and busy ports. The industrial city created an inhospitable environment for its inhabitants and social reformers stepped in to right the wrongs of industrialization. Parks and playgrounds were developed with funds from socially minded philanthropists. Wholesome recreation opportunities were provided to increase the quality of life of North Americans. This was the beginning of the organized parks and recreation system—a system to help disadvantaged people cope with their inhospitable environment. According to Murphy (1975, p. 43):

> ...in 1906, there were 41 cities that were maintaining municipally supported and operated playground programs. By 1915, 83 communities reported public recreation departments, and the number had increased to 465 by 1920.

Even though this movement had its roots in providing programs for socially disadvantaged people, as community recreation grew, the original focus on meeting the needs of people who were disadvantaged gave way to the demands of more affluent citizens of cities who made their own demands for community recreation services. As Kennedy, Smith, and Austin (1991) put it:

> As community recreation and parks departments attempted to spread their resources to meet everyone's recreational needs, concern for people with special needs has been lost as a central feature of public recreation and parks (p. 6).

Post World War II History of Recreation and Therapeutic Recreation

The modern history of therapeutic recreation actually began following World War II. It was during that time that an increase occurred in the number of Red Cross recreation personnel available in military and veterans hospitals. By 1945, the Veterans Administration had initiated a hospital social service division that included recreation services and recreation personnel being assigned to all hospitals. But what were they doing? Were they providing diversional recreation services or treatment-oriented therapeutic recreation services? Evidence that exists suggests that the services provided were called therapeutic recreation services were thought to be both largely diversional and treatment-oriented. Consider the following quote by Rensvold, Hill, Boggs, & Meyer (1957, p. 88):

> To the hospitalized, recreation can bring a refreshment of the spirit as well as encouragement toward therapy...Recreation can alleviate the boredom of living under the confines of hospital routine; it can minimize anxieties, abate loneliness, renew a sense of values, and supply the patient with healthful activities and motivation to get well...It (recreation) can help create new interests and develop present ones. These may be useful to the patient both while in the hospital and after his discharge. Finally, as an integral part of the patient's treatment, recreation helps him to greater confidence in and a better relationship with himself, the hospital staff, and with his fellow patients.

Rensvold et al. (1957, p. 89) continue about the *therapeutic benefits* of recreation in hospitals:

> Here (in the hospital), the ultimate purpose (of recreation) is to enlarge the patient's range of physical and mental activity to assist him in his difficult adjustment to the limitations set by his injury or illness. For the chronic patient, recreation must make him feel useful and wanted again. For the neuropsychic patient, recreation aids the doctor in his efforts to help the patient return into group activities and community living. For the long-term patient, recreation is a morale builder, offering him methods and means of occupying his time with entertaining and interesting activities as he becomes physically and emotionally prepared for eventual return to community living. For the child patient, there is a particular need for healthful and happy play activities. For the patient undergoing rehabilitation, recreation can be instrumental in counteracting his discouragement and relaxing him after his strenuous day of treatments.

As you will remember from Chapter 2, at about this same time, deinstitutionalization was getting underway. As a result, there were a lot more people with disabilities who were present in communities. The horrors of institutionalization were being recognized and the move to deinstitutionalize proceeded quickly and without much thought to what previously institutionalized people would do once they returned to live with their families or in group homes. Suddenly, a lot of people who had always lived in the structured environment of institutions were now living in much less structured environments. There were few work and school opportunities, and not surprisingly, even fewer recreation opportunities. Individuals who had been previously institutionalized entered a world that provided them little.

Not unlike the development of special education and special work, special recreation opportunities were demanded by parents and advocates as well. These, too, were segregated recreation programs in which only people with disabilities were permitted to participate. They began at a time when there were few opportunities. In 1957, Rensvold et al. (p. 87) stated:

> ...the non-institutionalized ill and handicapped are beginning to be provided with services...recreation specialists have been extending new areas of service to segments of the population who may virtually be said in the past to have been condemned to endure time rather than to enjoy it. Applying the principle of recreation for all, the recreation movement is developing patterns of specialized service which are not only refreshing to the spirit, but therapeutic and educational in their outcomes.

In describing the kinds of services that were available, Rensvold et al. (1957) described services and a philosophy that were ahead of the times. They designed programs "to meet the needs as indicated by the handicapped themselves" (p. 88). They provided such programs as:

> ...a visiting program for homebound children and adults, carried out by a corps of selected and trained volunteers; a club program for orthopedically handicapped adults; a similar program for orthopedically handicapped teenagers; a training program in home recreation activities for orthopedically handicapped children to be given to parents of handicapped children and other interested lay people; and television programs directed to the orthopedically handicapped (p. 88).

Although these early recreation programs attempted to listen to the desires of consumers, and in that sense were person-centered, the programs and services were provided exclusively for people with disabilities and with little attention to concerns of mainstreaming, integration, and inclusion. Since the post-war time, inclusive recreation, specialized recreation, and therapeutic recreation services have expanded. With the similarities in target population, these recreation services have often been confused by both its practitioners and observers. In the following section, we will try to define and explain these sometimes confused and confusing terms.

Recreation, Special Recreation, and Therapeutic Recreation

First, we will offer three definitions adapted from Bullock (1987) that we feel accurately describe the services:

1. **Recreation** is activities or experiences freely chosen for the intrinsic benefit. Recreation services, as referred to in this text, involve the provision of recreation programs and services for all people. No one is excluded and accommodations are made to facilitate and support participation. Recreation programs are staffed by general recreation professionals.
2. **Special Recreation** is the provision of recreation programs and services that are provided for people who require special accommodations because of unique needs they have owning to some physical, cognitive, or psychological disability (Kennedy, Smith, & Austin, 1991). These programs are usually provided in segregated settings—exclusively for people with disabilities. Special recreation programs are often staffed by therapeutic recreation professionals.
3. **Therapeutic Recreation** is the purposive use of recreation/recreative experiences by qualified professionals to promote independent functioning and to enhance optimal health and well-being of people with illnesses and/or disabling conditions. Therapeutic recreation programs are staffed by certified therapeutic recreation specialists.

Although recreation (inclusive recreation) is the type of service that we advocate as the most self-determining and person-centered, in the following section we will focus on special recreation and compare it to therapeutic recreation because special recreation is more prevalent today and because it is often confused with therapeutic recreation. We will start with an explanation of therapeutic recreation.

As is clear from the definition already stated, therapeutic recreation is concerned with recreation and treatment. It is not just recreation or just treatment; rather, it is recreation *and* treatment or recreation *as* treatment. As such, both words are important to an understanding of therapeutic recreation and neither should be de-emphasized.

Recreation refers to a state or condition of an organism or entity—its re-creation, renewal, restoration—a return to its appropriate state of mind, body or soul. The term *therapeutic* refers to remedies/treatments (healing, curative agents) to restore/remediate an organism to its appropriate state of physical, mental, or social functioning. As such, the phrase therapeutic recreation, taken at face value, leads logically to the truism that "all recreation is therapeutic." People say, "It makes me feel better to go to the movie," or "I feel ready for work after I play a little." They are saying "recreation is restorative—it is therapeutic." And it is, but that does not make it therapeutic recreation. It does, however, provide an irrefutably sound conceptual base for the use of recreation as a treatment modality.

The field of therapeutic recreation embraces the phrase "recreation is therapeutic" and goes on to say, "How can we use this curative agent (recreation/recreative experience) in the treatment of this or that person?" It is this purposiveness, when provided within a setting and program mandated to provide treatment, that defines *therapeutic recreation*.

Does that mean that therapeutic recreation only occurs within traditional inpatient settings (hospitals, institutions, etc.), which is where most treatment occurs? Not exactly! It would be more accurate to say that it occurs within agencies/organizations that have a clear *mandate* to provide treatment. That may be a traditional inpatient psychiatric unit, or a variety of community-based treatment options such as halfway houses, independent living programs, and other transitional community treatment programs. Therapeutic recreation could also occur through a municipal recreation department that is under contract with a bona fide treatment agency to provide treatment services. For the community recreation department, the phrase "under contract from a bona fide treatment agency" must be stressed. Public recreation programs, by their enabling legislation, are in the business of providing recreation programs and services, not treatment. That is not to say that they cannot provide good services unless there is a contractual arrangement for that type of treatment service. Considering the litigious society in which we live and the increased importance on accountability, when we define therapeutic recreation, we must place an insistence on the treatment mandate for not only logical but also prudent reasons. [1] Therapeutic recreation may occur in a variety of settings other than traditional inpatient settings as long as there is a clear treatment mandate.

Therapeutic recreation is not any and all recreation services for people who have disabilities. Just having a disability does not quantify a person to receive ***therapeutic*** recreation services. The person with a disability may receive therapeutic recreation services, or she simply may receive recreation services (usually called special or adapted recreation—which usually occurs in a segregated community-based setting). The determination between recreation and therapeutic recreation is made on the basis of need and mandate for treatment rather than on disability. To call recreation services ***therapeutic*** because they involve a person or group of people with disabilities or because they are in a hospital setting is not only inaccurate but also patronizing and stigmatizing to a person who happens to have a disability.

As such, it is not accurate to call a municipal or county recreation program or a girls club program for people with disabilities ***therapeutic recreation***. Such programs are not therapeutic recreation (treatment) programs—at least not by virtue of their service mandate. They are recreation programs for people with disabilities that are often staffed by people trained in therapeutic recreation. Most people, however, who are served by these special recreation services are requesting and receiving recreation services, not therapeutic recreation services—even though they may be receiving services from a certified therapeutic recreation specialist. Participants might need assistance or a lot of instruction but they usually do not need treatment nor did they come to a recreation program in the community recreation agency for treatment.

Participants with disabilities in special (sometimes *called* community therapeutic recreation) programs often improve their confidence and self-esteem. The same could be said though of the girl who makes the little league team and improves all season. Therapeutic recreators have assessments, written goals, and individualized plans. The little league coach does an assessment, has goals, and may have a different plan of action for each of his players—he just may not write them down. It is not the assessment, goals, and individualized plans—nor even the arduous task of writing them down and constantly documenting them—that make those recreation services into ***therapeutic recreation services***, just as it is not the setting or the people with disabilities that make it ***therapeutic recreation***.

The agency mandate to provide treatment to help people improve physical, intellectual, emotional, and social functioning through recreation is what makes it ***therapeutic recreation***. Treatment facilities, whether institutional or community-based, are mandated to provide treatment. Municipal/county recreation programs are mandated through enabling legislation to provide recreation programs and services, not treatment.

Conclusion

The very nature of the health care system (and other human services) already have and will continue to dictate a closer relationship between therapeutic recreators and other providers of recreation services (for people with disabilities) in the future. Shorter hospitalizations, as well as more community-based treatment services, will contribute to this closer relationship. *Treatment* will become more and more of a community-based phenomenon. The two groups of professionals must become more interdependent if the best interests of the people being served are to be realized. However, practitioners on both sides have to give up their long-held preconceptions about the field in order to more accurately understand the needs of the people whom they purport to serve. After all, it is the person, not the professional, who is at the center of recreation or therapeutic recreation programs and services!

Learning Activities

1. To make sure you understand the material in this chapter, tell your mom, siblings, boy/girlfriend, roommate, or someone else the difference between therapeutic recreation and special recreation. Encourage them to ask questions and to probe for more detail. Not only will you see how clearly you understand, but you may also discover issues or questions that were neither covered in class nor in the text. This is one way that you can become a more active participant in your learning.
2. Ms. Hortense Williams was cited in this chapter as an early advocate for recreation services for people with disabilities. Go to the library and try to find evidence of other early advocates (prior to 1940) for recreation services for people with disabilities. Look in magazines, journals, newspapers, newsletters, etc. How many examples did you find? Where did you find them? What was the general message?
3. Conduct a mini-research project during spring/fall break or on a weekend. Ask members of your family and some of your friends and their families the following questions:
   a. When you introduce yourself to someone, how do you do it?
   b. If you could do anything right now, what would it be?

Pay attention to the way work and leisure come up or do not come up. What can you infer from your "research"? Are the responses different for different members of your family (i.e., your grandmother and your sister)?

4. Based on your reading of the text so far, why would the authors prefer inclusive rather than special recreation services? How could therapeutic potentially not be person-centered?

References

Austin, D.R., & Crawford, M. (1991). *Therapeutic recreation: An introduction*. Englewood Cliffs, NJ: Prentice Hall.

Avedon, E.M. (1974). *Therapeutic recreation service: An applied behavioral science approach*. Englewood Cliffs, NJ: Prentice Hall.

Bullock, C.C. (1987). Recreation and special populations. In A. Graefe & S. Parker (Eds.), *Recreation and leisure: An introductory handbook* (pp. 203-207). State College, PA: Venture Publishing.

Coleman, D., & Iso-Ahola, S.E. (1993). Leisure and health: The role of social support and self-determination. *Journal of Leisure Research, 25* (2)

Godbey, G. (1989). *The future of leisure Services; Thriving on change*. State College, PA: Venture Publishing, Inc.

Kelly, J.R. (1996). *Leisure*. Needham Heights, MA: Alyn and Bacon.

Kennedy, D.W., Smith, R.W., & Austin, D.R. (1991). *Special recreation: Opportunities for persons with disabilities*. Dubuque, IA: Wm. C. Brown, Publishers.

Kraus, R., & Shank, J. (1992). *Therapeutic recreation services: Principles and practices*. Dubuque, IA: Wm. C. Brown, Publishers.

Lindeman, E.C. (1935, December). Recreation and the good life. *Recreation, 29*(9), 431-437, 468.

Murphy, J.F. (1975). *Recreation and leisure services*. Dubuque, IA: Wm. C. Brown, Publishers.

Navar, N.H. (1979). The professionalization of therapeutic recreation in the state of Michigan. Unpublished dissertation. Bloomington, IN: Indiana University.

Rensvold, V., Hill, B.H., Boggs, E.M., & Meyer, M.W. (1957, September). Therapeutic recreation. *The Annals of the American Academy of Political and Social Science* (Vol. 313), 87-91.

Sessoms, H.D., & Henderson, K.A. (1994). *Introduction to leisure services*. State College, PA: Venture Publishing, Inc.

Shivers, J.S., & Fait, H.F. (1985). *Special recreational services: Therapeutic and adapted*. Philadelphia: Lea and Febiger.

Williams, H.L. (1932, June). Recreation for crippled children. *Recreation, 26* (3), 139-140, 162.

Footnote

[1] For this insight, the authors acknowledge numerous personal communications with Dr. Lee Meyer, associate professor (retired), University of North Carolina at Chapel Hill.

Related Websites

http://www.islandnet.com/~riv/homepage.html
(Recreation Integration Victoria)

http://www.nssra.org/about/index.htm
(Northern Suburban Special Recreation Association)

http://www.abilitiescouncil.sk.ca/recreation.html
(Saskatchewan Abilities Council)

http://www.co.fairfax.va.us/rec/info19.htm
(Welcome to Therapeutic Recreation)

http://www.vwc.edu/vrps/tr/tr.htm
(Virginia Recreation and Park Society — Therapeutic Recreation Section)

http://www.pacificnet.net/computrnet/history/atra.htm
(American Therapeutic Recreation Association Code of Ethics)

http://inet.ed.gov/offices/OSERS/RSA/PGMS/RT/carhrec.html
(Therapeutic Recreation)

Section II
Chapter 7

Cross Disability Topics

If a man does not keep pace
with his companion,
perhaps it is because he hears
a different drummer.
Let him step to the music he hears,
however measured or far away.
-Thoreau

Introduction

Every recreation professional can benefit from some information about disabling conditions. That is why we have included Section II this book. In the chapters within this section we will discuss a variety of disabling conditions that affect the lives of many people in both the United States and Canada. Before you read the chapters on specific disabilities, you should consider some of the issues that have application to the variety of disabling conditions that will be discussed. As we have indicated throughout Section I, it is always important to consider the person as opposed to the assumed needs of a group of people with similar disabilities. You must never assume that because two or more people have the same disability, they are alike. As you know from your own experiences, just because you may fall into the category of student or recreation professional does not mean that you are the same as other students or other recreation professionals. None of us wishes to be categorized based on a single label and assumed to have specific skills, abilities, aspirations, and challenges because of that ascribed label. Hutchison and McGill (1992, p. 20) summarize this by saying:

> People working in the field of leisure must resist the temptation to view a diagnosis as the important truth and begin to look for other ways to determine people's interests and abilities. They can begin by building relationships with people and providing supports based on people's assessment of their own situation.

Hutchison and McGill call for all recreation and leisure professionals to listen to people with disabilities as a means of determining their aspirations and needs. This is consistent with Condeluci's (1995, p. 93) first action within the interdependent paradigm. He says that:

> Interdependence...suggests that the consumers must have the rights and privileges to determine their own situation. Most often this is done by being listened to. Regardless of situation, they are quite capable of recognizing their own reality. Even if the expert does not agree with their assessment, it seems that common sense should dictate this is where the process starts. Perception is reality, and if the person perceives his problems a certain way, then this is his reality.

Taken together, both quotes underscore the need to listen to people with disabilities and not to assume that we know much about the person simply based on disability. Just because a person has a physical disability does not mean he will not want to try skateboarding or will not be capable of it. Just because a person has mental retardation does not mean that she will not want to learn how to play chess. We must not assume based on a label.

You may be asking yourself the question that we grappled with for many months: Should we/ why have we included general and categorical information about specific disabling conditions in this text? If recreation and therapeutic recreation specialists should always program based on the needs of the person, why do we need to know about specific disabling conditions? We will discuss this in the section on labeling.

Following a more extensive discussion on the pros and cons of labeling, the remainder of this chapter covers a number of issues that we feel cut across the various disabling conditions that will be discussed in subsequent chapters in Section II. That is, rather than talking about each of these issues related to mental retardation, physical disabilities, etc., we will discuss them as they relate to people with disabilities. The issues that we will discuss are labeling and classification; severe multiple disabilities; lifespan and disability; diversity, including culture and gender; poverty and unemployment; friendships; and families.

Labeling and Classification

In previous chapters, we discussed in detail the importance of focusing on the uniqueness of each individual. In particular, we discussed a ***person-centered*** approach. Because language is powerful and capable of communicating both very positive and very negative images related to people with disabilities, we must pay close attention to the ways in which we refer to people with disabilities. Even though we will discuss categories and labels, the use of people first language is central to this goal.

Labeling is a way to designate or distinguish one thing from another. Since the beginning of time, human beings have classified similarities and differences in individuals as a way to understand themselves and their surroundings. In other words, humans have "labeled" as a way to describe an object, person, or act in a systematic manner so that others in that specific society will be able to understand what is being communicated.

Various ***labels*** have been used throughout history to describe different conditions. One of the earliest known classification systems for people with mental disorders was made by Hippocrates (460-377 B.C.), who named three syndromes: mania, melancholia, and phrenitis, to differentiate the syndromes that he had witness in Greek society (Ysseldyke & Algozzine, 1982). Since that early classification system, there have been countless medical, psychological, and more recently, educational schemes used to label or classify different levels and types of disabilities. However, in today's western society, when used in the context of naming or distinguishing an individual rather than an object, "labeling" has negative connotations and implications. In many ways, labels have been helpful, yet in other ways they have been problematic. In this section, we will review the controversy that surrounds labeling.

Opposition to Labeling

Those in opposition to the use of categorical labels suggest that labels stigmatize, stereotype, and reflect a prejudicial attitude toward individuals with disabilities (Morozas & May, 1988; Hallahan & Kauffman, 1997; Tam, 1998). Hallahan and Kauffman (1982, 1997) suggest that categorical labels often lead to the assumption that all people in a category have the same personality type and behavioral characteristic. In support of this notion, Mercer (1970) notes that a label may often be viewed as an inherent attribute of the person, rather than as a means of categorizing a person as a part of the larger social environment. In essence, labels tend to homogenize people.

Morozas and May (1988, p. 164) also note that "labeling is a form of intellectual laziness" that indicates a reluctance to make difficult decisions regarding how best to meet the needs of the individual. Rather than striving to determine what is best for the person, we fall into the trap of programming based upon a disability. We become ***intellectually lazy.*** We assume we know enough to program because we know general information about the category—the label.

Kennedy, Smith, and Austin (1991) suggest when categorical labels are assigned to people with disabilities, often the label creates a self-fulfilling prophesy; that is, the individual to whom the label is assigned may often exhibit behaviors considered stereotypical of that particular disability. The concept of self-fulfilling prophesy emerged from a study by Rosenthal and Jacobsen (1968). In their study, they found that when teachers were told that particular students had good potential, those students achieved higher scores on tests than the rest of the students. Often termed the ***Rosenthal effect,*** the concept of self-fulfilling prophesy has provided the basis for a good deal of research over the years.

How do stereotypes form in the first place? For the most part, stereotypes are born out of recollections of behaviors that have been displayed by a person with a particular disability. For example, a stereotype may emanate from a person seeing someone with a disability present a specific physical movement that might be considered "unusual" for the setting or period of time. This behavior is then associated with the disability, as opposed to the person. This association is transmitted to others through conversation until eventually the behavior is considered to be strongly associated with the disability. Because the behavior is considered stereotypic of the given disability, people come to expect it to occur. Often these expectations become ***self-fulfilling*** because they result in individuals with disabilities emitting the expected behavior.

According to Kennedy, Smith, and Austin (1991), the self-fulfilling prophesy may result from the individual with a disability focusing too much on his disability and not enough on who he is as an individual. As a result, the individual with a disability comes to expect that he should behave in the same manner as other people with similar types of disabilities. Though this is likely true, it is important to note that the reason a person with a disability may focus on his disability is because society has taught him to do so.

For many decades, professionals were trained to program for people with disabilities based upon disability labels and the general expectations or "rules of thumb" that had been developed for working ***with the disabled,*** not "people with disabilities." A good example of this is the concept of ***mental age.*** Though the practice of using the term has declined in more recent times, for decades professionals used intelligence tests to determine the mental age of a person with a disability. Once a person's mental age was established (for example, a 20-year-old man might have been classified as having a mental age of 6), whether consciously or unconsciously, expectations were based upon that as opposed to who he was as a ***person.*** This practice has all but disappeared among professionals, although it is still common among the general population; it continues to underscore the problems that labels can create.

One other important consideration related to the negative use of labels is the impact on the self-concept of people with disabilities and attitudes of non-disabled children and adults. The very label "disability" implies that there is something lacking or wrong. People with disabilities experience constant disability related environmental and social stresses that may bar them from a satisfactory integration into society (Tam, 1998). When a person is labeled according to a disability, that disability becomes the dominant factor in that person's life. They are set apart. Labeling creates a situation where people's identities are derived from being disabled. They are grouped together and feel as though they loose their individuality. Yet people whose characteristics fit a certain label often do not necessarily identify themselves as that label. In interviews with people with mental retardation for example, Chalifoux and Fagan (1997, p. 537) found that most interviewees did not say that they were retarded and never really thought of themselves as retarded. Marsha, a person with a disability says on behalf of other people with disabilities, "we reject any scheme of labeling or classifying us that encourages people to think of us as having diminished value. We are not diagnoses in need of a cure or cases to be closed. We are human, with human dreams and ambitions" (Woodward, p. 23). Dunn (1968) published a historic article in this area on the negative effects of labeling on the self-concept of people with mild disabilities. Since Dunn's article there has been a plethora of research that has focused on the impact of labeling (Gottlief & Leyser, 1981; Hallahan & Kauffman, 1982; MacMillan, Jones, and Aloia, 1974). The evidence has, however, been inconclusive. It is safe to say that depending upon the setting and circumstances, the impact of labels will vary.

Support for labeling

Given the negative implications that can be associated with labels, we must again ask the question, "Why use a label?" The answer to this question is complicated, and in some ways, even to us, not always completely satisfactory. It is a conundrum! One reason often cited in support of labels is that they provide a useful starting point for understanding people with disabilities (Labanowich & Hoessli, 1979). If we understand the nature of different disabilities, we can dispel stereotypes that have been formed about those disabilities. For example, understanding the nature of visual impairments enables us to dispel the myth that all people who are sight impaired have supernatural powers of hearing.

Secondly, also noted is that knowledge of disabilities will enable us to be more in tune with services for people with disabilities and, therefore, will allow us to direct people to the most appropriate types of services. According to a group of parents, "practically speaking, ***good labels*** are those that a parent can use to open doors for his child and maximize chances of marshaling resources on his behalf" (Gorham, Des Jardins, Page, Pettis, & Scherber, 1976). Gallagher (1976) described labels as passports to the improvement of services for people with disabilities. In other words, if a child has a label of mental retardation, her mother can insist on getting specialized services that the parent thinks are needed to enhance her daughter's education. Similarly, insurance companies only pay if there is a documented diagnosis or disability.

A third reason for the use of labels is to enable us to develop programs and services that will be accessible to people with various types of disabilities. If we use a municipal recreation department as an example, the fact that a programmer has some knowledge of various disabling conditions may ensure that the programs developed are as user friendly as possible. Such knowledge may lead the programmer either to look for a site that is accessible to people with physical impairment or to advertise the program using various media to ensure that people with sensory impairments can become aware of the availability of the program. We discuss this more in Section III.

Buildings and public transportation were once inaccessible to those who possessed physical disability but by defining that there was a problem posed on those individuals with an inability to use the facilities, laws were passed and improvements were made to make environments and programs accessible. Labeling in this case leads to and continues to lead to positive outcomes. Similarly, when a label is given to a certain group, it means that the existence of that group is recognized. Through recognition comes the hope of awareness and ultimately action and education. The awareness that society has attained from the labeling of individuals with disabilities has been great. The World Health Organization (WHO) acknowledged that there was a need for the labeling of conditions of individuals before anything could be done to provide equal and efficient care for them (Bickenbach, 1993). Through this labeling came the International Classification of Impairments, Disabilities, and Handicaps: A Manual of Classification Relating to the Consequences of Disease (ICIDH), which gave descriptions of conditions that would aid physicians and other professionals that were involved in giving care to those affected by disabilities. Also, labeling led to the passage of the Americans with Disabilities Act, the most pervasive piece of civil rights legislation ever passed.

Kennedy, Smith, and Austin (1991, p. 51) provide a useful term for summing up our feelings on the use of labels. They suggest that labels are ***paradoxical***. On the one hand they tend to imply that all people with disabilities are the same; they can lead to negative stereotypes. But in contrast, labels can help people with disabilities and their families to access needed services and may allow practitioners to become more familiar with the needs of people with disabilities, thereby ensuring that people with disabilities have many different recreation opportunities available to them. In any case, we should use labels as little as possible to refer to people with disabilities. In addition, we must ensure that we do not allow labels to develop expectations in our own mind regarding the potential of people with disabilities. We must strive to ensure that we focus on the person who happens to have a disability. Knowledge of a particular disability should be used as one small piece of the pie, the pie representing the many aspects of a person. In addition to having some understanding of the nature of different disabling conditions, the recreation practitioner needs to know that many individuals have severe and/or multiple disabilities. We will discuss the implications of this in the next section.

Severe Multiple Disabilities

In the subsequent chapters in this section we will discuss categories of disabling conditions, such as hearing impairments, mental retardation, and others. Within each of these chapters, we point out that a disability can vary quite dramatically in terms of severity. For example, individuals can experience mild hearing loss, complete deafness, or anything in between. What we do not discuss in these chapters is that a person can have multiple disabilities; he can have two or more disabilities at the same time. This is an issue that truly cuts across all disabilities.

Within the last decade there has been an increased interest in providing opportunities for individuals with multiple disabilities within community-based settings as opposed to institutional ones. This is in large measure due to the increased incidence of people living with severe disabilities. A recent American survey indicated that almost two thirds of adults with disabilities describe their disability as very (26%) or somewhat severe (37%), compared to only six out of ten in 1994, and just over half in 1986 (NOD/Harris, 1998). According to Schleien (1991), however, there is often a lack of consensus as to the meaning of the term severe and/or multiple disabilities. He indicates that under the broad rubric of ***severe multiple disabilities*** fall generic terms such as severe disability, severe multiple handicap, dual sensory impairment, and multiple disabilities as Deaf-blind and dual diagnosis (of which there is mentally-retarded-blind, cerebral palsied-deaf, and mentally retarded-mentally ill). The variety of terms is created by different classification systems used by various agencies, including recreation, education, residential, and vocational. Schleien (p. 191) suggests the following definition as being both general enough to include all of those identified above, yet specific enough for service providers:

> Severe multiple disability refers to those individuals with a profound disability or a combination of disabilities that so limit their daily activities that they require services and programming that is more innovative, extensive, and intensive than common programming for individuals with disabilities provides. This population is characterized as—but is not exclusively—nonambulatory, non-independently mobile, needing to be fed, needing assistance in toileting, and needing daily occupational or communication therapy.

Until recently, there have been few recreation and leisure opportunities for individuals with severe multiple disabilities. This was in part due to the lack of such people living within the community, thus little demand arose for such services, and the lack of awareness of the most effective strategies for facilitating such opportunities. However, during the past decade, an increased interest has emerged in determining the most salient strategies for enabling people with severe multiple disabilities to enjoy recreation participation. Some of these techniques will be covered in future chapters that focus on the process and techniques used in community recreation programming and therapeutic recreation interventions.

Prior to discussing specific techniques or strategies for working with people with severe multiple disabilities, we need to understand certain guiding principles that have surfaced from the literature and practice. First, it has become very clear that self-determination and decision making are as important for people with severe multiple disabilities as for those with less severe disabilities. For decades, a widely held assumption was that people with severe multiple disabilities were not capable of making choices or expressing preferences. This assumption was based on the fact that many people with severe multiple disabilities are not able to verbally communicate a choice preference. However, the work of Dattio and others has clearly demonstrated that people with severe multiple disabilities can and indeed want to make choices (Dattilo, 1986; Dattilo & Rusch, 1985; Dattilo & Barnett, 1985; Dattilo & Mirenda, 1987). Through the use of technology, these researchers have demonstrated that individuals with severe multiple disabilities can choose such things as their own music, video games, and meals. As a result of this work, we have come to accept the challenge of promoting decision making into recreation programs for people with severe multiple disabilities.

Just as self-determination has only recently become a priority for those supporting people with severe multiple disabilities, inclusion, and in particular social inclusion, is an area that has lacked attention. As with decision making, people with severe multiple disabilities were thought incapable of being included within regular recreation programs. Though it is true that many people with disabilities have been excluded from the mainstream, people with severe multiple disabilities have tended to experience greater constraints related to inclusion. However, research and demonstration projects have clearly established processes that can lead to full inclusion for people with severe multiple disabilities (Schleien, Olson, Rogers & McLafferty, 1985; Schleien, Ray Soderman-Olson, & McMahon, 1987; Wuerch & Voeltz, 1982).

One final area that has received some attention relative to recreation and leisure and people with severe multiple disabilities is communication. Dattilo (1994) suggests that providing people with severe multiple disabilities with alternative forms of communication is only the first step toward enhancing communication within a recreation environment. Practitioners must learn to be as responsive as possible when people with severe multiple disabilities are communicating. This accepting behavior must be modeled by practitioners in order to ensure that others begin to also practice such inclusive behaviors. Dattilo and Light (1993) demonstrated that professionals could be taught to decrease their dominant conversation to allow for opportunities for initiation by people with severe multiple disabilities.

We have discussed the issue of labeling and severe multiple disabilities in order to provide some context for the chapters you will read on specific disabilities. While we should try to understand the nature of a person's disability, it is equally important to try to gain some sense of the social system within which that person may live.

Life Span and Disability

Leisure scholars have long recognized the importance of viewing leisure within the context of life course or life span (Kelly, 1996; Neulinger, 1981; Rapoport & Rapoprot, 1978). According to Horna (1994), any analysis of leisure is incomplete if it does not take into account major life events. She indicates that though life stages may vary somewhat, a consensus has been reached among leisure scholars that life cycle stages can be divided into "the preparation (childhood and adolescence), establishment (adult, 'second age'), and culmination ('later years', 'third age') periods" (Norna, 1994, p. 91).

An analysis of the literature related to people with disabilities and recreation and/or therapeutic recreation reveals only bits and pieces that have been written related to life cycle, leisure, and people with disabilities. The majority of literature has centered on stages of the life cycle, such as childhood (Bullock, Mahon, & Welch, 1992; Dattilo, Light, St. Peter, & Sheldon, 1995) or old age (Hawkins, 1993; Mahon &* Searle, 1993; Wilhite, Keller, & Nicholson, 1991).

Similarly, within the broader field of disability, only more recently has there been some focus on issues related to the life cycle. This literature has tended to concentrate on transitions, such as the transition from adolescence to adulthood (Agran & Moore, 1987; Chang, 1988) and from adulthood to older adulthood (Ansello, 1988; Brown, 1989). Neither the broad area of disability nor that more specifically related to leisure and recreation or therapeutic recreation appears to have tackled issues related to disability across the life span.

A great deal has been written on childhood, disability, and play. Lewis (1987), in her text *Development and Handicap*, underscores the fact, however, that different disabilities have differential impact on the development of play skills.

According to Kelly (1996, p. 140):

> the early years are a time for learning, anticipation, and of being evaluated for later opportunities. Thus, these years must be understood within the context of societal expectations that the child become somewhat different in time as he or she grows up. During the early stages of this period, children strive to gain control, while at the same time they try to learn how to share control with others. Play helps them to move from the concrete to the abstract and also helps them to improve their physical ability, strength, endurance, and skill (Barnett, 1991; Corsaro & Eder, 1990).

Adolescence can be characterized as the period during which one identifies one's social identity. Adolescents are caught up with trying to answer the question: "Who am I?" (Kelly, 1996). This tends to result in a great deal of experimentation with different identities. Horna (1994) suggests that the primary focus on leisure during this period is its significance in the search for identity and testing one's abilities. Within the disability literature, a great deal of attention has been given to the issue of transition from school to work and from adolescence to adulthood for people with disabilities. In addition, the area of sexuality for adolescents with disabilities is also gaining attention.

Changing values of society make sexuality a much more complex issue (Ferguson, Ferguson, & Edwards, 1991). Society's lack of expectations for individuals leads to inappropriate sexual expression (Duncan & Canty-Lemke, 1986). Society's perceptions of individuals with mental retardation as sexual misfits makes integration a more difficult process (Mitchell, 1985). The issue of choice creates problems related to sexual expression, marriage, and having children. The issue is do we treat individuals as children or as adults (Mitchell, 1985; Ferguson et al, 1991)? We must consider the principles of normalization related to this, but we must also be rational. Blatt (1987) suggests that freedom is the most important concern. Ferguson et al. (1991), on the other hand, suggest that this issue must be treated on an individual basis.

According to Horna (1994), most adults in their second stage join the labor force, establish careers, find a spouse, and start a family. People tend to be occupied with productivity and performance, and in the later establishment period—evaluation (Rapoport & Papoport, 1978). For the majority of people who have children, this stage of life also tends to be occupied with family and parenthood obligations, such that one can trace the changes during an adults establishment period using the ages of the children.

For the most part, one can assume that many people with disabilities have the same preoccupations with work during this period of life as people without disabilities. Unemployment figures among people with disabilities are very high. Only three in ten people with disabilities, who are of working age, work full or part time, versus eight out of ten non-disabled adults (NOD/Harris, 1998). Forced free time/ leisure is of great concern among adults with disabilities. Given this, the leisure of some adults with disabilities may be somewhat different than those of the general public. They may have more free time, but with less discretionary income; they may also have far fewer opportunities to experience diversity in their leisure.

A variety of terms has been used to describe one's later life stage. Culmination, retirement, the third age, old age, and older adulthood have all been used to describe this period of life. As with other stages of life, the third age is one of transition. Aging is a lifelong process. The culmination period is marked by a number of life changes, such as retirement, possible movement to warmer climates, loss of spouse and friends, and changes in health status. Older adults are no more homogeneous than people of any other age, so there are far fewer generalizations one can make about this population than one might expect.

As has been noted by so many demographers, ours is an aging population. We are staying healthier and living longer than ever before. This same trend is evident within the population of aging adults with disabilities (Mahon, Mactavish, Mahon, & Searle, 1995).

With this trend has come a call by many to attend to the leisure needs of older adults with disabilities. One population that has received some attention in this area are older adults with mental retardation. Hawkins (1993) has studied the relationship between leisure activities and life satisfaction in older adults with mental retardation. She found leisure and life satisfaction and leisure activities to be significantly related in later life. Mahon and his colleagues at the University of Manitoba have begun to explore issues related to social integration, independence, and leisure in older adults with mental retardation. In addition, Mahon has also begun to investigate the utility of using leisure education and personal futures planning as the basis for retirement planning for older adults with mental retardation.

What is evident from this analysis of life course and disability is that most of the issues that people without disabilities face over the course of their lives are similarly experienced by people with disabilities. However, in some cases this is not true. The challenge is to understand where life-span changes may vary for people with disabilities and where they may have more severe impact on people with disabilities. Recognition of these differences can help to ensure quality of life and, in particular, will help leisure service providers to address the leisure needs to people with disabilities across their life span.

Diversity

The demographics of North America have changed dramatically during the 20th century. With the changes in demographics have come a much more diverse population and concomitantly, a much more diverse population of people with disabilities. Little attention has been paid to the issue of disability and cultural diversity.

The National Easter Seal Society has recently identified diversity as an important issue that must be addressed in relation to the provision of services for people with disabilities. They indicate that a focus on diversity:

> ...will mean that Easter Seal affiliates serve people with disabilities whose demographic characteristics such as disability, race, ethnicity, age, religion, gender, marital status, sexual orientation, and cultural background reflect the general population of their community (National Easter Seal Society, 1994, p. 24).

As is evident from this quote, diversity is a very broad issue. In order to provide examples of the relationship between disability, diversity, and recreation and leisure, we will highlight two areas related to diversity: Ethnicity and gender.

Ethnicity

As with the broader topic of diversity, there has *not* been a great deal of attention focused on ethnicity and disability.

One area that has been extensively studied im the United States is the question of whether there is an over-representation of minority students receiving special education services. Dunn (1968) is credited with one of the earliest comprehensive analyses of this question. Dunn contended that an overwhelming proportion of students (80%) served in programs for students with mental retardation were from minority groups (Latino, African-American, and native American groups) and lower socioeconomic families. Twenty-five years later, Artiles and Trent (1994) reviewed the status of this question. Though they readily admit there can be problems with how data have and can be used in answering the question of over-representation, Artiles and Trent conclude that the problem continues to exist. For example, they cite literature from the U.S. Department of Education that indicates that the proportion of minority youth in special education programs is greater than that in regular education. In particular, African-American youth are more highly represented in all disabilities categories; Hispanic youth are close behind.

What is at the root of the over-representation problem? Artiles and Trent (1994) indicate that the problem is multivariate in nature. First, litigation has led to a greater identification of students in general in special education. Second, a great debate continues about constructs such as intelligence and how they are assessed. For example, it is still unclear whether IQ tests are able to differentiate one's abilities with such challenges as language and cultural differences thrown into the mix. Many argue that they cannot. Third, in many cases the thought is that there may be biases in the referral and assessment process. Lastly, changing demographics may have an impact on this area. The number of white children being born in the United States is declining, while minority groups are the youngest and fastest growing.

If over-representation of ethnic minorities is a problem, what is the solution? Because the problem is multifacted, the answer must be as well. Artiles and Trent (1994) present the following as initiatives that could lead to a resolution of this problem:

1. Continue to refine the constructs of mental retardation and learning disabilities;
2. Develop a sound, culturally sensitive research agenda;
3. Restructure and refine systems so that they are more culturally sensitive;
4. Reform professional preparation programs to ensure that they are culturally sensitive; and
5. Advocate for policy changes relative to individuals from different minorities.

Though little has been achieved related to ethnicity, recreation, and disability, the five initiatives listed above have important implications for the recreation service delivery system. All can be adopted.

Gender

A search of the disability literature on the issue of gender results in a very brief list of references. This body of literature has almost exclusively focused on women with disabilities. It concludes that women with disabilities are members of two separate minority groups, often described as a multiple minority group. Deegan (1981, p. 276) defines a multiple minority group as:

> ...any group of people who are singled out from the others in society in which they live for differential and unequal treatment because they are defined as members of more than one minority group, and who therefore regard themselves as objects of this combination of collective discriminations.

According to Deegan (1981), the significant difference between those of a single versus multiple minority group is that there are what she describes as interaction effects for the multiple minority group. By this she means that the two areas (e.g., gender and disability status) combine to create more severely limiting conditions for the individual. In addition, Deegan also notes that a person with multiple minority status is commonly discriminated against by both those who do not consider themselves to be in the minority at all, as well as individuals who are in the "single minority group." In addition, people commonly have more than two minority areas, multiple minorities are, according to Deegan, exposed to new patterns of discrimination. The issue becomes less of the *us* versus *them* debate, which in some ways is helpful.

According to Krotoski, Nosek, & Turk (1996), there are an estimated 26 million women living in the United States that have some type of disability, which is more than half of the estimated population of people with disabilities. This very significant portion of the U.S. population are among the poorest, and least employed of any sub-group of U.S. citizens. According to Altman (1996, p. 51), "even when women with disabilities are employed, their mean earnings are the lowest as compared to men with and without disabilities, and women without a disability."

Beyond the economic situation of women with disabilities, there are a number of other issues to which women with disabilities are confronted. Chief among these issues are health concerns. In May, 1994, a conference was held to begin to address such issues. The Health of Women with Physical Disabilities conference highlighted a number of health concerns for women with disabilities. These included health risk factors, sexuality and reproductive health, stress, bladder and bowel function, and physical fitness. In their summary of the key themes of this conference, Nosek, Turk, and Krotoski (1996, p. 441) make the following comments:

> . . . we see a shedding of old paradigms for the women in society and a gradual abandonment of standards and definitions developed for men. There is a new understanding of wellness and sexuality for women in general, and, as expressed in this volume, the door has cracked open to include women with disabilities. We need to promote actively the new definition of wellness and fitness in the context of disability, a new definition of sexuality that includes psychological and social as well as physical aspects, and a new definition of functioning that addresses the ability to fill social roles and deal with stress that accompanies living with disability.

What is clear from this quote, is that women with disabilities are challenged by many and very diverse constraints to achieving quality of life.

What are the implications of what we know about gender and disability for recreation and therapeutic recreation? According to some feminist scholars, the sense of entitlement necessary to experience leisure is often not felt by women (Henderson, Bedini, & Bialeschki, 1993). Many women do not believe that they deserve or that they should be able to experience leisure. Henderson et al. (p. 38) suggest that:

> the lack of traditional roles that women with disabilities may experience, even though traditional social roles may be perceived as oppressive by some feminists, suggests self-estrangement and powerlessness. Individuals with disabilities who have been indoctrinated with the work ethic and sense of value based on work and family, may feel guilt in undertaking leisure.

Accordingly, women with disabilities may be less able to engage in satisfying leisure experiences. They may not see leisure as a human right, but as something that one deserves if one works hard and cares for a family.

The manner in which women with disabilities view leisure has important implications for therapeutic recreation. As we will discuss later, the therapeutic process must be contextualized to the individual. Therefore, gender must be considered an important element within the overall context of an individual's life. Henderson et al. (1993, p. 40-41) provide a number of suggestions for ensuring that a therapeutic recreation process is gender-sensitive. We have summarized them into the following six key points:

1. Assist individuals in coming to terms with their multiple minority status;
2. Provide opportunities for the individual to practice assertiveness;
3. Help the individual in identifying the "connections" in her life between family, work, education, leisure, etc;
4. Assistant the individual in identifying a personal meaning for and value of leisure and leisure preferences;
5. Embody feminist principles by working as a consultant to people with disabilities, not as an expert; and
6. Work as an advocate for women with disabilities.

All of the principles identified above will be discussed further in the leisure education chapter in Section III as well as in the conclusion of this book.

Poverty and Unemployment

According to studies conducted in both the United States and Canada, people with disabilities experience unparalleled, chronic unemployment. A poll, conducted by Harris (1998), commissioned by the National Institute on Disability, reported that 71% of people with disabilities surveyed were not working. Of those who reported that they were not working, the vast majority indicated that their unemployment was due to their disability/health problems. In addition, 72% of those not working indicated that they would prefer to work. What is even more disturbing is that these unemployment statistics in the United States are slightly worse than in 1994.

Canadian statistics on the employment of people with disabilities are quite a bit different. Statistics Canada (1991) reported that 52% of working age Canadians with disabilities are unemployed, which was down from 60% in 1986. It is difficult to know why there is such a disparity between the U.S. and Canadian statistics. What is clear, however, is that unemployment is one of the most critical issues with which people with disabilities are faced. In particular, one of the most concrete results of such high levels of unemployment is the poverty that comes with it. Over one third of working age Americans with disabilities lived in households with less than $15,000.00 in total income in 1997, as compared to only 12% of those without disabilities (NOD/Harris, 1998). This gap has remained constant for over a decade. In many cases, the vicious circle of chronic unemployment and poverty for people with disabilities can lead to health problems and limitations of personal control. This is compounded by the fact that poverty often leads to a lack of equitable access to health care, particularly in the U.S. where quality health care and employment are often tied together. In 1998, one in four adults with disabilities postponed getting health care because of cost (NOD/Harris, 1998).

Little doubt exists that poverty and unemployment have a significant impact on the leisure of people with disabilities. Bender, Brannon, and Verhoven (1984) described the chronic unemployment situation of people with disabilities as *forced leisure*. They indicate that:

> In length of this profile, and little has changed since the 1980s, there is no doubt that the handicapped (sic) need a chance to use their leisure time wisely. Traditionally, American education has overemphasized the development of work-oriented behaviors and attitudes...This narrow perspective has been a disservice to many...

Bender et al. suggest that the realities of employment necessitate that schools prepare individuals with disabilities for both work and leisure.

Hutchison and McGill (1992) suggest that financial poverty often leads to *poverty of experience.* Leisure tends to be restricted to what an individual can afford or to what is free. This is especially true because in North America our leisure is largely purchased, and thus the possession of disposable income is often a precursor to enjoying one's free time. One significant result of this is that the leisure choices of people with disabilities, which are already often undermined by the system within which the person lives, are further limited by lack of financial means. As a result, the leisure pursuits of people with disabilities tend to be restricted to such home-based activities as watching television and listening to music, as opposed to more community-based activities.

The realities of unemployment and poverty must be understood by those facilitating recreation opportunities for people with disabilities. Hutchison and Lord (1979, p. 43) indicate that people with disabilities should be counseled to ask the following questions when selecting a leisure pursuit:

1. Does this activity or leisure experience cost money? If so, how much does it cost?
2. Is it affordable, and if so, how can money be found to make it happen?
3. Are there subsidies that are available that are not unnecessarily stigmatized? How can these subsidies be provided without further devaluation occurring?
4. Are there less expensive ways to participate in the same activity or experience?

Friendships

Parents, advocates, leisure service providers, educators, and many others have come to recognize the importance of friendships for people with disabilities. With the strong emphasis on integration and inclusion in this text, we may find ourselves asking, "With whom should people with disabilities make friends?" The problem with this question is that it assumes that we or others have the right to decide what sort of friends are best for people with disabilities. Given all that we have discussed related to choice and self-determination, we know that this assumption is dead wrong. We cannot emphasize enough the importance of remembering that it is the individual who must ultimately decide who her friends will be. Heyne et al. (p. 2) summarized our feelings best in their introduction when they wrote,

> In her book, *Among Friends*, Letty Cottin Pogrebin writes, "...although the centuries of wisdom have yielded...scores of friendship criteria...in

> the last analysis, friendship is what you say it is." . . . Children tell us who their friends are, what they like and do not like about their friends, what surprises them, and what they learn from their friends.

Heyne, Schleien, and McAvoy (1994) provide a very comprehensive picture of the issues related to friendships and people with disabilities in their manual ***Making Friends: Using Recreation to Promote Friendship Between Children With and Without Disabilities.*** Some of their quotes are also very instructive in answering the question: "Why consider friendships for people with disabilities?" The answers are as follows:

1. By playing and making friends with other children, Elise will learn how to act appropriately in a group. She will learn to listen to others, to wait to take her turn, and to pay attention to what is going on around her.
2. When our younger child (who does not have a disability) began to make friends earlier than our older daughter, Tracey (who does have a disability), we realized Tracey had missed some important milestones in learning to get along with and in relating to others. We hope that by being with nondisabled peers she can learn the give-and-take of social relationships and what it means to be and to have a friend.
3. As parents, it is important that we learn what are realistic expectations regarding friendships for our son. Should we expect the same kinds of interactions that our other (nondisabled) children enjoy with their friends? Or should we accept that Sam's friendships will be different and not pressure him—or ourselves—by expecting more than is realistic (Heyne et al., 1994, p. 5)?

These quotes from three different parents provide insight into the reasons that we must focus on facilitating friendships for individuals with disabilities, including children, adults, and older adults. One central reason is that often people with disabilities have greater difficulty making friends. This may relate to their social skills—the fact that they do not participate in many recreation activities that help to naturally cultivate friendships or possibly because they do not go to their neighborhood school. One parent suggested that often we are unsure of what to expect out of friendships between people with and without disabilities. This may be because we have not experienced such friendships ourselves or have not seen any develop between our children and other children with disabilities. What seems clear, however, is that friendships are important for people with disabilities.

While it may be clear that friendships are indeed important for people with disabilities, there is some debate regarding the nature and value of different types of friends. Harry, Park, and Day (1998) contend that the disability-related literature has had a powerful bias toward friendships which involve people with and without disabilities. They question whether the field has devalued friendships between people with disabilities, and in fact other types of friendships such as mentoring relationships, family-based friendships, and cross-age friendships. Our own review of the literature on disability, friendships, and recreation/leisure suggests that such a bias may indeed exist in our own field. For example, Schleien, Ray, and Green (1997) almost exclusively discuss strategies for facilitating friendships between people with and without disabilities.

Our recent research on social inclusion (Mahon, Lutfiyya, Mactavish, Rodrigue, Strain, and Studholme, 1998) suggests that people with disabilities do not distinguish between people with and without disabilities, when discussing friendships. They assign equal value to friends with and without disabilities. This point is underscored by Amanda's (a participant in our study on social integration) thoughts on having friends with and without disabilities:

> I go to school with other kids like me. But I also know other kids who aren't like me...don't have to go to special class—don't have a disability. To me, that isn't the same as being friends. Friends are people I like and like me...I guess anybody at school could be my friend...but only Dawn really is (a classmate with a disability). We hang around everyday. I like coming to school to be with Dawn.

Put another way, Amanda's thoughts suggest a sense of belonging is derived from friendships with people—independent of whether these people have a disability or not. Amanda's perspective is underscored by Harry, Park, and Day's (1998, p. 401) summary comments on this issue:

> Our attempts to assist in enriching the social lives of children and youth with disabilities should provide them with diverse social opportunities while offering support for the relationships that they initiate and to which they are attracted. Social inclusion should mean respecting and supporting a wide range of individual choices and values.

If it is more difficult for people with disabilities to make friends, just what are the barriers? Heyne et al. (1994) identify a number of common barriers to making friends. These are summarized in Table 7.1.

Table 7.1
Some Common Barriers to Making Friends

Families' Busy Schedules
At times within the busy life of a family, friendships for children with disabilities may seem like a luxury, or parents may assume they are not possible.

Lack of Knowledge about Recreation's Role
Parents may not understand that recreation can play a vital role in helping to facilitate friendships.

Inappropriate Social Skills
If children do not know how to join and behave in a group, meet other kids, take turns, etc., they may have difficulty making friends.

Table 7.1 cont.

Difficult Communication
Friendship development may be challenging if an individual has difficulty with expressive or receptive communication.

Distance Between Homes
If children with disabilities do not go to their neighborhood school they may have difficulty experiencing spontaneous play with their peers because they do not live close by.

Families Not Acquainted
Realistically, parents are the ones who often have to serve as catalysts for friendships between their family member with a disability and his peers. This may occur by contacting other parents; this can be difficult if you do not know the parents of your children's friends.

Lack of Transportation
As with so many aspects of the lives of people with disabilities, lack of transportation can negatively impact the development and maintenance of friends. In particular, if an individual relies on others for transportation, her ability to enjoy more spontaneous experiences with friends is curtailed. This can be a real problem with adolescents who may not want to rely on parents for transportation, but who cannot transport themselves.

Need for Information about Disabilities
Individuals without disabilities usually require some sort of disability awareness training to help them move beyond their potential lack of comfort with individuals with disabilities.

Lack of Common Interests
Most often we associate with people because we share a common interest. The challenge can be finding common interests between individuals. This is usually a minor barrier.

No Phone or Lack of Phone Skills
The telephone is a major tool we use to stay in touch with our friends and to arrange to meet. If an individual does not have a phone, or is not comfortable using one, this can pose a significant challenge.

Heyne and her colleagues have identified a number of ways to help people with disabilities develop friends. Their suggestions include tips for family members and recreation service providers. We have selected some of the key points they have identified and incorporated these into a list of suggestions in Table 7.2.

Table 7.2
Ways to Help Encourage Friendships

Families:
1. Make friendship development a priority.
2. Become acquainted with other families.
3. Schedule children's time together.
4. Invite children into the home and on outings.
5. Encourage children to talk about their friends at home.
6. Encourage positive social interactions.
7. Learn about community recreation resources.
8. Strengthen friendship/social skills.

Recreation Staff:
1. Welcome all children in recreation programs.
2. Ensure architectural accessibility.
3. Ensure program accessibility.
4. Educate staff to meet individual needs.
5. Provide cooperative activities that promotes positive peer interaction.
6. Strengthen friendship skills of participants without disabilities and participants with disabilities.
7. Prepare people as integration facilitators.
8. Promote inclusion as everyone's responsibility.

As we have discussed extensively throughout this text, the facilitation of quality of life for people with disabilities must be a shared goal. The suggestions summarized in Table 7.2 underscore the fact that families, recreation staff, and others must work together to help promote friendships.

Families

During the past quarter-century, a significant body of literature centered on family recreation has emerged (Orthner & Mancini, 1990; Rapoport & Rapoport, 1975). The vast majority of this literature has, according to Mactavish (1997), concentrated on typical families—those that do not include individuals with disabilities. Mactavish suggests that this literature has considered the nature of family recreation, including both the patterns (where and with whom the activity takes place) and forms (the activity). The family recreation literature has also articulated the benefits of family recreation.

A general conclusion that can be drawn from reading the literature on family recreation for typical families is that family recreation is valued and important in many families' lives. Much less literature exists on the recreation patterns and forms of families that include children with disabilities, the benefits they may receive from family recreation, and the constraints they can experience. As a result, though one might assume the same to be true for families that include children with disabilities, there is far less literature to help answer this question. What is clear, however, is that policymakers, service providers, and most importantly—families, have all begun to articulate the need to include families in all aspects of decision making, planning, and the facilitating opportunities for individuals with disabilities. Given the increased attention on people with disabilities and their families and our knowledge of the benefits of family recreation, we must understand how best to create environments conducive to family recreation.

The issue of recreation and families with children with disabilities has received little attention in the recreation and leisure literature until very recently. However, during the past few years there has been some effort to change this. Such authors as Ashton-Shaeffer, Shelton, and Johnson (1995), Bullock, Johnson, and Shelton (in press), and Mactavish (1997), have contributed to a relatively new, yet expanding body of literature.

Mactavish (1994) provides a comprehensive picture of the nature of family recreation people with developmental disabilities. According to Mactavish (p. 175), "Spending time together in mutually enjoyable activities was the primary objective parents reported for shared recreation." Thus, meeting this objective was the most significant benefit families cited for family recreation. According to Mactavish (1997, p. 75), family recreation experiences were characterized by three different patterns:

> 1) an all family pattern, which involved everyone in the immediate family; 2) a subunit/subgroup pattern, whereby small groups within the family engaged in activities together; and 3) an equal combination pattern, in which participation alternated between small-group activities and those involving the entire family . . . Overall, small-group (i.e. subunit pattern) activities tended to dominate the recreation experiences of the families in this study.

Most of the small-group activities involved the mother, the child with a disability, and sometimes other siblings. Families in this study identified a number of benefits to family recreation including the opportunity to re-establish what is important in life, bringing the family closer together, and providing opportunities for the children with disabilities to become integrated into their community. In contrast, the most common constraints cited by families were work responsibilities, and lack of time.

Past experiences, and in particular—past benefits, tended to influence the degree to which families negotiated through constraints. Typically, families used various combinations of whole family and subunit participation patterns as a way to negotiate such constraints.

In addition to the work of Mactavish (1994) and others at the University of Minnesota, Bullock and his colleagues at the University of North Carolina at Chapel Hill conducted a five-year research study designed to study the effectiveness of incorporating families into a leisure education process as a means of facilitating self-determination in individuals with disabilities. Ashton-Shaeffer et. al. (1995) and Bullock et al. (in press) both describe initial outcomes from this federally funded, efficacy study titled "Family Link in Leisure Education." The findings these authors reported suggest that families can play a crucial role in enhancing the leisure education process, thereby creating greater opportunity for self-determination for individuals with disabilities. At the same time, however, the authors also present some interesting comments from the families involved win their study. Most of the families indicate that they think that parental/family involvement in leisure education is important. However, some parents/family members also indicated that they have always had to facilitate recreation experiences for their children with disabilities. In some ways the leisure education process created more work for them; work that they could do without. So, though the family-centered leisure education process is effective at meeting its central goal, it may present additional perceived constraints for the families that have to be negotiated in various ways.

Conclusion

In this chapter we have discussed a number of issues that cut across the field of disability and relate to people with various disabling conditions. Hopefully, you have come to understand that there are many things to consider when you include individuals with disabilities within recreation programs. The severity of the person's disability and her socioeconomic status and culture have significant implications for a recreation or therapeutic recreation programmer. In many ways, most important is that the community recreation specialist be aware of these issues. She is the one who will help to determine whether programs are sensitive to gender, culture, age, degree of disability, family on text, and the like.

The remaining chapters within this section of the book will discuss specific disabling conditions. More specifically, we will discuss the following general disability categories: mental retardation, physical disabilities, visual impairments, hearing impairments, and mental illnesses. These do not represent an exhaustive list of disabilities. However, they do represent the most common disability groupings. Each of the five chapters contains the same sections. The chapters begin with a section on "Some Things You Might Want to Know." This section provides an overview of such things as the definition of the disability, the scope of severity for the disability, prevalence, and etiology. "Some Things You Might Want To Do" is the second section within each chapter. We have tried to provide a brief review of what are considered to be some best practices for working with individuals with the specific disability, keeping in mind that all individuals have their own unique needs. The third section discusses "Implications for Recreation" from a disability-specific perspective. These sections tend to be very brief, as most of what we know about recreation programming tends to relate to all people with disabilities.

The last section of each of these chapters highlights "Health and Safety" information for people with the specific disabling conditions.

Each of the chapters within this section is purposefully short. We do not think it is important that you have a detailed knowledge of disabling conditions at this point in your educational program. For those of you who are interested in therapeutic recreation, you will acquire more detailed knowledge as you are exposed to future course work, practicums, and further reading. As you begin to read these chapters, keep in mind that the knowledge you gain will help you understand just one small aspect of individuals with disabilities you may meet in the future. At the same time, try to recall the issues we have discussed in this chapter. How might the information related to families be helpful related to including a child with a hearing impairment in a swimming program? What might be some constraints to making friends for an older adult with mental retardation? Finally, remember, a label can be both positive and negative; much depends upon how you as a student/ professional use it.

Learning Activities

1. Identify some recreation programs within your community. Discuss how they could be made to be more sensitive to gender and ethnicity for both people with disabilities and people without disabilities.
2. Think of a situation in your life when you have treated someone a certain way based on who you thought he was, based on prior knowledge of that person's family, that person's appearance, etc. Discuss this with your classmates.
3. Discuss how some movies are good examples of stereotyping and labeling. Can you think of examples of labeling in books?

References

Agran, M. & Moore, As. (1987). Transitional programming: Suggesting an adaptability model. ***Advances in mental retardation and developmental disabilities, 3***, 179-208.

Altman, B.M. (1996). Causes, risks, and consequences of disability among women. In D. Krotoski, M. Nosek, & M. Turk (Eds.), ***Women with Physical Disabilities: Achieving and Maintaining Health and Well-Being***. Baltimore, MD: Brookes.

Andrze, H. (1999). "Stereotyping." Online. Internet, retrieved 2 January 1999. Available: HYPERLINK http://cvn.strath.ac.uk/mscit/sanmugav/EX3_3/

Bickenbach, J. E. (1993). ***Physical Disability and Social Policy***. Toronto: Unniversity of Toronto Press.

Ansello, E.F. (1988). The intersecting of aging and disabilities. *Educational Gerontology*, 14 (5), 351-364.

Artiles, A.J., & Trent, S.C. (1994). Over-representation of minority students in special education: A continuing debate. *Journal of Special Education,* 27 (4), 10-37.

Ashton-Shaeffer, C., Shelton, M. & Johnson, D.E. (1995). The social caterpillar and the wallflower: Two case studies of adolescents with disabilities in transition. *Therapeutic Recreation Journal*, 29 (4), 324-336.

Barnett, L.A. (1991). Developmental benefits of play for children. In B.L. Driver, P.J. Brown, and G.L. Peterson (Eds.), *Benefits of Leisure*. State College, PA: Venture, pp. 215-247.

Bender, M., Brannon, S.A., & Verhoven, P.J. (eds.). (1984). *Leisure education for the handicapped: Curriculum goals, activities, and resources*. San Diego, CA: College Hill Press.

Blatt, B. (1987). Life, eugenics, euthanasia, and sterilization. In B. Blatt, *The Conquest of Mental Retardation*. Austin, TX: Pro-Ed.

Brown, P.J. (1988). *Effects of self-advocacy training in leisure on adults with severe physical disabilities*. Unpublished doctoral dissertation, Virginia Polytechnic Institute and State University, Blacksburg, Virginia.

Bullock, C.C., & Johnson, D.E. (1997). Recreation as a related service. In F.M. Brasile (Ed.), *Recreation therapy: Perspectives of a dynamic profession*. Raven Sword, WA: Idyll Arbor.

Bullock, C.C., Johnson, D.E., & Shelton, M. (In press). *Kids in context: Exploring the potential of children with disabilities*. Cresshill, NJ: Hampton Press, Inc.

Bullock, C.C., Mahon, M.J., & Welch, L.K. (1992). Easter Seal's progressive mainstreaming model: Options and choices in camping and leisure services for children and adults with disabilities. *Therapeutic Recreation Journal, 27* (3).

Chalifoux, L. M. & Fagan, B. (1997). Labeling children who are visually impaired "Disadvantaged." *Journal of Visual Impairment and Blindness*., 91 (6), 531-538.

Chang, M.K. (1988). Follow-up students of graduates with mental retardation: A review. *The Illinois Schools Journal, 67* (2), 26-30.

Condeluci, A. (1995). *Interdependence: The route to community*. Winter Park, FL: GR Press, Inc.

Dattilo, J. (1986). Computerized assessment of preference for severely handicapped individuals. *Journal of Applied Behavior Analysis, 19* (4), 445-448.

Dattilo, J. (1994). *Inclusive leisure services; responding to the rights of people with disabilities*. State College, PA: Venture Publishing Inc.

Dattilo, J., & Barnett, L.A. (1985). Therapeutic recreation for individuals with severe handicaps: An analysis of the relationship between choice and pleasure. *Therapeutic Recreation Journal, 19*, 79-91.

Dattilo, J., & Light, J. (1993). Setting the stage for leisure: Encouraging reciprocal communication for people using augmentative and alternative communication systems through facilitator instruction. *Therapeutic Recreation Journal, 27* (3), 156-171.

Dattilo, J., & Mirenda, P. (1987). An application of a leisure preference assessment protocol for persons with severe handicaps. *Journal of the Association for Persons with Severe Handicaps, 12* (4), 306-311.

Dattilo, J., & Rusch, F. (1985). Effects of choice on leisure participation for persons with severe handicaps. *Journal of the Association for Persons with Severe Handicaps, 10*, 194-199.

Dattilo, J., Light, J., St. Peter, S., & Sheldon, K. (1995). Parents' perspective on leisure patterns of youth using augmentative and alternative communication systems. *Therapeutic Recreation Journal, 29* (1), 8-17.

Deegan, M.J. (1981). Multiple minority groups: A case study of physically disabled women. *Journal of Sociology and Social Welfare, 8*, 274-297.

Driedger, D. & Gray, S. (1992) *Imprinting our image: An anthology by women with disabilities*. Gynergy Books, Canada.

Duncan, D., & Canty-Lemke, J. (1986). Learning appropriate social and sexual behavior: The role of society. *The Exceptional Parents, 16* (3), 24-26.

Dunn, L.M. (1968). Special education for the mildly retarded: Is much of it justifiable? *Exceptional Children*.

Ferguson, D.L., Ferguson, P.M., & Edwards, J. (1991). Parent and professional perspective: Sexuality and culture in the lives of people with severe disabilities. *TASH Newsletter; 16* (3), 9-10.

Fine, M., & Asch, A. (1982). Disabled women: Sexism without the pedestal. *Journal of Sociology and Social Welfare, 8* (2), 233-248.

Gallagher, J.J. (1976). The sacred and profane uses of labeling. *Mental Retardation, 14*, 3-7.

Gorham, K.A., Des Jardins, C., Page, R., Pettis, E., & Scherber, B. (1976). Effect on parents. In N. Hobbs (ed.), *Issues in the classification of children, 2.* San Francisco, CA: Jossey-Bass.

Gottlieb, J., & Leyser, Y. (198). Facilitating the social mainstreaming of retarded children. *Exceptional Education Quarterly, 1* 57-69.

Hallahan, D.P., & Kauffman, J.M. (1982). *Exceptional children: Introduction to special education*. Englewood Cliffs, NJ: Prentice-Hall.

Hallahan, D. P., & Kauffman, J. M. (1997). Exceptional Learners. (7th ed.) Boston: Allyn & Bacon.

Harris, L., & Associates (1994). N.O.D./*Harris Survey of Americans with Disabilities*. New York, NY: Lou Harris and Associates, Inc.

Harry, B., Park, H., & Day, M. (1998). Friendships of many kinds: Valuing the choices of children and youth with disabilities. In L. Meyer, H. Park, M. Grenot-Scheyer, L. Schwartz, & B. Harry (Eds.), *Making Friends*. Baltimore, MD: Brookes.

Hawkins, B. (1993). Leisure participation and life satisfaction of older adults with mental retardation and Down's Syndrome. In E. Sutton, A.R. Factor, B.A. Hawkins, T. Heller, & G.B. Seltzer (eds.), *Older adults with developmental disabilities: Optimizing choice and change* (pp. 141-151). Toronto, Ontario: Paul H. Brookes.

Henderson, K.A., Bedini L.A., & Bialeschki, M.D. (1993). Feminism and the client-therapist relationship: Implications for therapeutic recreation. *Therapeutic Recreation Journal, 27* (1), 33-43.

Heyne, L.A., Schleien, S.J., & McAvoy, L.H. (1994). *Making friends; Using recreation activities to promote friendship between children with and without disabilities*. Minneapolis, MN: Publications Office, Institute on Community Integration.

Horna, J. (1994). *The study of leisure: An introduction*. Toronto, Ont.: Oxford University Press.

Hutchinson, P., & Lord, J. (1979). ***Recreation integration: Issues and alternatives in leisure services and community involvement.*** Ottawa, Ontario: Leisure ability Publications, Inc.

Kaplan, M. (1975). ***Leisure: Theory and policy***. New York, NY: Wiley.

Kely, J.R. (1996). ***Leisure: Third edition***. Englewood Cliffs, NJ: Prentice-Hall, Inc.

Kennedy, D., Smith R., & Austin, D. (1991). ***Special recreation: Opportunities for persons with disabilities***. Dubuque, IA: William C. Brown, Publishers.

Krotoski, D. Nosek, M. & Turk, M. (1996), ***Women with Physical Disabilities: Achieving and Maintaining Health and Well-Being***. Baltimore, MD: Brookes.

Labanowich, As. & Hjoessli, P. (1979). Module 2: Knowing the campers. In D.A. Vinton & E.M. Farley (Eds.), ***Camp staff training series***. Lexington, KY: University of Kentucky.

Lewis, V. (1987). ***Development and handicap***. New York, NY: Basil Blackwell.

MacMillan, D.L., Jones, R.L., & Aloia, G.F. (1974). The mentally retarded label: A theoretical analysis and review of research. ***American Journal of Mental Deficiency, 79***(3), 241-261.

Mactavish, J.B. (1994). ***Recreation in families that include children with developmental disabilities: Nature, benefits, and constraints***. Unpublished doctoral dissertation, University of Minnesota.

Mactavish, J., Schleien, S., & Tabourne, C. (1997). Patterns of family recreation in families that include children with a developmental disability. ***Journal of Leisure Research, 29***(1), 21-46.

Mahon, M.J., & Searle, M.S. (1993). Leisure education: its effect on older adults. ***Journal of Physical Education, Recreation, and Dance, 65***, 36-41.

Mahon, F., Mactavish, J. Mahon, M., & Searle, M. (1995) ***Older adults with mental disabilities: Exploring the meaning of independence***. Winnipeg, MB: University of Manitoba.

Mahon, M., Lutfiyya, Z., Mactavish, J., Rodrigue, M., Strain, L., & Studholme (1998). "Transitions: Building communities through social integration." The 7th Annual Conference on Developmental Disabilities, Winnipeg, MB, October, 1998.

Marozas, D.S., & May, D.C. (1988). ***Issues and practices in special education***. White Plinas, NY: Longman, Inc.

Mercer, J.R. (1970). Sociological perspectives on mild mental retardation. In H.C. Haywood (Ed.), ***Socio-cultural aspects of mental retardation***. New York, NY: Appleton-Century-Crofts.

Mitchell, L.K. (1985). ***Behavioral intervention in the sexual problems of mentally handicapped individuals: In residential and home settings***. Springfield, IL: Thomas.

National Easter Seal Society. (1994). ***Diversity and inclusion: Implications for Easter Seal Society.*** Chicago, IL : National Easter Seal Society.

Neulinger, J. (1981). ***The psychology of leisure*** (2nd ed.). Springfield, IL : Charles C. Thomas, Publisher.

Nosek, M., Turk, M., & Krotoski, D. (1996). Conclusions. In D. Krotoski, M. Nosek, & M. Turk (Eds.), ***Women with Physical Disabilities: Achieving and Maintaining Health and Well-Being.*** Baltimore, MD: Brookes.

Orthner, K.D., & Mancini, J.A. (1990). Leisure impacts on family interaction and cohesion. *Journal of Leisure Research, 22* (2), 125-137.

Pal, D. (1992). Catch 22 for unemployed disabled adults: Ontario March of Dimes survey. *Abilities*, 12, 52-53.

Rapoport, R., & Rapoport, R.N. (1975). *Leisure and the family life cycle*. Ondon: Routledge and Kegan Paul Limited.

Rapoport, R., & Rapoport, R.N. (1978). *Leisure and the family life cycle*. London: Routledge and Kegan Paul Limited.

Rosenthal, R., & Jacobsen, L. (1968). *Pygmalion in the classroom: Teacher expectation and pupils' intellectual development*. New York, NY: Holt, Rinehart, & Winston.

Schleien, S.J., Olson, K.D., Rodgers, N.C., & McLafferty, M.E. (1985). Integrating children with severe handicaps into recreation and physical education programs. *Journal of Park and Recreation Administration, 3*(1), 50-66.

Schleien, S.J. (1991). Severe multiple disabilities. In D.R.Austin, & M.E. Crawford (eds.), *Therapeutic recreation: An introduction*, 189-223.

Schleien, S., Ray, M.T., & Green, F.P. (1997). *Community recreation and people with disabilities*. Baltimore, MD: Paul H. Brookes.

Schleien, S.J., Ray, M.T., Soderman-Olson, M.L. & McMahon, K.T. (1987). Integrating children with moderate to severe cognitive deficits into a community museum program. *Education and Training in Mental Retardation, 22* (2), 112-120.

Statistics Canada (1991). Online. Internet, retrieved 24 January 1999. Available: HYPERLINK http://www.statcan.ca/english/freepub/92-125-GIE/html/act.htm

"Stereotyping is essential." (1999). Houghton Mifflin Company. Online. Internet, retrieved, 18 February 1999. Available: http://www.hmco.com/college/communication/ohair/ch03/sld0004.htm

Stodden, R.A. (1991, June). *Panel-focus on outcomes*. A paper presented at the Transition Project Directors' Sixth Annual Meeting, Washington, D.C.

Tam, S. F. (1998). Comparing the self-concepts of persons with and without physical disabilities. *The Journal of Psychology,* 132(1), pg. 78-86.

Wilhit, B., Keller, M.J., & Nicholson, L. (1991). Integrating older persons with developmental disabilities into community recreation: Theory to practice. *Activities, Adaptation & Aging, 15* (1-2), 111-129.

Witt, P.A., & Goodale, T.L. (1981). The relationships between barriers to leisure enjoyment and family stages. *Leisure Sciences, 4* (1), 29-49.

Woodward, J. R. (1999). "A disabled manisfesto." Online. Internet, retrieved February 27, 1999. Available: HYPERLINK http://www.fedupfeds.org/dismanifesto.htm

Wuerch, B.B., & Voeltz, L. M. (1982). *Longitudinal leisure skills for severely handicapped learners: The Ho'onanea curriculum component*. Baltimore, MD: Paul H. Brookes.

Ysseldyke, J.E., & Algozzine, B. (1982). *Critical issues in special education and remedial education*. Boston, MA: Houghton-Mifflin.

Related Websites

http://www.une.edu.au/eeo/talk.html#talk6
(Language and Disability)

http://www.soton.ac.uk/~psyweb/staffpages/rer/BJCPLABS.html
(An Analysis of Labels for People with Learning Disabilities)

http://www.mentalhealth.org.uk/ldchoice.htm
(The Choice Initiative: Working with People with Severe, Profound, and Multiple Learning Disabilities)

http://www.dpa.org.sg/DPA/publication/dpipub/winter96/dpi11.htm
(International Day of the Disabled Person — poverty)

http://web.syr.edu/~thechp/nrc.htm
(National Resource Center)

http://www.ncd.gov/publications/minority.htm
(Meeting the Unique Needs of Minorities with Disabilities: A report to the President and the Congress)

http://www.dinf.org/pres_com/pres-dd/intro.htm
(Disability and Diversity: New Leadership for a New Era)

http://www.ablelink.org/public/default.htm
(The Ability OnLine Support Netork)

http://www.nau.edu/~wst/access/disab/disabart.html
(Disability — Women, Gender, and Disability)

http://www.usc.edu/go/awd/RTC.html
(Rehabilitation Research and Training Center (RRTC) on Aging With a Disability)

http://www.chmc.org/departmt/sibsupp/
(The Sibling Support Project)

Chapter 8

People with Mental Retardation

Introduction

The condition of mental retardation[1] was for a long time considered an incurable disability that afforded the individual with little potential for growth and development, yet today people with mental retardation are seen as individuals with tremendous potential. Mental retardation is no longer viewed as an absolute trait but as a condition that can be improved with the right supports. Previously, a diagnosis of mental retardation was often determined by a single IQ test score. Now, mental retardation is diagnosed by looking at IQ *and* behavior.

Much of this shift in attitude has been due to research and innovative programs that have demonstrated significant gains by individuals with mental retardation in all life spaces, including academic settings, vocational/work placements, integrated living, and recreation. Much of what has been developed for such persons can be credited to a shift from a deficit approach to understanding the condition of mental retardation toward a learning potential orientation. In this chapter we will highlight some basic information related to mental retardation, including its definition, levels, prevalence, and etiology. Following this, within the section "Some Things You Might Want to Do," we highlight some suggestions for working with persons with mental retardation within a recreation setting. Finally, we discuss some implications for recreation and health and safety.

Some Things You Might Want To Know

In May of 1992, the American Association on Mental Retardation (AAMR) revised their 1983 definition of mental retardation. The new definition is a significant departure from the old:

> Mental retardation refers to substantial limitations in present functioning. It is characterized by significantly subaverage intellectual function-

> ing, existing concurrently with related limitations in two or more of the following applicable adaptive skill areas: communication, self-care, home living, social skills, community use, self-direction, health and safety, functional academics, leisure and work. Mental retardation manifests before age 18.

The new definition departs from the old in at least three ways:

1. The new definition refers to substantial limitations in only certain personal capabilities. These specific capabilities include cognitive, functional, and social abilities.
2. The necessity for disabilities to be identified in at least two adaptive skill areas for the diagnosis of mental retardation is probably the most significant departure from the old definition. In the 1983 definition, mental retardation was diagnosed solely on the basis of intellectual functioning.
3. The new definition clearly states that the disability must now be identified before page 18. In addition, it indicates that the disability may not be a lifelong condition. This addition underscores the emphasis placed on adaptive skills in the new definition. If an individual who has been identified with the condition mental retardation develops her adaptive skills to the point where two (adaptive skills) are no longer considered underdeveloped, in effect, she would no longer be considered to have mental retardation. This point clearly demonstrates the shift toward a learning potential orientation to persons with mental retardation (Auxter, Pyfer, & Huettig, 1993).

Given the focus on adaptive skills within the present definition, we must have some understanding of this term. According to Grossman (1983, p. 1) adaptive behavior refers to "the effectiveness or degree with which individuals meet the standards of personal independence and social responsibility expected for age and cultural group." Expected adaptive behavior varies with the age of the individual. Adaptive behavior is usually not measured directly. Instead, the individual's teachers, parents, and significant others are used as informants (McLoughlin & Lewis, 1990). Table 8.1 describes the cluster of skills expected at different age levels.

Levels of Mental Retardation

Prior to the introduction of the 1992 definition of mental retardation by the AAMR, mental retardation was described as having four levels: mild, moderate, severe, and profound. Each of the levels was based upon the intellectual functioning or IQ of the individual. The new classification system includes only two levels: mild and severe. In contrast, these two levels are based on the adaptive skills of the individual, suggesting that mental retardation is environmentally determined. Given this, then, IQ is only used in the first stage of diagnosis in the new definition.

In addition to adaptive skills, levels of functioning are also based on the levels of support required. The four levels of support described by Luckasson et al. (1992) include the following:

Table 8.1
Cluster of Adapted Skills Identified With Various Age Levels

Infancy and Early Childhood	1. Sensorimotor Skill development 2. Communication skills (including speech and language) 3. Self-help skills 4. Socialization (development of ability to interact with others)
Childhood and Early Adolescence	5. Application of basic academic skills in daily life activities 6. Application of appropriate reasoning and judgment in mastery of the environment 7. Social skills (participation in group activities and interpersonal relationships
Late Adolescence and Adult Life	8. Vocational and social responsibilities and performance.

(Adapted from Grossman, 1983)

1. **No support.** The person is either self-sufficient or can procure needed supports on his or her own.
2. **Minimal support.** The person needs intermittent help or supports in areas such as case management, transportation, home living, physical health, employment, and self-advocacy.
3. **Substantial/extensive support.** The person needs regular ongoing supports that includes instruction, assistance (such as attendant care), and/or supervision within a designated adaptive skill area.
4. **Pervasive/consistent support.** The person needs constant care on a 24-hour basis, which may include the maintenance of life-support function/systems.

Prevalence and Etiology

The prevalence of mental retardation in the population is generally estimated to be 2.5 % (Batshaw & Shapiro, 1997). This estimate is based on a statistical interpretation of intellectual functioning within the population. Estimates of the percentage of persons to have either mild or severe mental retardation based on the 1992 AAMR definition are not yet available. However, most persons with mental retardation fall within the range of mild mental retardation. Batshaw and Shapiro also estimate that the prevalence is about half of the predicted 2.5% (.8%-1.2%) if individuals who score low on IQ due to cultural or social disadvantage are removed. Also generally estimated (again based upon the old definition of mental retardation) is the incidence of severe mental retardation in developed countries at about 3 to 5 per 1000 births (Sherrill, 1993).

The etiology, or origin, of mental retardation is most typically described as either organic (known medical causes) or nonorganic (unknown or familial/environmental causes). We generally estimate that about 75% of known cases of mental retardation are nonorganic in nature (Zigler & Hodapp, 1986). What has been suggested, however, is that an increasing trend toward a higher occurrence of organic etiology is emerging as a result of alcohol and drug abuse and a higher occurrence of traumatic brain injury from such things as car accidents. Another way that the causes of mental retardation are often grouped is according to the onset of the disability. In this case, the causes are generally grouped into the following three categories: prenatal, perinatal, and postnatal. ***Peri-*** refers to the period between the 28th day following conception to the 28th week of pregnancy (Sherrill, 1998).

The biological etiologies identified by the Batshaw and Shapiro (1997) are as follows:

- Cromosomal (35%)
- Multiple congenital anomalies (16%)
- Early pregnancy problems (11%)
- Perinal insults (10%)
- Single-gene defect (10%)
- Postnatal brain damage (5%)
- Other (13%)

During the past decade, the issue of aging has gained prominence as it related to people with mental retardation. As with the general population, people with mental retardation are living longer (Sison & Cotton, 1989). With this increase in life expectancy, a number of health-related problems have come to the surface. One of the most notable areas of concern relates to people with Down syndrome. People with Down syndrome have higher rates of Alzheimer's disease. Although about 20 to 40 percent of people with Down syndrome exhibit the symptoms of dementia, autopsy's show that almost all older adults with Down syndrome show brain changes associated with Alzheimer's disease. There is also growing evidence that people with Down syndrome experience premature aging (Hawkins & Eklund, 1994). They are often in their mid to late 40s when symptoms of Alzheimer's disease first appear, compared to the late 60s for the nondisabled population.

Mental retardation usually results in a developmental disability. Since the terms are sometimes used interchangeably, they can cause confusion for parks and recreation practitioners. A ***developmental disability*** is defined as:

> A severe chronic disability of a person five years of age and older that (1) is attributable to a mental or a physical impairment or is a combination of mental and physical impairments; (2) is manifested before the

> person attains age 22; (3) is likely to continue indefinitely; (4) results in substantial functional limitations in three or more of the following areas of life activity: (a) self-care (b) receptive and expressive language, (c) learning, (d) mobility, (e) self-direction, (f) capacity for independent living, and (g) economic self-sufficiency; and (5) reflects the person's need for a combination and sequence of special, interdisciplinary, or generic care, treatment or other services that are of a lifelong or extended duration and are individually planned and coordinated. Developmental disabilities also apply to infants and young children from birth to age five, inclusive, who have substantial developmental delay or specific congenital or acquired conditions with a high probability of resulting in developmental disabilities if services are not provided (North Carolina Council on Developmental Disabilities (1993).

In addition to mental retardation, other disabling conditions such as cerebral palsy and head injuries that meet the above stated criteria are also considered developmental disabilities (North Carolina Council on Developmental Disabilities, 1993). It is important to note that the definition of developmental disability varies somewhat from state to state. Canada does not have an official definition of the term.

Recreation students and practitioners should take note that an IQ score may give a general idea about the intellectual level of a person, but it does not indicate that all people with the same score share specific characteristics or abilities. Intelligence test scores are only one part of the assessment process. The daily functioning of the individual within the environment is also considered. Ultimately, this is how we are al viewed—by what we do and how we function everyday. ***Mental retardation*** is defined as the interaction between the individual and his or her environment—meaning both have a role. Supports provided to an individual can improve how she functions (or even change the diagnosis of mental retardation) and can come from the environment or the individual.

The environment can change. Mechanical or technological devices or personal care assistance can improve an individual's functioning in one or more behavior skills. A change in the personal, educational, or work situation can improve functioning or learning new skills or coping mechanisms that can improve his level of functioning (The Arc of the U.S., 1993).

People with mental retardation may have problems in learning. They may learn at a slower rate and may have limited ability to comprehend abstract ideas. Many have socially appropriate behavior; however, some individuals may exhibit inappropriate or immature social interaction skills because of limited opportunities to learn such skills and restricted experiences in using them. Some people with mental retardation have problems in communication. Some may have a limited vocabulary, while others may be nonverbal and rely on sign language or on some form of a communication board for expression. However, most people with mental retardation can generally communicate without modification.

Some persons with mental retardation also have accompanying physical disabilities that may require support in some tasks. An important consideration is to decide whether support will be needed in an activity so that a person can participate. If so, be sure that you, a friend, volunteer, or family member understands the support needed and how to provide it. We discuss people with physical disabilities in another chapter. Some of the information in that chapter is applicable to persons with mental retardation who have associated physical disabilities.

Some Things You Might Want To Do

Throughout this text we have discussed the importance of focusing on the unique challenges and needs of the individual. At the same time, it is possible to learn from the past experiences of parents, professionals, and others regarding best practices for working with persons with mental retardation in the area of recreation and leisure. Following are some suggestions:

Focus on Abilities

It is important to determine and to concentrate on the abilities of each individual. Do not underestimate abilities and interests. Often, people with mental retardation have not met their unique potential because of a lack of expectations.

Make it Understandable

Break down directions into simple steps or basic concepts that can be learned sequentially. A number of resources exist that provide information on how best to task analyze recreation activities for persons with mental retardation (Schleien, Ray, & Green, 1997; Dattilo & Murphy, 1987). Directions may need to be repeated. Demonstrate, where possible, what is expected. Use hands-on learning techniques and visual aids. Be creative in the teaching methods you use for activities. Consider substituting color codes for numbers, using partners or team groupings rather than individual participation, etc.

Ensure Dignity

Speak to participants, regardless of the severity of disability, with respect and dignity. Do not talk "down" to the person. Often a person's ability to understand speech is more developed than his speaking vocabulary. Do not talk about a person in front of him. A speech problem or lack of speech does not indicate that a person cannot understand. If you think a person needs help, offer to assist, but wait until your offer of assistance is accepted. The person may prefer to do the activity by himself, even if it is not at the level you would do it.

Recognize Individual Constraints

Recognize that some people with mental retardation have real limitations. Do not lose your composure or patience if they are not able to comprehend or perform what you think is important. Consider other adaptations that will allow inclusion of a person with these limitations in the program or activity.

Facilitate Decision Making

Allow each individual a choice of activities in which she wishes to participate or wishes to learn. As we discussed in Chapter 3, Mahon (1994) has pointed out that decision making can occur on different levels for people with mental retardation. Mahon suggested that a hierarchy developed by Yates (1990) is instructive when attempting to facilitate decision making by persons with mental retardation. When working to facilitate increased decision making in people with mental retardation, we must go beyond the facilitation of simple choices. Whenever possible, we should work toward people making constructive decisions where they devise their own alternatives, weigh the consequences of each, and choose one that meets their needs.

Provide Feedback

Provide positive feedback for successful experiences. Be supportive and encouraging during a failure situation. Be specific when offering suggestions for improvement (i.e., demonstrate choking up on a bat). Do not give praise or positive feedback when it is not deserved. At the same time, do not bribe individuals for their attention and participation. A person with mental retardation may be eager to please you and gain approval. Do not take advantage of anyone's willingness to work and do favors for you.

Look to the Experts for Support

The parents, teachers, guardians, and friends of a person with mental retardation may be good sources of information about the person's abilities and background. Some persons with the mental retardation take medications or use special equipment. Do not be intimidated by this. If you work interdependently with the individual and members of his social support network, you will soon feel at ease with these new challenges.

Structure the Environment

Structure of activities is important. Some people with mental retardation have a difficult time focusing attention on a single topic or activity for lengthy periods. Provide a variety of activities—active and passive, easy and challenging. Allow plenty of time for learning and for completion of a task; repetition is important to learning. Allow opportunity for participants to independently try new skills, and provide some noncompetitive games and activities that emphasize group cooperation and group building. Try to avoid activities that eliminate participants from the game or action.

Set Clear Behavioral Expectations

Discuss the type of conduct expected and accepted for the situation or activity. Be consistent and firm when discipline is required. Treat the participant with mental retardation like all others in the group. Schleien and Ray (1988) provide a useful overview in their text of behavioral principles that can be used in a recreation environment. Those interested in working with people with mental retardation may want to take courses in behavioral and/or cognitive behavioral psychology to expand knowledge in this area.

Ensure Safety

Before beginning an activity, review safety rules with all participants. A person with mental retardation may not have the judgment to understand which situations are dangerous.

Implications for Recreation

Many people with mental retardation can easily participate in community recreation programs. Other people with mental retardation may need supervision in daily activities and may require increased attention and modifications in recreation environments. There is no prescribed list of activities to be offered for persons with mental retardation. They take part in a wide variety of activities. Some challenges that may be encountered when a person with mental retardation chooses to participate in a regular program include a slower performance speed, an inability to handle more than one instruction at a time, fluctuating rates of progress, and a resistance to changes in routine. Difficulties can be minimized by providing appropriate support and careful attention to skill teaching strategies. Extra time may b needed for the person with mental retardation to adjust to a new situation or to learn a new task. It may be useful for the person to be paired with a buddy or companion—someone (such as another participant) who can ensure that initial difficulties can be overcome, thus allowing the person with mental retardation to fully use her abilities.

You will need to get to know the individual with mental retardation as a person, and then you can provide support, assistance, and guidance, if required, in order for him to participate in recreation activities.

Health and Safety

Persons with mental retardation take part successfully in all types of sports, games, and other recreation activities. Most persons with mental retardation function independently in the community and require no special consideration regarding safety in recreation programs. Other individuals may have lower ability levels, and the degree of supervision required will depend on both the type of activity in which they choose to take part and their skill levels in that particular activity.

Down syndrome is a specific category of mental retardation caused by an extra chromosome. Individuals can often be identified by physical appearance—a broad round face, close-set slanted eyes, high cheekbones, and short fingers. Some people with Down syndrome have a condition called atlantoaxial instability, which is greater than normal mobility of the two upper cervical vertebrae. Those with the condition are exposed to possible serious injury if they forcibly flex the neck because the vertebrae may shift and thereby squeeze or sever the spinal cord.

If you are leading fitness, sports, or athletic programs that include an individual with Down syndrome, it is important that:

1. The individual be temporarily restricted from all activities placing stress on the neck (i.e., gymnastics, swimming, some exercises).
2. The person is examined for atlantoaxial instability by a physician knowledgeable of the condition (x-rays with views of the neck are required).
3. Anyone with the condition be permanently restricted from programs that put stress on the neck.

Conclusion

We have provided you with an overview of the condition of mental retardation. As you have come to understand, mental retardation is a developmental disability that has numerous causes. The onset of this disability can occur prior to birth, at birth, or following birth. Mental retardation may not be a lifelong condition. A significant addition to the new definition of mental retardation introduced by the American Association on Mental Retardation is that adaptive skills form the basis of a decision as to whether a person has the condition of mental retardation, and if so, to what degree of severity. This is a very significant change, as it moves away from using IQ as the sole determinant of this disability. As we discussed, significant advances have been made in the field of mental retardation regarding instructional practices that can help people to become very independent. In Section III, we will highlight some strategies such as leisure education, which can be used to facilitate leisure and life satisfaction for people with mental retardation.

Learning Activities

1. Discuss some challenges that might result in trying to integrate an adolescent with mental retardation into a community recreation activity such as a soccer league. How would you go about overcoming these challenges?

2. How could you go about including an adult with mental retardation in a weekly chess group?

3. Discuss in a group any contact you have had with people with mental retardation. What was your initial reaction to the individual(s)? What were the circumstance? What were other people's reactions?

4. How could the principle of normalization be applied to people with mental retardation to ensure dignity for all people? Is there any way the application of this principle might backfire? If so, how?

References

American Association on Mental Retardation. (1992) ***Mental retardation: Definition, classification, and systems of support.*** Washington, D.C.: Author.

Auxter, D., Pyfer, J., & Huettig, C. (1993). ***Adapted physical education and recreation***. St. Louis, MO: Mosby-Year Book, Inc.

Batshaw, M.L., & Perter, Y.M. (1987). ***Children with handicaps: A medical primer*** (2nd ed.). Baltimore, MD: Paul H. Brookes.

Batshaw, M.L. & Shapiro, B.K. (1997). "Mental retardation." In M.L. Batshaw (ed.), ***Children with Disabilities*** (4th ed.). Baltimore, MD: Paul H. Brookes.

Grossman, H.J., (ed.). (1983). ***Classification in mental retardation.*** Washington, D.C.: American Association on Mental Deficiency.

Hawkins, B.A., & Eklund, S.J. (1990). Planning processes and outcomes for an aging population with developmental disabilities. ***Mental Retardation,*** 28, 35-40.

Mahon, M.J. (1994). The use of self-control techniques to facilitate self-determination skills during leisure in adolescents with mild and moderate mental retardation. ***Therapeutic Recreation Journal, 28*** (2), 58-72.

McLoughlin, J.A., & Lewis, R.A. (1990). ***Assessing special students*** (3rd ed.). Columbus, OH: Merrell Publishing Company.

North Carolina Council on Developmental Disabilities. (1993). ***Fact Sheet.*** Raleigh, NC.

Schleien, S.J., & Ray, M.T. (1988). ***Community recreation and persons with a disability: Strategies for integration.*** Baltimore, MD: Paul H. Brookes.

Schleien, S., Ray, M.T., & Green, F.P. (1997). ***Community recreation and people with disabilities.*** Baltimore, MD: Paul H. Brookes.

Sherrill, C. (1993). ***Adapted physical activity, recreation, and sport*** (4th ed.). Madison, WI: Brown & Benchmark Publishers.

Sison, G. F. P., & Cotten, P. D. (1989). The elderly mentally retarded persons: Current perspectives and future directions. ***Journal of Applied Gerontology,*** 8, 151-167.

Yates, J.F. (1990), ***Judgment and decision making***. Englewood Cliffs, NJ: Prentice-Hall, Inc.

Zigler, W.G. & Hodap, R. (1986). ***Understanding mental retardation***. Cambridge, Eng.: Cambridge University Press.

NOTE: Significant portions of this chapter are adapted from Bullock, C.C., McCann, C.A. & Palmer, R.I. (1994). ***LIFE resources: The LIFE resources manual*** (2nd ed.). Published by the Center for Recreation and Disability Studies, Curriculum in Leisure Studies and Recreation Administration, University of North Carolina at Chapel Hill. The authors would also like to thank Carrier McCann for her significant contributions to this chapter.

Footnote

[1]The term mental retardation is commonly used in the United States. In Canada, the more commonly used terms are mental disability or intellectual disability. For consistency, mental retardation will be used throughout this text.

Other Sources of Information

Administration on Developmental Disabilities
Administration for Children and Families
U.S. Department of Health and Human Services
200 Independence Avenue, SW
Washington, DC 20201

http://www.acf.dhhs.gov/programs/add/

The Arc of the United States
500 East Border Street, Suite 300
Arlington, TX 76010
(817)261-6003 (Voice)
(817)277-3491 (FAX)
(817)277-0553 TDD
thearc@metronet.com (e-mail)

http://thearc.org/welcome.html

American Association on Mental Retardation (AAMR)
444 North Capitol Street, NW
Suite 846
Washington, D.C. 20001-1512
Telephone: (202) 387-1968 or (800) 424-3688
Fax: (202) 387-2193
e-mail: info@aamr.org

http://www.aamr.org

Related Websites

http://busboy.sped.ukans.edu/~music/resources/mr/mr.shtml
(Mental Retardation Resources)

http://www.icdi.wvu.edu/Others.htm#g6
(Resources on Mental/Learning Disability)

http://TheArc.org/welcome.html
(The ARC of the United States)

http://TheArc.org/misc/dislnkin.html#sources
(Additional Sources of Information Regarding Mental Retardation/Developmental Disability)

http://www.familyvillage.wisc.edu/lib_cdmr.htm
(Cognitive Disability/Mental Retardation)

http://www.libertynet.org/speaking/index.html
(Speaking for Ourselves)

http://serc.gws.uky.edu/www/resources/mr.html
(University of Kentucky—Mental Retardation Sites)

Chapter 9

People with Physical Disabilities

Introduction

In this chapter we will discuss a variety of physical disabilities that will provide you with some sense of the nature of physical disabilities. If you wish to learn more about specific physical disabilities, refer to "Other Sources of Information" at the end of this chapter. As we have discussed throughout this text, it is important to be aware of the abilities of the person and the level at which she is capable of functioning. Keep in mind that individuals with the same physical condition will differ in choice of activities and in the degree to which they can accomplish the skills associated with that activity. Many recreation leaders are uncomfortable with all of the technical information and medical jargon related to the specific impairments included within this disability class. In this chapter we have attempted to distill the large body of technical information related to physical disabilities into the most germane information for the recreation leader. As with the previous chapter, we will provide some basic information about a number of physical disabilities in the "Some Things You Might Want to Know" section, followed by some practical tips in the remaining sections.

Some Things You Might Want To Know

Thousands of people in the United States have some degree of physical disability. Physical disabilities may affect a person's coordination, mobility, balance, agility, strength, endurance, or a combination of all these capabilities. Because there is such a wide range of causes, definitions, and ranges of severity in considering physical disability, no recognized categorical system exists. Terms referring to physical conditions such as ***paraplegia, cerebral palsy, and muscular dystrophy*** are often used in an attempt to categorize a physical disability. However, such terms are not always helpful to the practitioner, since the individuals with the same condition differ greatly in their level of ability. In the following sections we briefly review information on the most prevalent types of physical disabilities.

Arthritis

The term arthritis includes more than 100 different diseases that cause inflammation of the joints, frequently resulting in pain, swelling, discoloration, and in more serious cases, loss of mobility and tissue and bone damage. The word arthritis is derived from two Greek roots, Arthro-, meaning joint, and -itis, meaning inflammation (Auxter, Pyfer, & Huettig, 1993). Arthritis limits daily activities for nearly 37 million Americans. It is the leading cause of industrial absenteeism and the second leading reason (after heart disease) for receiving disability benefits (Samples, 1990). Arthritis is neither infectious nor contagious.

Osteoarthritis is a disease of unknown origin that attacks weight-bearing joints such as the knees, hips, and ankles. The cartilage at the bone ends of the joint wears thin and fragments, making it more difficult for the joint to be moved. Although the condition may become worse in cold or wet weather, to a large extent it is predictable from day to day and changes occur over an extended period of time.

Rheumatoid arthritis is a chronic, systemic disease of unknown cause. It may not affect all joints, or it may affect different joints at different times. It is a progressive disease that may be characterized by a series of remissions, in which symptoms subside for a period of weeks to years, and exacerbations, in which symptoms become worse. In addition, the individual (more often females than males) may feel unwell, may tire easily, and may be anemic. Juvenile rheumatoid arthritis can affect children as young as age two.

Arthritic diseases are most often unpredictable; people with arthritis seldom know for sure when pain, stiffness, or deformities may occur. Arthritis is frequently an invisible disease, and this invisibility contributes to adverse social and psychological side effects encountered by many people with arthritis. Friends, coworkers, and the general public may often misperceive an individual with arthritis as faking the symptoms and severity, thinking he craves attention and lacks initiative.

Disabling effects arising from arthritis come in numerous varieties and combinations. Those with arthritis in the legs will find it difficult to walk any distance. Some, particularly those with arthritis in the hips, cannot climb a bus step or a flight of stairs. They often cannot reach their toes and may have difficulty rising from a low seat (including a toilet). Many will find an activity involving prolonged standing very difficult. Even so, only a very few will need a wheelchair, although this can become necessary either occasionally or permanently.

In instances of spinal arthritis (the degeneration of the lumbar discs) difficulty may be experienced in lifting heavy weights. Those with cervical spondylosis (another variation) may have renewed pain when carrying heavy loads, whereas those with arthritis of the shoulders will have problems with lifting and in reaching outwards and upwards. When the wrists and fingers are painful and swollen, they will experience difficulty in gripping small items, grasping articles, picking up heavy objects, and applying sustained pressure to small pieces of equipment (National Institute on Disability and Rehabilitation Research, 1993).

Cerebral Palsy

Cerebral palsy is commonly used term for a group of conditions characterized by an inability to fully control motor function.The condition may involve one or more limbs and is a result of nonprogressive brain damage at either the prenatal state or from shortly after birth. Other disabilities are often associated with the condition. It is difficult to establish incidence and prevalence rates for cerebral palsy because of the controversy over diagnostic criteria. However, it has been estimated that there are approximately 1.4 to 2.4 per 1000 live births (Pellegrino, 1997).There are three types of cerebral palsy. Each is briefly discussed.

1. *Spastic cerebral palsy* is the most common type of cerebral palsy. In this condition, one or more areas of the body may be involved, such as these involving posture, lying, sitting, standing, and walking. Poor hand function with sensory loss may also be involved in spastic cerebral palsy.Voluntary movement is present but is rather labored or jerky instead of smoothly coordinated. Speech, chewing, and swallowing may be difficult.There may also be retardation of growth in affected limbs.
2. *Dyskinetic cerebral palsy* is characterized by tonal abnormalities that involve the whole body. The muscle tone of the individual can change from hour to hour over the course of a day. Individuals most often will exhibit rigid muscle tone during their waking hours, and normal or decreased muscle tone when asleep. Involuntary movements are the most common characteristic of this form of cerebral palsy.
3. *Ataxic cerebral palsy* involves a disturbance of balance and sense of direction. Voluntary movements are present but may be clumsy or uncoordinated. Poor fine hand movements are evident as well. Nystagmus (eye jerking involuntarily) may occur.

Cerebral palsy takes many forms and no two people with this condition are precisely alike.The term mixed cerebral palsy is used when more than one type of motor pattern is present, and one pattern does not clearly predominate. Some are so mildly affected that they have no obvious disability. Others who are more seriously affected may have difficulty with walking, with manual manipulation, or with speech. Some even experience perceptual difficulties. Most people with cerebral palsy have average or above average intelligence.

Head Injury (Traumatic Brain Injury)

Brain injury often results from a trauma to the head and/or brain.Traumatic brain injury can result from a blow to the head, such as one that occurs in a motor vehicle crash. Other conditions can cause brain damage as well, including heart attacks, aneurysms, chemical and drug reactions, lack of oxygen to the brain, and others. In most cases, an injury sustained as a result of one for these causes will result in an increased need for support in the following areas: physical capacities (the way we move and manipulate things); behavioral and emotion capacities (the way we eat, tolerate, and feel); and cognitive capacities (the way we think and process information) (Golden, 1993).

A brain injury is different from many other disabilities because the onset of the injury can be traumatic and can occur suddenly. Brain damage can result in permanent, irreversible damage that can affect one's abilities to perform tasks that were once performed with ease. There is no cure for brain injury and prevention is the best option. Approximately two million head injuries occur per year, or approximately one every 15 seconds. Most occur in motor vehicle accidents, with young males (average age 25) composing the majority of this group (Golden, 1993).

Different areas of the brain are responsible for specific functions. When these different areas are damaged, a variety of disabilities may result. For example, the part of the brain that controls speech may be damaged, leading to communication problems, or the area that regulates movement may be damaged, leading to someone needing a wheelchair for mobility. However, not all people who have head injuries have speech problems or use wheelchairs. Each person is affected in a different way.

Depending upon which areas of the brain are damaged, head injury can produce losses in movement, sensation, communication, intellect, and memory. There is no such thing as a typical brain injury. The effect of brain damage and the extent of handicap varies from person to person. Difficulties with memory, judgment, movement, and inappropriate behavior may continue for several months or years or can last permanently.

Multiple Sclerosis

Multiple sclerosis (MS) is a chronic, sometimes progressive disease of the central nervous system (brain and spinal cord) that most often affects young adults. The onset of symptoms occurs most often between the ages of 20 and 40 years, with women affected twice as often as men. In approximately 50% of persons with multiple sclerosis, there are deficits in intellectual functioning, though this is often difficult to accurately assess because of the presence of depression and anxiety (National Institute on Disability and Rehabilitation Research, 1994).

Symptoms result from multiple areas of patchy scarring (sclerosis) of the insulation that surrounds nerves in the central nervous system. This scarring is comparable to the loss of insulating material around an electrical wire that interferes with proper transmission signals. Symptoms may vary from a mild alteration of sensation to paralysis of limbs and interference with speech, walking, and other basic functions.

Multiple sclerosis is variable and unpredictable. The majority of people with multiple sclerosis do not become severely disabled and continue to lead productive and satisfying lives. MS is not a fatal disease, and individuals can be expected to have normal or near-normal life expectancy. Multiple sclerosis is neither contagious nor hereditary, although there may be a familial predisposition.

Although a cure has not yet been found, many symptoms can be relieved. Treatment may take many forms, including medication for pain, physical therapy, diet control, and exercise. Foley, Millker, Traugott, LaRocca, Scheinberg, Bedell, &

Lennox (1988) have found that anxiety and distress can have a negative impact on the immune system of persons with multiple sclerosis, independent of the age of the person or the severity of the disability. Some people with multiple sclerosis use adaptive devices such as eating utensils, clothing, wheelchairs, and crutches. Others have catheters because of a lack of muscle control and an inability to void properly. In more serious cases, attention is to be given to minimizing secondary effects. For example, heavy physical effort or intense mental strain may make existing symptoms worse. In severe cases of multiple sclerosis, an individual may have poor physical coordination.

Muscular Dystrophy

The muscular dystrophies are a group of progressive diseases of voluntary muscles characterized primarily by weakness and fatigue. The heat and breathing muscles may also be involved, causing further problems. The most severe type is Duchenne muscular dystrophy (also known as childhood muscular dystrophy), which affects young boys, few of whom reach the third decade of life. There are, however, other childhood and several adult varieties of muscular dystrophy that may result in a person having mild to severe physical impairment (Davies, 1982).

Other varieties of muscular dystrophy include myotonic, limbgirdle, and facioscapulohumeral syndromes, among others. People with these disorders may have a normal life expectancy but, nonetheless, become severely disabled by middle life. The acioscapulohumeral type is uncommon and affects the facial muscles, causing the sufferer difficulty in closing his eyes and giving him a pouting appearance of the lips. (Other participants may need to be aware of this.) In cases that affect the arms, lifting is likely to be difficult. When legs are affected, individuals experience *foot-drop*, which causes individuals to catch their toes on the edge of carpets. The diseases cause physical limitations and generally do not involve mental impairment.

Depending on the type, muscular dystrophy may be either rapidly or slowly progressive. People with slowly progressive types may be employed and take part in community activities. The main difficulties experienced by individuals with less severe handicaps include lifting heavy objects, climbing stairs, getting out of a low chair, and in carrying out tasks requiring rapid movement. Those more severely affected use wheelchairs. Many people, even those with the most severe disabilities, retain some finger control and are thus able to operate light-touch equipment (e.g., computers, video games).

For many children, the inevitability of death carries a special set of challenges. Parents and families experience a great amount of stress and guilt. Since it is also very difficult for families not to overprotect their children, facilitating independence in children with muscular dystrophy is particularly challenging. Parents are also faced with the question of how long to keep their child in school. As a child's health deteriorates, keeping him in school becomes more difficult, yet withdrawing him may be perceived as giving up (Halliday, 1989). Leisure and recreation can play a vital role in the life of a child with muscular dystrophy, as it can add fun to a life often associated with the health care system.

Poliomyelitis

Poliomyelitis is an acute infection of the central nervous system. The infection (once known as infantile paralysis) is caused by a virus that enters the system through the nose or mouth. It attacks the nerves controlling muscles, resulting sometimes in paralysis or partial paralysis of one or more limbs. If the trunk and lower limbs are paralyzed, the person may need to use a wheelchair, but he may be able to walk with the aid of crutches. Polio attacks the nervous system and causes paralysis of limbs. It does not affect intellectual capacity. Polio can attack people of any age, particularly those who live or work overseas. In the United Sates and Canada, vaccination has eliminated new cases of the disease.

Probably about 300,000 people in the United States are disabled because of polio. The extent of their handicaps varies. Some have very minor handicaps, such as a weak finger, while others may need to use respirator equipment. Polio is a static disability that does not progress or grow worse; however, in recent years a returning of symptoms has affected some individuals. (See the next section on post polio syndrome.)

Post Polio Syndrome (Sequelae)

Post polio sequelae is thought to be caused by chronic overuse of undamaged muscles that are compensating for weak ones. The central factor is overloading of the anterior cells of the spinal cord that control the muscle movements. The polio virus attacks and destroys these cells. People with polio who have been able to lead fairly typical lives with work and exercise are discovering recurring symptoms of poliomyelitis and are having to deal with this on a psychological and a physical basis. Support groups are being developed to assist with the trauma of psychological readjustment, of having to "relearn" all over again, and not being self-sufficient. Recent statistics indicate that about 25% of the individuals with polio are thought to be affected from this syndrome. The symptoms include extreme fatigue, muscle weakness, debilitating joint pain, breathing difficulties, and intolerance of cold.

The situation is complicated by the fact that although there is a vaccine to prevent polio, a treatment has never been developed. Some doctors believe that these debilitating effects can be minimized or reversed by decreasing activity, using devices such as braces or wheelchairs, and following specifically tailored exercise programs. There is no evidence to indicate that post polio sequelae could lead to death.

Spina Bifada

Spina bifada is the most common form of neural tube defect (Liptak, 1997). It is a congenital deformity of the vertebrae in which some of the vetebral arches fail to close. About 80% of those born with the most severe forms of spina bifida also develop hydrocephalus. This condition occurs when the natural flow of cerebrospinal fluid within the brain is obstructed, and the resultant pressure within the brain causes severe or even fatal brain damage. However, since 1960, surgical treatment has been available in the form of the insertion of a plastic one-way valve called a shunt, which allows the fluid to drain away. A small number of people may have hydrocephalus without spina bifida, either as a congenital defect or as the results of a childhood illness.

Damage to the spinal cord or spinal nerves causes varying degrees of paralysis and lack of sensations below the level of damage. There may also be incontinence, but each individual should have worked out with her doctor the most suitable method of controlling it, so this will not likely affect recreation participation.

The effect of spina bifida on the individual can vary from mild difficulty with walking to severe physical disability. In addition, if hydrocephalus is also present, the individual may have limited intellectual capacity. In its mildest form (spina bifada occulta), where in the spinal cord and nerves are undamaged, spina bifida is unlikely to cause any handicap. In fact, many people born with spina bifida oculta are not even aware of it, and the only outward sign of it may be a dimple in the skin and perhaps a tuft of hair along the spinal column.

In people born with more severe forms of spina bifida (meningocele and myelomeningocele), some of the nerves surrounding the spinal cord, and sometimes the cord itself, are affected. This can limited the ability to walk, and persons affected by these forms of spina bifida may need a cane or crutches to compensate for the weak muscle in their legs. Many people born with myelomeningocele will need to use a wheelchair in adult life, either occasionally or permanently. Also, because of the spinal abnormality, a person with spina bifida may only grow to around 4' 9" in height.

In spite of the success of surgical techniques in controlling hydrocephalus, some people may still sustain brain damage that can limit intellectual abilities or give rise to epilepsy. Hydrocephalus may also affect coordinator and fine finger movement.

Spinal Cord Injuries

When the spinal cord (i.e., the bundle of nerves that passes down the spine) is damaged through accident or disease, the individual may become paralyzed below the level of injury. Below this level, the person either has no feeling or voluntarily function or, at least, has somewhat impaired sensations and function. The amount of sensations and function depends upon the completeness of the injury. Spinal cord injuries can range from minor bruises to actual severs.

The extent of the paralysis depends on where the spinal cord is injured. Paraplegia is a condition in which the lower extremities and/or lower torso are paralyzed from injury to the sacral, lumbar, and thoracic areas of the spine (see Figure 9.1). Injury to the thoracic area often results in the need for a wheelchair, while those to the sacral or lumbar parts of the spine may result in some loss of sensation in the legs, so that leg braces may be required for mobility. Quadriplegia, which causes the greatest amount of disability, additionally involves paralysis of the arms and/or hands, which results from an injury to the cervical area in the neck. Individuals with injury to the upper region (C2-4) can control some neck muscles but will likely require assistance with many daily living skills; an injury to C5-7 often means that the person is quite capable of living independently. A spinal cord injury causes a loss of sensation and/or function because messages sent by the brain are blocked or interrupted at the injury site as they travel down the spinal cord. In a spinal cord injury, the brain is unaffected, thus cognitive skills are unaffected.

Figure 9.1
Spinal Section

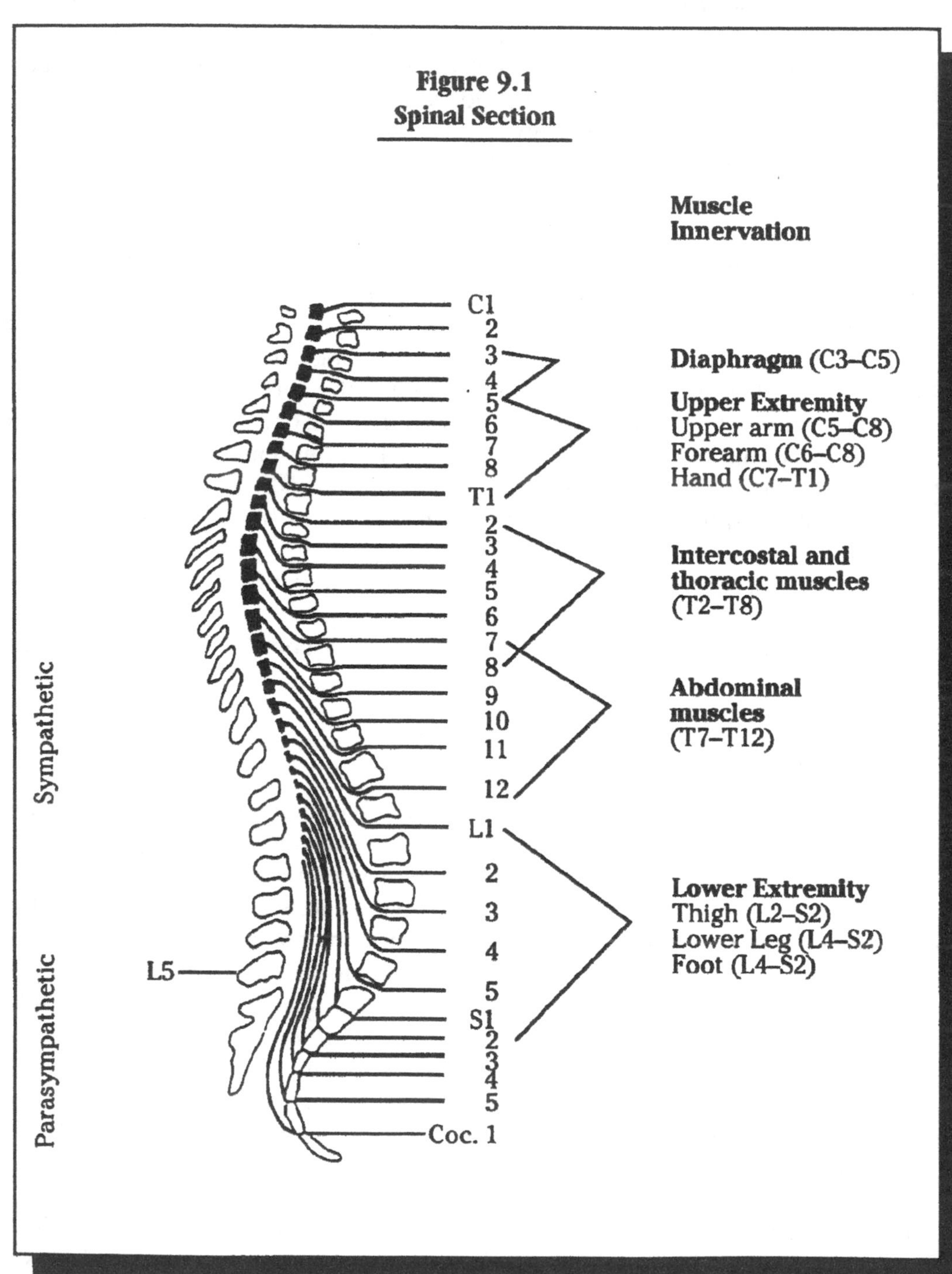

Most people with spinal cord injuries use wheelchairs for mobility. The most important thing to remember is that a person who uses a wheelchair is just like everyone else! A person with a spinal cord injury faces more difficulties in activities such as dressing, bathing, and eating than does a nondisabled person. However, with adaptive equipment and personal care assistance, these obstacles can be overcome. For a person with a spinal cord injury, the disability itself is often not a handicap; barriers such as stairs, inaccessible restrooms, and narrow doorways are the handicaps, making an activity difficult or even impossible. The use of a wheelchair imposes some challenges, but these can be lessened by providing access to and around the recreation area.

Some Things You Might Want To Do

Ask Before Helping

If you think a person may need help, offer assistance and then wait for a reply. If a person with a physical disability falls, wait for the person to indicate whether or not help is required. If assistance is required, the person can tell you what method of help is needed. Do not automatically assume that a person in a wheelchair needs you to drive it, but if the person wants assistance, provide it.

Consult the Experts

People with disabilities are the most knowledgeable of their disability. In addition, professionals working with and providing services to people with disabilities often are quite knowledgeable of disabling conditions. To determine potential programs, activities, and ideas for adaptation, ask the experts—the people with the disabilities. Following this, talk to the professionals who are familiar with the needs of people with disabilities.

Exercise Patience

Be patient without being overprotective or overindulgent. A person may not move quickly but may want to complete a project or activity independently. Some people with physical disabilities may have problems with speech. It may be necessary to ask them to repeat a word or phrase until you become familiar with their speaking style.

Respect Individual Differences

Crutches, walkers, prosthetic devices (artificial limbs), and wheelchairs are necessary accessories for some people. Do not take them away from participants unless they ask. Taking away such assistive devices can leave a person stranded. Help to sensitize others to the fact that people with disabilities consider such accessories to be part of who they are as people.

Do Not Assume

Allow participants to take part in all activities that you offer to the group. Let these individuals make their own decisions regarding what they can and cannot do. Do not impose your assumptions or anticipated limitations on the capabilities or interests of someone else. The best rule of thumb is to assume inclusion until told otherwise by the person with a disability.

Be Aware of Skills and Challenges

Make sure that programs offer opportunities for success and new experiences and are a challenge to all participants. Be creative and ready to try new games or old games with a different twist. Your role is to help people with disabilities identify activities and experiences that provide the best match between skill and challenge.

Adapt When Necessary

Ask people with physical disabilities about special equipment, aids, or techniques they may use to assist them in daily living that may be useful in the recreation environment. Provide adaptive equipment when necessary to include an individual with a physical disability in an activity. Recreators or people with disabilities can modify existing equipment or can obtain commercially available adaptive equipment. Refer to the sections on technology in Chapters 13 or 17 for further discussion on this topic.

Reduce Impact of Barriers

Minimize environmental barriers that limit functioning. A hard, firm surface is usually easier than grass or soft dirt for maneuvering a wheelchair. Plan ahead for field trips in order to assess a facility for potential barriers, using a person with a physical disability or a professional who is knowledgeable as the evaluator.

Some Things You Might Need To Know

Personal Aids and Devices

Individuals with physical disabilities usually depend on personal aids and devices to increase their functional abilities. These aids and devices can range from those easily available, such as a standard wheelchair, to the very personalized types of aid, such as a form-fitted hand strap to assist in holding a pen. Typically, aids and devices become as personal to the individual as clothes do to some other people. Consequently, any handling or assistance concerning aids should be done carefully and considerately.

Mobility aids (wheelchairs, crutches, walkers, and braces) are the most visible and easily recognized devices. Aids to body function include prostheses (artificial limbs), ileostomy or colostomy bags (body waste collection devices), and breathing assistance devices. In most situations, the individual has mastered the use and care of the aid or device and will not need assistance. If assistance is required, the individual can usually direct the correct kind and level of help needed. It is not only entirely proper, but usually essential to ask for guidance when assisting an individual with his aid or device. For children, be sure to ask a parent or guardian about correct assistance with the device.

It is also important to ask if there are any implications for recreation activity associated with the device, such as where and when the device can or cannot be used, under what conditions the device might be problematic to the owner or to others, special storage considerations, etc. Following are some common do's and do not's in the use of wheelchairs.

Wheelchairs

There are right and wrong ways to handle a wheelchair. This checklist of actions to do and not to do may be helpful to someone who is asked for assistance by a person who used a wheelchair.

Folding a Wheelchair

To fold most wheelchairs, remove the cushions first and pull upward on the seat fabric at the center front and back. Do not lift the chair by the armrests—they will probably come right out in your hands.

Opening a Wheelchair

Keep fingers turned toward the middle of the seat and press with the heels of the hand on the two sides of the seat. Do not put fingers between the chair frame and the seat, they will be crushed.

Putting a Wheelchair Into a Car Trunk

Position the folded wheelchair close to and parallel with the trunk. Do not bend your back, keep it straight and bend knees and hips. Grasp struts of chair, not the wheels, armrests or movable parts. Keep one hand well forward, the other well back. Lift the chair vertically by straightening your legs. Balance the chair on the edge of a trunk. With the full weight being taken by the wheels resting on the trunk edge, tip the chair up. When it is almost horizontal, slide it into the trunk.

Pushing a Wheelchair Down a Curb

Place your foot on the tipping lever. Take firm hold of the handgrips, then tip the chair backwards. Gently lower the chair down the curb. You must now take some of the weight, so be sure to arch your back and bend your knees. Also important is that both rear wheels hit the ground at the same time. Another method is to turn the back wheels to ground level, then lower the front wheels.

Pushing a Wheelchair Up a Curb

Place foot on tipping lever and lift the chair off its front wheels, moving them forward into the curb. Gauge the distance to the curb carefully; avoid forcing the front wheels against any ridge or unevenness. A second person can help to lift the chair by grasping one handle of the wheelchair and the bar below the armrest. Movements should be made together on an agreed signal. Sometimes the wheelchair passenger can help to control the chair by steadying the rear wheels.

Carrying a Wheelchair Up Stairs

Although a child or a very light adult with a disability can be lifted by one helper, two helpers are usually required. Position the wheelchair squarely at the foot of the stairs with its back toward the steps. Tip the chair backward. Take a firm grip, place one foot up on the first step, throw the same shoulder slightly backward and pull the chair up onto the first step. A second helper stands in front to steady and lift the chair when it rises upward over the steps, holding the chair frame below the armrests. Repeat for the second step. Make sure you are solidly balanced, throw your weight back, and pull up again.

Carrying a Wheelchair Down Stairs

Do not try to take a wheelchair down a flight of stairs unless you are absolutely sure you can hold the weight of the person in it and maintain full control. Grasp handgrips, slowly move the chair forward, control the forward and downward movement against the step's edge. Use your body as a brake at the top of the step. Do not wait until the chair drops to do so. Stop for a rest between steps. Use another assistant, perhaps a passerby, whenever available. The second assistant stands below in front, holds the chair frame under the armrests, slowing and steadying the descent.

Implications for Recreation

Remember that a physical disability may have no bearing on a person's ability to participate in a specific recreation program. For example, using a cane for assistance in walking or using a wheelchair will have little or no impact on taking part in a photography class. Mobility is the major limitation for many people with physical disabilities. Increasing the number of people on a team or shortening boundaries in a game can result in successful participation by such individuals. For example, in volleyball, nine-person teams, rather than six, could be used to reduce the amount of court space that each player must cover.

Low strength level is another limitation for some people with physical disabilities. Adaptive equipment allows the individual to take part in many sports and games. For example, bowling ramps and handle-grip bowling balls can allow a person to participate in a bowling league or to bowl recreationally. Another example is a spring-loaded billiard cue that can be used by a person with limited upper arm strength.

In considering how a potential participant can take part in a particular activity, you must look at the physical requirements of the activity and the abilities of the person. Often, the person can take part without adaptation, but for some, adaptation may be necessary. The one primary authoritative source for information on the recreation implications of a particular person's specific disability is the person himself. Because of the individual nature of a physical disability, you will not be able to specifically outline its effects upon a person's recreation participation. An activity suitable for one person may not necessarily be suitable for another.

Some people with physical disabilities will have full movement of hands and arms so there is little need for any special aids. Some will use a wheelchair for moving, and they may need adjustments to the height of activity areas, table games, etc. People who lack sensation in their lower limbs may require some protection in some activities, such as wearing socks when swimming.

The major barrier to recreation participation for a person who uses a wheelchair is often in inaccessibility of facilities. Adequate means of access is of paramount importance if the individual is to realize his full recreation potential. For example, steps may need to be replaced by ramps, door may need to be widened, and perhaps an elevator may need to be provided to allow a wheelchair user to move from one floor to another. A toilet stall may need to be modified to afford access for a wheelchair and privacy for the individual. Also, it will be important to ensure that activity rooms, theaters, ball parks, etc. are accessible, and that features such as telephones and water fountains are usable.

Adaptive techniques have been developed for teaching persons with physical disabilities the skills for sports such as horseback riding, skiing, and swimming. Instructors who are teaching these activities to classes that include people with physical disabilities may want to gather resources that provide information on adaptive techniques.

Adaptive equipment exists for many sports and arts and crafts activities. Card holders, card shufflers, utensils, and tools with built up handles are forms of adapted equipment that can be useful. People with physical disabilities can offer suggestions for adapting activities and/or equipment. Some sports teams exist specifically for people who use wheelchairs. Wheelchair basketball, wheelchair football, and other sports are played with minor modifications of the rules.

Conclusion

In this chapter we have reviewed a number of disabling conditions that fall under the broad heading of physical disabilities. By now, you should understand that the term physical disabilities does not provide the level of description necessary for understanding the individual needs of a person with cerebral palsy or spina bifida. What should also be evident is that even terms like cerebral palsy refer to a diverse group of disabling conditions with some basic similarities. Given this, it is clear that we must try to understand disability at the level of the person. We must go beyond knowing that a person has cerebral palsy and learn about the specific challenges he faces with his specific disability. Nonetheless, it is useful to now have a basic starting point: a general knowledge about physical disabilities. In addition, the information we presented in the sections "Some Things You May Want to Do" and "Some Things You Might Need To Know" will serve as a starting point for understanding the needs of people with physical disabilities. We sign off this chapter with the reminder not to assume; always ask the person with the disability.

Learning Activities

1. Choose one specific physical disability (e.g. muscular dystrophy). Discuss the considerations for including a person with your selected disability in a community recreation program of your choice.
2. Discuss how the recreation needs of a person with a spinal cord injury might change from childhood to adulthood.
3. Discuss how the concept of social role valorization could be applied when developing recreation programs that would include people with physical disabilities.
4. Try to identify areas where advances in technology would serve to assist people with physical disabilities and where it might present barriers.

References

Auxter, D., Pyfer, J., & Huettig, C. (1993). ***Adapted physical education and recreation.*** St. Louis, MO: Mosby-Year Book, Inc.

Davies, B. (1982). ***The disabled child and adult.*** London: Bailliere Tindall.

Foley, F., Millker, A., Traugott, U., LaRocca, N., Scheinberg, L., Bedell, J., & Lennox, S. (1988). ***Psychoimmunological dysregulation in multiple sclerosis.*** Psychosomatics, 29 (4), 398-403.

Golden, T.P. (1993). ***Managing and working effectively with employees who have sustained a brain injury.*** Ithaca, NY: Program on Employment and Disability at Cornell University.

Halliday, P. (1989). ***Special needs in ordinary schools: Children with physical disabilities.*** London: Cassell.

National Institute on Disability and Rehabilitation Research (1993). ***Arthritis: An overview of research findings.*** Washington, D.C.: Author, Department of Education.

National Institute on Disability and Rehabilitation Research (1994). ***Multiple sclerosis research update.*** Washington, D.C.: Author, Department of Education.

Samples, P. (1990). Exercise encouraged for people with arthritis. ***The Physician and Sports Medicine, 18*** (1), 122-127.

Thompson, G., Rubin, I., & Bilenker, R. (Eds). (1983). ***Comprehensive management of cerebral palsy.*** New York, NY: Grune & Stratton.

NOTE: Significant portions of this chapter are adapted from Bullock, C.C, McCann, C.A., & Palmer, R.I. (1994). LIFE resources: The LIFE resources manual (2nd ed.). Published by the Center for Recreation and Disability Studies, Curriculum in Leisure Studies and Recreation Administration, University of North Carolina at Chapel Hill. The authors would also like to thank Carrie McCann for her significant contributions to this chapter.

Other Sources of Information

Arthritis

Arthritis Foundation, National Office
1330 West Peachtree Street
Atlanta, Georgia 30309
(404)872-7100.
http://www.arthritis.org/

Missouri Arthritis Rehabilitation, Research Training Center
http://www.hsc.missouri.edu/~arthritis/marrtctp.html

The McCaig Centre for Joint Injury and Arthritis Research
The University of Calgary
3330 Hospital Drive N.W.
Calgary, Alberta T2N 4N1
(403) 220-8666.
http://www.ucalgary.ca/UofC/faculties/MED/Surgery/mccaig_hs.html

National Arthritis and Musculoskeletal
and Skin Diseases Information Clearing House
http://www.nih.gov/niams/

The Arthritis Society of Canada National Office
393 University Avenue, Suite 1700
Toronto, ON M5G 1E6
416-979-7228
Fax: 416-979-8366
http://www.arthritis.ca/home.html

Cerebral Palsy

United Cerebral Palsy Association
1660 L Street, NW, Suite 700
Washington, DC 20036
1-800-872-5827
Fax: 1-800-776-0414
E-mail:ucpnatl@ucpa.org
http://www.ucpa.org/

National Easter Seal Society
http://www.seals.com/

Cerebral Palsy Association of British Columbia
15-3683 East Hastings Street
Vancouver, B.C. V5K 4Z7
(604) 205-9455
http://www.bccerebralpalsy.com/index.htm

Head Injury

The Brain Injury Association Inc.
105 North Alfred Street
Alexandria, VA 22314
703-236-6000
Fax: 703-236-6001.
http://www.biausa.org/

THINK FIRST Foundation
22 S. Washington Street
Park Ridge, IL 60068
http://www.thinkfirst.org/

National Institute of Neurological Disorders and Stroke
National Institutes of Health
Bethesda, MD 20892
http://www.ninds.nih.gov/

Brain Injury Rehabilitation Clinic
University of Washington
Department of Rehabilitation Medicine
Box 356490
Seattle, WA 98195-6490
206-543-7374
http://weber.u.washington.edu/~rehab/bi/index.html

Journal of Cognitive Rehabilitation
http://www.neuroscience.cnter.com/nsp/default.htm

Multiple Sclerosis

The American National Red Cross
http://www.redcross.org/donate/donate-now.html

The National Multiple Sclerosis Society
http://www.nmss.org/

The Amyotophic Lateral Sclerosis Association, National Office
21021 Ventura Blvd., Suite #321
Woodland Hills, CA 91364
Patients: 800-782-4747
All Others: 818-340-7500
alsinfo@alsa-national.org
http://www.alsa.org/

Multiple Sclerosis Association of America
National Headquarters
706 Haddonfield Road
Cherry Hill, NJ 08002
1-800 LEARN MS
Fax: 1-609-661-9797
http://www.msaa.com/

Multiple Sclerosis Foundation, Inc.
Cliff Orer, Program Services Administrator
Kitty Burofsky, Program Services Administrator
6350 North Andrews Avenue
Fort Lauderdale, FL 33309
(800) 441-7055
(954) 776-6805
FAX: (954) 938-8708
http://www.msfacts.org/

Muscular Dystrophy

Muscular Dystrophy Association
MDA Headquarters
3300 East Sunrise Drive
Tucson, AZ 85718-3208
(520) 529-2000
(800) 572-1717
FAX: (520) 529-5300
http://www.mdausa.org

Research and Training Center on Progressive Neuromuscular
Department of Physical Medicine and Rehabilitation
UC DAVIS, CA 95616-8655
(530) 752-2903
http://disability.ucdavis.edu/

Poliomyelitis

Sister Kenny Institute
800 East 28th Street
Minneapolis, MN 55407
(612) 863-4400
http://www.sisterkennyinstitute.com/

Post Polio Syndrome (Sequelae)

The Post-Polio Task Force Information Center
http://www.post-polio.org/

Gazette International Networking Institute
4207 Lindell Blvd., #110
Saint Louis, MO 63108-2915
314-534-0475
Fax: 314-534-5070
E-mail: gini_intl@msn.com

Spina Bifida

Spina Bifida Association of America
4590 MacArthur Boulevard, NW, Suite 250
Washington, DC 20007-4226
(800) 621-3141
(202) 944-3285
Fax: (202) 944-3295

National Easter Seal Society
230 West Monroe Street, Suite 1800
Chicago, IL 60606
(800) 221-6827
(312) 726-4258
Fax: (312) 726-1494
http://www.easter-seals.org/

Spinal Cord Injuries

American Paralysis Association
500 Morris Avenue
Springfield, NJ 07081
(800) 225-0292
(973) 379-2690
Fax: (973) 912-9433
Paralysis@aol.com
http://www.apacure.org

American Paralysis Association-Spinal Cord Injury Hotline
2200 Kernan Dr.
Baltimore MD, 21202
(800) 526-2456

Rehabilitation Research & Training Center
on Secondary Conditions of Spinal Cord Injury
1717 6th Avenue South
Birmingham, AL 35233-7330
205-934-3334
TDD: 205-934-4642
FAX: 205-975-4691
http://www.sci.rehabm.uab.edu/docs/rrtchome.htm

National Spinal Cord Injury Association
8300 Colesville Road, Suite 551
Silver Spring, MD 20910
(800) 962-9629
(301) 588-6959
Fax: (301) 588-9414
mailto:nscia2@aol.com
http://www.spinalcord.org/

Sports Organizations By and For People with Disabilities
http://etcs.ext.missouri.edu:70/info/maa/sports.html

Paralyzed Veterans of America
801 18th Street, NW
Washington, DC 20006
(800) 424-8200
(202) 872-1300
http://www.pva.org/

WHEELCHAIR SPORTS, USA,
3595 E. Fountain Blvd., Suite L-1
Colorado Springs, Colorado 80910—USA
719-574-1150
Fax: 719-574-9840
E-mail: wsusa@aol.com
http://www.wsusa.org/directry.htm

Mainstream Magazine
http://www.mainstream-mag.com/

Related Websites

http://www.arthritis.org/
(Arthritis Foundation)

http://www-hsl.mcmaster.ca/tomflem/cp.html
(Illness Health Care Information Resources — Cerebral Palsy)

http://curry.edschool.virginia.edu/go/specialed/categories/tbi.html
(Office of Special Education — Traumatic Brain Injury)

http://aspin.asu.edu/msnews/indexa.htm
(International Multiple Sclerosis Support Foundation)

http://www.mdac.ca/
(Muscular Dystrophy Association of Canada)

http://www.santel.lu/SANTEL/diseases/polio.html
(Poliomyelitis)

http://www.eskimo.com/~dempt/polio.html
(Polio Survivors' Page — Polio and Post-Polio Resources)

http://www.spinabifida.net/
(SpinaBifida.Net)

http://www.spinalcord.org/
(The National Spinal Cord Injury Association's Spinal Cord.Org)

Chapter 10

People with Visual Impairments

Introduction

Historically, people with visual impairments have been identified by a confusing array of terms—***blind, legally blind, visually impaired, partially blind, and partially sighted.*** To add to the confusion, although blindness is one of the most well-known disabilities, people rarely realize that only a small percentage of the approximately one half-million people in the United States who are legally blind have absolutely no vision. The term legal blindness was established in 1932 and is still quite commonly used by government and other agencies to determine eligibility for services (National Institute on Disability and Rehabilitation Research, 1994). The remaining individuals have some visual acuity varying from ability to read print (although the field of vision may be restricted) to the ability to just distinguish light from dark. Individuals who have some limits in terms of visual acuity, but who are not classified as legally blind, are most often described as having a visual impairment. As you will recognize, however, millions of people in North America have some level of visual impairment that results in the need for glasses or contact lenses, but these same people would never describe themselves as having a visual impairment. In this chapter we will present information on the levels of visual impairment as well as on some of the more common types and causes. Following this, we provide tips that will ensure that your first and/or future encounter(s) with people with visual impairments is positive.

Some Things You Might Want To Know

The quality of vision, and therefore visual impairment, is most often referred to in terms of acuity (clearness) and field (the angle of vision). It is important to remember, however, that there are visual impairments that affect vision in ways that are not indicated by measurements of these two characteristics, such as difficulty in the perception of colors and extreme sensitivity or insensitivity to light.

The most common way of referring to the quality of vision is in terms of the 20/20 method, which is used to measure the ***visual acuity*** of a single eye. The term 20/20 vision means the ability to see at 20 feet what a person with perfect vision can see at 20 feet. Another level of visual capability is the ***field of vision***. This is the diameter, in degrees, of the arc within which a person has perceptive ability when looking straight ahead. A person with perfect vision can perceive things about 90 degrees in all directions while looking straight ahead, making a visual field about 180 degrees in diameter. People with ***tunnel vision***, the result of several visual impairments, can see only straight ahead and not to the sides. They have no peripheral vision, only central vision. Some people are just the opposite. They can see to the sides but not straight ahead. They have no central vision, only peripheral vision (Hernigan, 1992).

A person who is ***legally blind*** is one whose vision in the better eye, even with glasses or contact lenses, is no better than 20/200 or whose visual field has a maximum diameter of 20 degrees. A person who is ***totally blind*** has complete loss of vision and light perception. People with this level of blindness are actually a small minority of people with visual impairments, even of those people classified as legally blind. Most of such people retain some measure of shape and/or length perception capability. Recently, the term low vision has gained wide acceptance. According to the National Institute on Disability and Rehabilitation Research (1994, p. 1):

> Low vision is a general term that describes a serious loss of vision which may be hereditary and whose onset may be congenital or adventitious. The condition may results from genetic causes, from eye disease or accidents, or it may result from health-related conditions commonly associated with the aging process...By definition, a person with low vision cannot be adequately corrected medically, surgically, or with conventional spectacles or contact lenses.

Blindness can be caused by diseases, aging, or accident; however, the most predominant cause is aging. Approximately 1.5 million people in the United States are classified as having some form of visual impairment (Jernigan, 1992). Each year about 50,000 more people become blind. Using the estimate of 1.5 million people in the United States having visual impairments, researchers have approximated that 700,000 of them are 65 years of age or older (Chiang, Bassie, Javitt, 1991). Among those of working age, the most common causes are diabetes and accidents. It is important to realize that blindness or partial vision does not imply the presence of any other physical, intellectual, or psychological disability.

There are many types of visual impairments. Some of the more common ones are cataracts, glaucoma, retinitis pigmentosa, diabetic retinopathy, and retrolental fibroplasia. Each is briefly described:

1. **Cataracts** are a primary cause of blindness, especially for older people. The normally clear lens in the eye becomes milky or cloudy because of some disturbance to the nutrition of the lens, most commonly caused by a lack of oxygen.

Cataracts can be removed easily through surgery, providing good vision after the operation for most people.

2. **Glaucoma** is a condition that often results in permanent blindness. More fluid enters or is formed in the eyeball than can escape through the canal that ordinarily removes it, causing increased pressure inside the eyeball. A simple test can detect glaucoma, which can usually be controlled through medication in the form of eye drops. If not controlled, glaucoma can result in a tiny spot of vision in the immediate center and eventually total blindness.
3. **Retinitis pigmentosa** is a hereditary condition in which there is dystrophy (or wasting) of the rod-shaped cells in the retina. This results in a small central area of vision (tunnel vision) and sometimes total blindness.
4. **Diabetic retinopathy** is one of the more common causes of visual impairment and total blindness. People with diabetes may undergo vascular changes that cause hemorrhaging in the retina. Quite often the blood reabsorbs and fairly good vision returns for a long period of time. Depending on the condition, blindness may come on suddenly and be permanent.
5. **Retrolental fibroplasia** is a condition that causes blindness in newborn infants. The disorder, which is caused by oxygen poisoning, results in spasms of the retinal vessels. Both eyes are affected, and it may produce complete or nearly complete blindness. The condition has been attributed to the use of a high concentration of oxygen in incubators of premature babies.

People with visual impairments are able to obtain varying amounts of visual information about their environment. However, it is important to realize that while vision provides people with a great deal of information about their environment, it is not the only source of information. People with visual impairments have usually learned to rely on other senses to fill in the gap created by their restricted ability to obtain visual information. Smell, touch, hearing, and the perception of movement all become more important sensory channels. Some people have adapted to the loss or unreliability of one information source by relying more heavily on others. This increased reliance often results not in an actual physical change in the acuity of other senses but in an enhancement of them. Such enhancement is likely the effect of the increased use of, and attendance to, senses that ordinarily occupy a secondary position in information gathering. Contrary to common belief, blindness does not give a person magical hearing or an exceptional memory.

Many people who are blind have received mobility training and are able to move around with ease. Some pursue recreation activities that require considerable outdoor mobility. Clerical jobs, even if reading is required, can be done by people who are blind with the use of special equipment such as closed-circuit television reading aids and Optacons (Optile to TACtile CONvertorsS), which transpose visual images such as print into tactile "images" that a person can feel. It is very unusual for adaptations to be required either to the furniture or to the premises where a person who is blind is to participate. However, it is helpful if visual warnings and information signs are supplemented with audio or tactile signs.

This increased reliance on nonvisual information gathering is a key element in making activities accessible to a person who has impaired vision. Adapting activities for people with visual impairments may mean taking advantage of the adaptations they have already made for their inability to see clearly. That can mean using other sensory channels instead of, or at the same time as, visual channels.

The only way to know for sure the extent of a person's visual disability, the methods he uses to adapt, and his specific needs in a recreational environment, is to ask him. Do not make assumptions. One common assumption is that most people who are legally blind can read Braille. This is simply not the case. Less than 10% of people who have severe visual impairments can read Braille. Many people prefer to use audio cassettes. Above all, use your imagination. That is the sense, more than any other, that will help ***you*** to provide accessible programs for recreation participants who are visually impaired.

Some Things You Might Want To Do

Ask Before Helping

If someone with a visual impairment seems to need assistance, offer your help but do not give it unless your offer is accepted. If it is accepted, ask for an exact explanation of how you can help.

Do Not Shout

Loss of sight does not affect a person's hearing. Do not shout at a person with a visual impairment. Similarly, it does not affect a person's mental ability. Talk directly to him, not to others on his behalf.

Use Your Typical Expressions

Do not be afraid to use words like ***see, look, or blind***. Such words are a part of our everyday vocabulary and people who are blind use them, too. At the same time, if you find yourself looking at something interesting, make sure you include the person who is blind in your experience by describing it to her as clearly as possible.

Identify Yourself

When you meet a person who is blind, be sure to identify yourself. Remember to let her know when you leave, too. In addition, if things change in the setting you are in, let the person who is blind know.

Remember, Guide Dogs Are Often "On Duty"

Do not pet a guide dog unless you have the owner's permission. When the dog is in harness, he is "on duty." If he is distracted, the owner may be placed in jeopardy.

Be Descriptive

Use specific, descriptive language when giving directions, explaining things, or describing a place, an event, or an activity to a person who is blind. Colors, textures, movements, and directional indicators in a description can make it more vivid for someone with a visual impairment.

Provide Orientation

Orient people with visual impairments to new environments. Describe the size, shape, distances, boundaries, and any obstacles or potential hazards. During activities, orient them to the placement of objects around them that they will use. The military analogy of a clock face to explain position is often used by people with severe visual impairment. For example, say the lanyard strips are at 3 o'clock and the hooks are at 9 o'clock.

Guide and Describe

If a person who is blind accepts your offer of assistance, you should ask, "Would you like to take my arm?" Brush your forearm against hers so she can grip your arm above the elbow. The grip should be firm enough to maintain while walking and should not be uncomfortable. Children will grip the same as above, except will do so at the wrist. Some older adults or those who have ambulatory problems may not want to walk arm-in-arm. This offers more support than the grip. They may also wish to travel at a slower pace.

IMPORTANT: Do NOT attempt to lead the individual by taking his arm! Your arm should be relaxed along your side and the person who is blind will provide his arm bent at the elbow. With his right hand he will grip to your left elbow. Be sure to keep your arm close to your body. This is called the sighted guide method.

While using the sighted guide method, the person who is blind should travel a half-step behind you. Pick a comfortable walking pace for both of you. If the person pulls your arm back or tightens his grip, you are probably going too fast. Never try to push or steer a person who is blind ahead of you. You should also try to keep the person aware as conditions or surroundings change. Remember to mention curbs, steps, doorways, narrow passage, ramps, etc. Let her know if the stairs go up or down and when she reaches the last step. When guiding a person who is blind to a seat, simply place her hand on the back of the chair and let her seat herself. Explain what you are doing as you do it.

Think Before You Open

When you are approaching a door, say so. Have the free hand side of the person who is blind on the hinged side of the door. You should stop and change arms if not positioned correctly. Place your hand on the knob and let the person who is blind follow your arm to the door knob. Tell her whether the door opens toward or away from you. Allow the person who is blind to hold the door open for both of you.

Cut Down on Noise

Minimize background noises when instructing individuals with visual impairments. Extraneous noises can be very distracting and create confusion for people who rely on auditory information in their environment.

Allow for Manipulation and Explanation During Instruction

When you are demonstrating a skill, people with visual impairments may want to hold your hands as you work. Explain graphically in concrete terms what you are doing as you do it. Sometimes it is best to stand behind the participant, reaching through his arms, with his hands on yours, so he can follow your exact movements.

Implications for Recreation

People with visual impairments cannot see to catch or hit objects or detect boundaries. Sound source balls and audible goals may be used in games for persons who are blind, and bright yellow or orange objects can be used with persons who are partially sighted. Providing different textures and using smooth ground vs. grass or wood vs. carpet can indicate lines and boundaries.

Adapted devices that are used in certain sports, such as guide rails in bowling and raised print added to games and equipment, can provide access for participation to people with visual impairments. Braille playing cards, dominoes, and board games as well as measuring cups and oven dials are available. Also available are "talking" typewriters, computers, and calculators that may be of use to people with visual impairments in some types of educational or recreational programming.

Leaders should try to give clear and concise directions to groups that include people who have visual impairments. They may need to be at the front of a group or class to take advantage of any vision problems that may exist. Written materials or directions for an activity may need to be put into Braille or large print or recorded on audio cassette. Orienting persons to the activity room, gym, field, or swimming pool is important in order for them to know the size and layout of the space. Placing any materials or equipment so that they are easily accessible and always in the same location is useful.

In an arts and crafts project it is helpful to have a completed object for the person to feel. In a sport, exercise, or dance activity the person may wish to be physically guided through the action first in order to feel the type of movement required.

Health and Safety

There is no evidence to suggest that people who are blind or partially sighted are any more likely to have an accident at a recreation facility than their sighted peers, providing that sensible precautions are taken. For example, corridors and passageways should be kept clear, and no unnecessary obstacles should be placed in them. Contrasting colors can also assist people who are partially sighted. Thus, a door and a wall should ideally be different colors. The top and bottom steps should be clearly marked and, if possible, the texture of the top and bottom steps altered so they are identifiable by foot or cane. These provisions will, of course, also be helpful to sighted people and may reduce accidents in general.

Most people who have a visual loss are perfectly healthy apart from their lack of vision and should not be overprotected. In the event of an emergency, provisions may need to be made to help evacuate participants who are visually impaired.

Conclusion

People with visual impairments are presented with some unique challenges in their lives. They must function within a world that is becoming increasingly visually oriented. At the same time, advances in technology have resulted in new opportunities for such individuals. Advancements in computer technology have resulted in people who are blind being able to use computers and related technology. The role of the recreation practitioner is to help create an environment that is accessible to people with visual impairments. As with all adaptation initiatives, the best way to achieve accessibility is to use people who are blind as part of your accessibility assessment team. As we have discussed previously, this means looking at not only existing facilities but also programs, marketing processes and information, and the like. The facilitation of inclusive programs for people with visual impairments must be a very conscious process. In this chapter we have outlined some considerations for working with people with visual impairments. The challenge for all recreation service providers is to ensure that you translate the information we have provided you to all staff and consumers of your services.

Learning Activities

1. To practice guiding techniques, blindfold a partner. Guide your partner in various settings, such as outdoor trails, swimming pools, and recreation facilities.
2. Obtain information from your local parks and recreation agency. Review the material to determine whether it is accessible to people with visual impairments (e.g., large print, audio tape, etc.). If it is not accessible, decide how it could be made to meet the needs of people with various levels and types of visual impairments.
3. Choose four or five games or activities that you feel a person who is blind would have difficulty participating in. Discuss how the games or activities could be modified to include a person who is blind while still providing the experience sighted people would expect.

4. Construct a log of one of your recent days. Analyze how much of your activity required sight. Discuss how/if these activities could be modified for a person who is blind.

References

Chiang,Y., Bassie, L.J., & Javitt, J.C. (1991). Federal budgetary cost of blindness. *The Milibank Quarterly, 70* (2), 319-338.

Jernigan, K. (Ed.) (1992). ***What you should know about blindness, services for the blind, and the organized blind movement.*** Maryland: the National Federation of the Blind.

National Institute on Disability and Rehabilitation Research. (1994). ***Rehab Brief***, 16 (1), 1.

NOTE: Significant portions of this chapter are adapted from Bullock, C.C., McCann, C.A., & Palmer, R.I. (1994). ***LIFE resources: The LIFE resources manual*** (2nd ed.). Published by the Center for Recreation and Disability Studies, Curriculum I Leisure Studies and Recreation Administration, University of North Carolina at Chapel Hill. The author would also like to thank Carrie McCann for her significant contributions to this chapter.

Other Sources of Information

American Council of the Blind
1155 15th Street, NW, Suite 720
Washington, DC 20005
(202) 467-5081
(800) 424-8666
Fax: (202) 467-5085
http://acb.org/

American Foundation for the Blind
http://www.afb.org/index.html

Related Websites

HYPERLINK http://www.icdi.wvu.edu/Others.htm#g4 http://ww.icdi.wvu.edu/Others.htm#g4
(Resources on Visual Disability)

HYPERLINK http://omni.cc.purdue.edu/~alps/visual_sites.html http://omni.cc.purdue.edu/~alps/visual_sites.html
(Visual Impairment Related Sites)

HYPERLINK http://www.spedex.com/resource/links/general.htm http://www.spedex.com/resource/links/general.htm
(Special Education Exchange General Links)

HYPERLINK http://curry.edschool.virginia.edu/go/specialed/categories/vi.html http://curry.edschool.virginia.edu/go/specialed/categories/vi.html
(Office of Special Education — Visually Impaired)

HYPERLINK http://eisc-prise.mciu.k12.pa.us/EISC/Selected_Sites/Sites_blindvi.html http://eisc-prise.mciu.k12.pa.us/EISC/Selected_Sites/sites_blindvi.html
(Blind/Visual Impairments)

HYPERLINK http://serc.gws.uky.edu/www/resources/vi.html http://serc.gws.uky.edu/www/resources/vi.html
(University of Kentucky — Visual Impairment Sites)

Chapter 11

People with Hearing Loss

Introduction

Hearing impairment is the general term used to describe and encompass all types of loss, ranging from very mild to profound deafness. Services for people with hearing losses have the longest history of any services related to people with disabilities in North America and around the world. The first school for people who were deaf was founded by Charles Michel abbe de l'Eppe in Paris in 1755 (Valentine, 1991). In the United States, Thomas Gallaudet founded the American School for the Deaf in Hartford, Connecticut, in 1817. Gallaudet attracted Laurent Clerc, and intellectually gifted deaf man who had been teaching at the Paris Institute to help pioneer deaf education in the Untied States, Clerc adapted his native French sign language for use in the United States. By adding new words and modifying the meaning of expressions to accommodate differing cultural idioms of France and America, Clerc created American Sign Language (ASL), a new distinct language. In 1856, the institution now known as Gallaudet University was established in Washington, D.C. (Sherrill, 1998). More recently, the issues of education and community living for people with hearing impairments have become quite controversial. In particular, a great debate in North America has emerged as to whether the concept of inclusion has a place within the deaf community. We will highlight the issues of this debate later in the chapter. In this chapter we will define hearing impairment and deafness. We will also describe the nature and magnitude of hearing loss different people experience and the different forms of communication people with hearing losses may use. Beyond this, we will provide our thoughts on ways to ensure that people who are deaf are treated with respect and are included in recreation programs.

Some Things You Might Want to Know

Hearing loss is the most common disability among Americans. More than 24 million people in the United States have a hearing loss that can hinder daily communication (Ross, 1990). As is the case with all disabilities, there are different degrees of hearing loss.

Hearing impairments are typed according to the location of the damage or deficit (Steinberg & Knightly, 1997):

- **Conductive hearing loss** is caused by damage or obstruction in the outer or middle ear.
- **Sensorineural hearing loss** is caused by a malfunction of the cochlea or auditory nerve.
- **Mixed hearing loss** occurs when conductive and sensorineural factors combine to cause hearing loss.
- **Central hearing loss** occurs when the hearing centers of the brain are unable to interpret signals correctly.

A person who is deaf may also have impaired speech to a degree because he may not be able to hear well enough to correct phonetic errors in his own speech. Anyone who becomes deaf after about the age of seven usually has normal language and vocabulary. On the other hand, those who become deaf at any earlier age may have a more restricted command of language and vocabulary, which may cause some difficulty with communication.

Hearing loss may be congenital or the result of an accident, certain drugs, or illness. It may also be caused by prolonged exposure to excessive levels of noise. Whatever the cause, the presence of a hearing loss implies a breakdown in the physiological mechanisms of hearing (Glolas, 1981). Accidents are the leading cause of conductive hearing loss. They include the rupture of the ear drum by a blow or by an explosion that causes sudden pressure in the outer ear.

Hearing loss is classified as mild, moderate, or severe, based on the degree of loss as measured in decibels. A decibel is a unit used to measure the intensity of sounds. A sound of zero decibels is the softest sound that an acute ear can hear. Ordinary conversation is measured at 60-70 decibels. The chart in Table 11.1 illustrates the various degree and effects of hearing loss (Turkington & Sussman, 1992).

Table 11.1
Degree and Effects of Hearing Loss

Decibel Level (db) and Associated Terms	Effects of Loss on the Understanding of Language and Speech	Program Implications and Needs
26-40 db Slight	May have difficulty hearing faint or distant speech	A hearing aid may be beneficial
	May experience difficulty with vocabulary and speech articulation	Proper lighting and close proximity to speaker will help

Controversy within the Deaf Community

Controversy exists within the deaf community related to the terminology used to describe people with hearing losses. A significant percentage of the deaf community reject "people-first" language, preferring the use of the term *Deaf people*. This portion of the deaf community considers the community of Deaf people to be a culture, with the capital D representing the culture (Dolnick, 1993). This argument is based on the deaf community representing a very large portion of Americans who share a common language—American Sign Language. The controversy that surrounds this assertion is that not all people who are deaf agree with this perspective. Many do not share the desire to be seen as a culture, but rather, they see themselves as a part of the broader community. Given the lack of consensus on this issue, it is important to be sensitive to the perspectives of the various people with whom you may come in contact.

Speech

Depending on the degree of hearing loss, the person actually may hear speech if it is clear and may also speak clearly. People with more severe hearing losses may be able to speak clearly. People with more severe hearing losses may be able to hear amplified speech with the assistance of a hearing aid and/or an assistive listening device. The speech of some people with severe hearing losses may be somewhat unclear. In contrast, some people who are deaf choose not to use their speech because they believe that sign language is their first language (Turkington & Sussman, 1992).

Speech-reading, or *lipreading*, is a technique learned by some people with hearing losses to assist them in understanding others' speech when they cannot hear it well or at all. Lip-readers watch a speaker's mouth and identify words by the shape and position of the lips and tongue. This is a difficult skill to master since less than 35% of English words are recognizable solely by mouth positions and movements. Context and nonverbal communications are essential adjuncts to this skill.

Signing

Signing is often used as a communication technique by people who are deaf. Signing involves using the position and movement of the hands, as well as other body language, to create predefined symbols for concepts. American Sign Language is a language with its own grammar and syntax. In comparison, the English sign systems (called signed English) follow the syntax of spoken English. One other form of sign language is the use of finger spelling. Finger spelling involves using hand shapes to create a predefined symbol for each letter in the alphabet. Words are literally spelled the way they are in written English (O'Grady, 1991).

Table 11.1 cont.

41-55 db	Will understand conversations within 3-5 feet if speaker is facing him	A hearing aid will be beneficial
	May exhibit speech errors and limited vocabulary	Proper lighting and placement of person in relationship to speaker is important
		Fatigue and extraneous noise will affect person's ability to comprehend speech
56-70 db Moderate	To comprehend conversation, speech must be loud and distance small; will have difficulty unless conversation is directed at her	Hearing aids and an assistive listening system needed
		Assistance to comprehend new vocabulary is needed; concrete examples and demonstrations are helpful
		Close proximity to speaker and proper lighting is essential; only minimum background noise
71-90 db Severe	Will understand only strongly amplified speech	In addition to the above points, balance may be a problem, depending upon what part of the ear is damaged
	May hear voices about one foot away	
	Has distorted speech; may be able to hear vowels but not all consonants	More difficulty in interacting in a group discussion, so someone will need to clue him into the topic and he will need to face the speaker
	Has speech and language errors	

Table 11.1 cont.

90+ db Profound (Dcaf)	Will not understand even maximally amplified speech	In addition to the above points, assistance of an interpreter may be needed, depending on the activity
	May not hear loud sounds but is aware of vibrations	Sign language or written messages may be relied upon
	Relics hcavily on vision to supplement any hearing	Demonstration and the use of visual aids are essential
		New vocabulary must be taught

(Adapted from *Closing the Gap*, Dept. of Leisure Studies, San Jose State University)

Other Methods of Communication

Cued speech is a phonemically-based system used by some people who are deaf. This method uses eight hand shapes and four positions around the face to show spoken language. Writing is the only mean of communication for some people with hearing losses and speech impairments. Some of them are not comfortable writing because their language does not follow standard English syntax.

Most people who are deaf have a keyboard device called a text telephone or TTY, which enables them to communicate with others who have the same devices. Many other persons with hearing loss use volume-controlled telephones that amplify the incoming sound. A telephone so equipped can be used by anyone by adjusting the volume. This type of phone allows a person with a hearing loss to be independent. Telephone relay systems that are necessary for the TTY system are now in place in most states. A deaf person with a TTY can contact a telephone relay operator who, in turn, contacts a person without a TTY and relays the message (Turkington & Sussman, 1992).

Many activities need not preclude the participation of people with hearing losses, no matter how severe if the communication component of the activity is addressed. Most often, the only adaptation necessary is to be sure that visual cues are incorporated into the activity to compensate for the participant's level of ability in responding to strictly verbal cues. If an interpreter will be needed, ask the participants which particular sign systems they use of if they are cued speech. Interpreters are familiar with different communication methods and can assist you in locating the appropriate one.

Hearing loss is not a disability that handicaps the ability to work or play, provided the activity does not necessarily require good hearing. Accommodations should be made whenever possible to allow for full participation.

People who have hearing losses may sometimes be difficult to understand when they speak because of speech sound errors and unusual intonation. With a little patience and practice, however, the hearing person can usually quickly achieve understanding. People with hearing losses will be at a disadvantage at meetings, classes, activities, or when answering the telephone unless accommodations are made. If fellow participants in a group take care to face the person when speaking, the opportunity for speech-reading is available.

Some Things You Might Want To Do

Ask Before Assisting

If people with hearing losses seem to need assistance, offer your help but do not give it unless your offer is accepted. Make sure you have the attention of people with hearing losses before you begin communicating with them, perhaps by touching their arm or gesturing.

Articulate

Speak clearly and distinctly at a normal rate and volume. Do not exaggerate the volume or speed of your own speech unless you are asked to. Do not exaggerate your lip movements. Try to avoid eating, smoking, or chewing while you talk; it makes your speech harder to understand. Be sure you have been understood before going to something else. Repeat yourself as often as necessary, perhaps rephrasing, because you may have been using some words that are difficult to understand.

Be Expressive!

Use facial expressions, hand gestures, and body movements to accentuate your speech. Subtle changes in tone or volume to indicate feeling or meaning may be missed by someone with a hearing loss. The more visual cues you use, the easier it will be for the person to understand you.

Prevent Distractions

When giving instructions or explanations, keep background noise to a minimum to prevent distractions and confusion concerning the activity in which the person is involved. If it is very loud, go someplace where it is quieter, or give instructions before entering a noisy area.

Position Yourself

Face people with hearing losses while you are speaking. They will not be able to "hear" the back of your head. Be sure that your face and upper body are clearly visible. Get close enough to be seen plainly, face the light-ensuring enough of it is illuminating your face—and avoid shadows on your face (like those cast by broad-rimmed hats and sunglasses). Avoid standing in front of a window or with your back to a bright light.

Do Not Exclude

Remember that having multiple speakers and creating activities that involve listening to tapes, turning out lights, or closing the eyes will automatically exclude people with hearing losses. Be careful to make accommodations.

Speak to the Person

Be sure to talk directly to a person with a hearing loss, not to an interpreter. Address yourself to whom you are sending your message. Table 11.2 provides some helpful hints when working with a sign language interpreter.

If at First You Don't Succeed...

If you are having trouble understanding someone's speech or he is having trouble understanding yours, try repeating what has been said. If that fails, try using a pencil and paper. Clear communication is what is important, not how it is accomplished. Visual aids such as diagrams, written instructions, pictures, or media, in addition to verbal instructions, assist individuals with hearing losses in comprehending directions and instructions.

Adapt, When Necessary

Some adaptations and modification may be needed to make an activity accessible to people with hearing losses if communication is an essential component. Incorporate visual cues into directions or instructions; some possibilities include using flags or lights to start or stop play and/or using hand signals.

Implications for Recreation

Communications difficulties can be minimized by the use of a hearing aid or other assistive device and by leaders using visual demonstrations with simple words and sentences. Training may take a little time, but once the recreation skill has been learned by the person with the hearing loss, his participation will be typical.

Speech-reading can assist the person who is hearing impaired to better understand a portion of what is said. Leaders and participants can learn tips to enhance communication by observing the following simple rules:

Table 11.2
How to Work with a Sign Language Interpreter

1. Always look at and speak directly to the person with a hearing impairment, not the interpreter.
2. Always speak in the first person. Do not say, "Tell him..." or "Ask her..." This excludes the person with a hearing impairment and is confusing for the interpreter.
3. Allow the interpreter to sit or stand near the hearing person. Make sure the person with a hearing impairment can clearly see both the interpreter and the speaker.
4. Do not use the interpreter to interpret select portions of what is said. The interpreter follows a professional code of ethics and therefore MUST interpret everything that is said or signed. The interpreter is also required to keep all assignment-related information confidential and to remain impartial.
5. Hand all materials and forms to the person with a hearing impairment, not the interpreter. This recognizes the person with a hearing impairment as the one who has the appointment; it also shows that the hearing consumer is comfortable dealing directly with the person with a hearing impairment.
6. Remember that the interpreter is the communication line. As such, he or she is responsible to give equal services to both the hearing consumer and the person with a hearing impairment.
7. Speak normally. Rely on the interpreter to let you know if there is a need to slow down or pause.
8. When giving directions or using visual handouts, be sure to allow time to review the printed materials either before or after the explanation. Remember that the person with a hearing impairment cannot look at the printed materials and the interpreter at the same time.

(Adapted from the Accessibility Consulting Group, Toledo, Ohio)

1. Make sure the person who is deaf is looking at you when you speak with him.
2. Speak with a clear voice (do not shout).
3. Move lips clearly to aid speech-reading.
4. Be ready to repeat your words or to write them down, if necessary.

People who are deaf often use sign language as well as speech. Although it is not necessary for hearing participants to learn sign language, some enjoy learning manual communication from their associates who are deaf. This is worth encouraging on an informal basis because it aids more fluent communication and fosters good relationships.

People may sometimes be nervous with respect to dealing with others with hearing losses because communication can initially be difficult. This may discourage casual conversation, although this phase generally passes. Experience has shown that a person with a hearing loss is usually accepted and communication becomes easy once other participants become accustomed to the individual and then follow the rules of visual communication.

The need for good acoustics and lighting cannot be overemphasized, and many hearing aid users can also benefit considerably from the installation of an assistive listening system.

Health and Safety

People with hearing losses are as healthy as anybody else and are quite able to take part in varied environments. A hearing loss does not necessarily affect mobility and has no adverse effect on participation in many kinds of activities.

Special safety arrangements may or may not be necessary. Although long-standing deafness trains people to use their eyes and to spot and avoid dangerous situations, fire and other alarms should incorporate a flashing light system or a vibrotactile alarm, particularly if a person with a hearing loss is taking part in an activity alone. Participants should be instructed to ensure that people with hearing losses are made aware of dangerous situations that arise unexpectedly.

Conclusion

Deafness and other hearing impairments are disabilities with a long history of services in the United Sates and Canada. Remarkably, given this long history, great debate regarding how best to integrate people with hearing losses into the mainstream still exists. Should they be forced to speak if they have the capability? Should they be educated separately or in mainstreamed classrooms? The debate continues. People who are not deaf cannot fully appreciate this debate. How should we as students and future practitioners respond to these questions? If we consider some of the guiding principles of this book—self-determination, interdependence, integration, and social role valorization—our response becomes clear. As with all people, we must treat people with hearing losses as individuals and respect their perspectives and personal choices. Given this, the services we deliver must be sensitive to this debate and must offer people who are deaf the opportunity to use various methods of communication when participating in recreation programs. In this chapter we have presented you with a brief overview of people with hearing losses. We have explained the various methods of communication and presented some things to consider when working with people with hearing losses. We have explained the various methods of communication and presented some things to consider when working with people with hearing losses. We encourage you to explore how you can become better able to communicate with people with hearing losses so that you can meet their needs as recreation consumers.

Learning Activities

1. Find out where you can take an American Sign Language (ASL) course. We encourage you to take such a course because it will help you to facilitate the inclusion of people with hearing losses into recreation programs.
2. Do a telephone survey of recreation-related agencies in your area. Determine which of them have TTYs and if any have people on staff who are able to speak ASL. Ask what the agencies' policies are relative to funding for interpreters so that people with hearing losses can be included in their programs.
3. Carry on a conversation in small groups, with each person taking a turn wearing ear plugs and the rest of the group speaking very quietly. After each turn, ask the person with the assumed hearing loss what the group did well to facilitate communication and what they could have done better.
4. Choose a few different recreation activities. Analyze what barriers to communication a person who is deaf might experience in trying to participate in the given activity. Identify some strategies for counteracting the barriers identified.

References

Accessibility Consulting Group. (1993). ***How to work with a sign language interpreter***. Available from the Ability Center, Accessibility Consulting Group, Toledo, OH.

Bambord, J., & Saunders, E. (1985). ***Hearing impairment, auditory, perception, and language disability***. Great Britain: Edward Arnold Publishers.

Department of Leisure Studies. (1980). ***Closing the gap***. San Jose, CA: Department of Leisure Studies, San Jose State University.

Dolnick, E. (1993). Deafness and culture. ***The Atlantic Monthly***, 272(3), 37-53.

Glolas, T.G. (1981). ***Hearing handicapped adults***. Englewood Cliffs, NJ: Prentice Hall.

Higgins & Nash. (1987). ***Understanding deafness socially***. Springfield, IL: Charles C. Thomas, Publisher.

O'Grady, J. (1991, June). ***A sign of the times***. Times Educational Supplement.

Ross, M. (1990). ***Hearing-impaired children in the mainstream***. Parkton: York Press.

Sherill, C. (1998). ***Adapted physical activity, recreation, and sport: Crossdisciplinary and lifespan*** (5th Edition). Boston, MA: WCB McGraw-Hill.

Steinberg, A.G. & Knightly, C.A. (1997). Hearing: Sounds and silences. In M.L. Batshaw (Ed.), ***Children with Disabilities*** (4th Ed.). Baltimore, MD: Paul H. Brookes.

Turkington, C., & Sussman, A.E. (1992). ***The encyclopedia of deafness and hearing disorders***. New York, NY: Facts on File.

Valentine, P.K. (1991). A nineteenth century experiment in the education of the handicapped: The American Asylum for the deaf and dumb. ***New England Quarterly***, 355-375.

NOTE: Significant portions of this chapter are adapted from Bullock, C.C., McCann, C.A., & Palmer, R.I. (1994). *LIFE resources: The LIFE resources manual* (2nd ed). Published by the Center for Recreation and Disability Studies, Curriculum in Leisure Studies and Recreation Administration, University of North Carolina at Chapel Hill.

The authors would also like to thank Carrie McCann for her significant contributions to this chapter.

Other Sources of Information

Alexander Graham Bell Association for the Deaf
3417 Volta Place, N.W.
Washington, DC 20007-2778
(202) 337-5220 Voice and TTY
http://www.agbell.org/

American Speech-Language-Hearing Association
10801 Rockville Pike
Rockville, Maryland 20852
Answer Line: 888-321-ASHA
Action Center: 800-498-2071
(301) 897-5700
TTY: (301) 897-0157
Fax: (301) 571-0457
http://www.asha.org/index.htm

National Cued Speech Association
4245 East Avenue
Rochester, NY 14618
http://bombur.mit.edu/CuedSpeech/ncsainfo.html

National Information Center on Deafness (NICD)
Gallaudet University
800 Florida Ave. NE
Washington, DC 20002-3695
(202)651-5051
TTY: (202)651-5052
Fax: (202)651-5054
http://www.gallaudet.edu/~nicd/index.html

National Association of the Deaf NAD
814 Thayer Avenue
Silver Spring, MD 20910-4500
(301) 587-1788 TTY: (301) 587-1789
Fax: (301) 587-1791
Email: NADHQ@juno.com website: http://www.nad.org/

National Technical Institute for the Deaf
52 Lomb Memorial Drive
Rochester, NY 14623-5604
(716) 475-6700
Fax: (716) 475-2696
http://www.rit.edu/~418www/index.shtml

Self Help for Hard of Hearing People, Inc.
7910 Woodman Ave. — Suite 1200
Bethesda, Maryland 20814
(301) 657-2248
TTY: (301) 657-2249
Fax: (301) 913-9413
http://www.shhh.org/

Chapter 12

People with Mental Illnesses

Introduction

Mental illness is one of the foremost public health problems within North America. It is estimated that during any one year period, up to 50 million Americans exhibit a clearly diagnosable type of mental disorder that interferes with employment, attendance at school, or daily life (American Psychiatric Association, 1998). Significant debate exists as to what constitutes mental health or mental illness. According to Compton (1994, p. 16),

> At the root of the issue...is how *illness* is defined. This term serves a vitally important role in declaring whether a behavior is deviation from some norm, a social construction, or a biological/physiological phenomena.

The *Diagnostic and Statistics Manual of Mental Disorders (DSM-IV)* (American Psychiatric Association, 1994, p. xxxi) describes mental disorders as:

> conceptualized as a clinically significant behavioral or psychological syndrome or pattern that occurs in a person that is associated with present distress (e.g., a painful symptom) or disability (i.e., impairment in one or more important areas of functioning) or with a significantly increased risk of suffering death, pain, disability, or an important loss of freedom. In addition, this syndrome or pattern must not be merely an expectable and culturally sanctioned response to a particular event, e.g., the death of a loved one. Whatever its original cause, it must currently be considered a manifestation of a behavioral, psychological, or biological dysfunction in the individual. Neither deviant behavior, e.g., political, religious, or sexual, nor conflicts that are primarily between the individual...There is no assumption that each category of mental disorder is a completely discrete entity with absolute boundaries dividing it from other mental disorders or from no mental disorder. There is also no assumption that all individuals described as having the same mental disorder are alike in all important ways.

The DSM-IV definition is in many ways quite comprehensive. However, as it quite obvious, its focus is decidedly medical. There are numerous definitions of mental health that take a different approach to mental illness—that take a less medical perspective (Mental Health Consumers Task Force, 1991; Boorse, 1982). All are not without their flaws. These definitions of mental health are useful for recreation professions because they in many ways provide a framework for establishing goals. By knowing what positive mental health can mean for a person, we are able to identify strategies for achieving such a state. Compton (1994, p. 18) suggests that mental health:

> ...is comprised of one's ability to: manage or control daily experience; interact in an acceptable manner with others; exhibit intellectual alertness and reasoning powers; derive a sense of meaning and value from life; achieve a sense of happiness and self-esteem; demonstrate resiliency during and after stressful life events; and develop a sense of maturity in introspective, prospective, and retrospective matters.

People with mental illnesses are often presented with very significant challenges with respect to their participation in recreation programs. In many ways, because mental illness is such a misunderstood disability, people with mental illnesses experience some of the most significant barriers to recreation participation and the greatest prejudice from both the general public and recreation service providers within the context of recreation. Given this, recreation students and professionals should see the importance of having a good understanding of mental illness and its implications for recreation. In this chapter we will provide a brief overview of some of the most common forms of mental illness. Given the large body of information on this topic, we have attempted to synthesize the information into key points. Following this, we present some common *myths* related to mental illness and some corresponding *facts*. As with all other chapters in this section, we also discuss some things you might want to do and implications for recreation, health, and safety for people with mental illnesses.

Some Things You Might Want to Know

Approximately two percent of the population is affected with a serious mental illness. The causes of these brain diseases remain unknown but are probably multiple and not the fault of the individuals or their families. In addition to having a brain disease, people with mental illnesses may be functionally impaired for an indefinite period of time in many of the primary activities of life: social interactions and relationships, concentration and decision making, self-care, employment, home making, education, and recreation. The problems of people with mental illnesses are compounded by stigma and discrimination, which may explain their limited involvement in community recreation experiences. In addition to stigma, many must also deal with the burden of poverty. A high percentage of people with mental illnesses are unemployed and economically disadvantaged. This is because of the interaction between the challenges they experience in work settings and the inability or lack of interest of employers to accommodate them in jobs.

People with mental illnesses may be the most under-represented group of people with disabilities to be served by community parks and recreation and commercial recreation providers. Society's misperception of these individuals' needs and abilities, consumers' reluctance to expose themselves to an unknown and potentially harsh environment, media misrepresentation, and a lack of accurate information on positive and reasonable ways to offer inclusive and accessible services all contribute to a pattern of exclusion for these citizens.

The first step to understanding people with mental illnesses is to realize that mental illnesses are indeed illnesses. The two main divisions are psychosis and neurosis. Psychoses are characterized by delusions, hallucinations, disturbances in the thinking process, serious limitations in judgment and insight, and the inability to objectively evaluate reality. Psychoses can be classified into organic or functional impairment. Some examples of psychoses include Alzheimer's disease (organic), manic-depressive disorder (functional), and schizophrenia (functional). Neuroses are more common and less severe than psychoses. It is sometimes quite difficult to distinguish between whether a disturbance is due to a neurosis or to problems coping with everyday life, such as fear or simple sadness. Some examples of neurosis include mild depression, feelings of tenseness or anxiety, phobias, and obsessional behavior (Nevid, Spencer, & Green, 1994).

The distinction between mental illness and mental retardation is an important one. Mental retardation is a developmental disability that delays the development of an individual's intellectual potential. Mental retardation can result in varying levels of intellectual ability. Though more recently it has been suggested that mental retardation does not need to be a lifelong disability, this speaks more to the individual's potential to live independently in the community rather than to intellectual capacities. At this point in time, there is no known cure for mental retardation. In contrast, mental illness is not a developmental disability and does not directly impact intellectual capacity. However, the associated characteristics of mental illness may render an individual less intellectually capable. Mental illness can be treated and often cured. With proper diagnosis and treatment, the symptoms of mental illness may disappear (APA, 1998).

Important to note are two frequent occurrences in people with mental illnesses. Often individuals experience *comorbidity,* which is the overlap of two or more medical disorders in a single patient. For example, a person who has mental retardation may also have mental illness. Secondly, during the process of treatment a person may go through a syndrome shift, which is a change in the individuals' primary diagnosis (Kocherty, 1993).

There are three main causes of mental illness. Mental illness is sometimes found to result from a biological disorder. In contrast, certain conditions are brought on by early childhood experience. Lastly, mental illness can occur when an individual cannot adequately cope with a stressful situation. Leading to a breakdown in coping mechanisms (Kalat, 1990). Richter (1984) suggests that mental illness develops not because of personal problems but as a response to environments created by society, within which certain individuals have a difficult time coping. We can identify both predisposing and precipitating factors in the environment that may result in the onset of mental illness. A predisposing factor is a condition that may cause mental illness. A precipitating factor is a specific even that causes onset. The existence of one or the other factor in the environment of a given person will not necessarily result in the onset of mental illness. For example, the death of a close friend might or might not be a precipitating factor. It is the interaction of the individual and various aspects of his environment that will determine whether or not an onset of mental illness will occur.

There are many different types of mental illness: depression, bipolar disorder, schizophrenia, anxiety disorders, and eating disorders. We will briefly discuss each of these disabilities. Though there are numerous types of mental illness, we will only highlight some of the most prevalent.

Depression and Bipolar Disorder

Depression is a mental illness that can seriously disrupt an individual's moods for long periods of time. Depression can affect people of all ages and can lead to suicide if left untreated. According to the DSM-IV (1994), there are two forms of depression: major depressive episodes and dysthymia. Major depressive episodes are characterized by at least five of nine symptoms displayed within a two-week period, with at least one of the symptoms being either depressed mood or loss of interest or pleasure. The nine characteristics are summarized in Table 12.1.

Depressive disorders are usually viewed as a continuum determined by the frequency, duration, and severity of the symptoms. Dysthymia is described as dysphoria (an emotional state characterized by anxiety, depression, and restlessness) that lasts for at least two years.

Most treatment of depression combines pharmacologic intervention combined with some level of psychotherapy. According to Patrick (1994), the use of leisure as a component of treatment for depression has advantages because individuals can self-prescribe, it can involve little cost, and there may be a number of forms of leisure that can be used successfully. We will discuss the use of leisure education with people with severe and persistent mental illnesses in Chapter 16.

Table 12.1
Symptoms Associated with Major Depressive Episodes

1. Depressed mood.
2. Significantly diminished interest in the pleasure of most activities.
3. Significant weight loss not associated with dieting.
4. Insomnia or hypertension.
5. Psychomotor agitation or retardation.
6. Fatigue.
7. Excessive guilt or feelings of worthlessness.
8. Reduced ability to reason or indecisiveness.
9. Recurrent thought of death or suicide ideation.

(Adapted from DSM-IV, 1994, p. 327)

Bipolar disorder (manic depression) is a mental illness characterized by mood swings from periods of extreme elation to severe depression. A manic phase involves hyperactive behavior, inflated self-esteem, distractibility, sleeplessness, and excessive and rapid talking. A depressive state has already been described in the previous section. Patrick (1994) suggests that manic depression lies on a continuum of mood disorders that range from minor dysphoria to manic depression.

Schizophrenia

Schizophrenia is a psychotic illness in which individuals experience hallucinations, abnormal emotions, impaired thinking, and behavioral changes. People with schizophrenia can exhibit ***positive*** symptoms, meaning in addition to or in excess of what is normal. In this case, their emotions are greatly exaggerated. However, more common is for a person with schizophrenia to exhibit ***negative*** symptoms, which is more of a deficit state. With it they can display a lack of enthusiasm, little enjoyment, and a marked loss of energy. Schizophrenia can develop gradually or can set in suddenly. The gradual onset can usually be traced back to early signs such as withdrawal from friends and family, lack of enthusiasm, more than the usual fears, etc. It is uncommon, however, to associate such indicators early on, as families are typically not aware of the significance of such signs in relation of mental illness.

The age of onset for schizophrenia is before adolescence and after age 45. Schizophrenia affects approximately one person in a hundred. There have been many attempts to subtype schizophrenia, and as knowledge of this disability continues to grow, information about subtypes is enhanced. To date, five subtypes have been identified:

1. **Catatonic** is associated with disturbances in movement. Individuals may exhibit everything from an almost complete absence of movement to extreme agitation.
2. **Paranoid** is associated with the predominance of one or more delusions or auditory hallucinations. These are typically quite consistent. Individuals tend to be less impaired than those with other subtypes.
3. **Disorganized** is characterized by verbal patterns that are very loose and disorganized; they do not have a consistent theme.
4. **Undifferentiated** is a label used to describe individuals who do not fit any of the characteristics of the other subtypes.
5. **Residual** is associated with a person who has one or more episodes of some form of schizophrenia, but who no longer displays any psychotic features. Individuals still do display some level of emotional blunting, social withdrawal, and illogical thinking.

The causes of schizophrenia are not known. Strong evidence suggests that some aspects of the illness are hereditary, though they do not seem to follow typical patterns. For example, there may be only one person in a family affected, or different symptoms may exist for different people in the same family. Schizophrenia is typically controlled through a combination of medication and social-psychological treatments.

Anxiety Disorders

Anxiety disorders include phobias, panic disorders, and obsessive-compulsive disorders. People with phobias feel extreme terror when confronted with a specific situation or object and may make adjustments in daily activities to avoid these situations or objects. Panic disorders are characterized by sudden, intense feelings of dread for no apparent reason. People who suffer from obsessive-compulsive disorders will attempt to cope with anxiety by associating it with repeated, unwanted thoughts or ritualistic behaviors.

There are two classes of behavioral theories that attempt to account for anxiety disorders: respondent, or cognitive theories and avoidance theories (Hickey & Baer, 1988). Cognitive theories suggest that anxiety is learned through classical conditioning; that is, that the individual learns to associate an object or experience with pain or other anxiety-producing stimuli. Some cognitive theorists also suggest that anxiety can be learned by observing other anxious people in certain conditions. Some people can develop anxiety with flying by watching other anxious people. Cognitive models of treatment emphasize altering the expectation of harm, often by replacing anxious thought or expectations with more positive thoughts. This may be achieved by using such strategies as self-talk, in which the individual learns to verbalize self-affirming statements.

Avoidance theories of anxiety disorders suggest that anxiety represents a drive for avoidance behavior (Hickey & Baer, 1988). These theories do not address the cause, but focus more on the outcome of the avoidance of the anxiety; i.e., the behaviors that result from the anxiety. Bandura (1977) suggests that avoidance behavior resulting from anxiety can be altered by improving one's sense of *self-efficacy*.

Eating Disorders

Eating disorders are serious, life-threatening illnesses in which people have a preoccupation with food and an irrational fear of becoming fat. The two most common eating disorders are anorexia nervosa and bulimia nervosa. The prevalence of eating disorders ranges somewhere between 1% and 4%, with 90% and 95% of those affected being females (American Psychiatric Association, 1993). The DSM-IV criteria for anorexia nervosa and bulimia nervosa are presented in Table 12.2. The DSM-IV has specified two types of anorexia nervosa: restricting type of anorexia nervosa does not regularly engage in binge eating or purging behavior (e.g., self-induced vomiting or the misuse of laxatives, diuretics, or enemas), whereas an individual with the binge-eating/purging type will engage in these behaviors during their current anorexia nervosa episode. Two types of bulimia nervosa are specified in the DSM-IV: the purging type and the nonpurging type. During the current episode of bulimia nervosa, an individual with the purging type has regularly engaged in self-induced vomiting or the misuse of laxatives, diuretics, or enemas, whereas an individual with the nonpurging type will engage in inappropriate compensatory behaviors such as fasting or excessive exercise.

Table 12.2
DSM-IV Criteria for Anorexia Nervosa and Bulimia Nervosa

Anorexia Nervosa

- Refusal to maintain a minimal normal weight
- Intense fear of weight gain or of "getting fat"
- Disturbance in the way one views his/her body (e.g., seeing fat where there is clearly none)
- In females, absence of at least three menstrual cycles when otherwise expected to occur

Bulimia Nervosa

- Recurrent episodes of binge eating characterized by both of the following: 1) Eating in a discrete period of time (e.g. within any 2-hour period, an amount of food that is definitely larger than most people would eat during a similar period of time and under similar circumstances; 2) a sense of lack of control in over eating during the episode
- Recurrent inappropriate compensatory behavior such a self-induced vomiting; the using of laxatives; and strict dieting or exercise to prevent weight gain
- Binge eating and inappropriate behaviors both occur, on average, at least twice a week for 3 months.
- Self-evaluation is unduly influenced by body shape and weight
- The disturbance does not occur exclusively during periods of anorexia nervosa

(Adapted from DSM-IV, 1994, p. 544-550)

Eating disorders present extremely complex challenges with respect to treatment because they typically involve medical, psychological, and interpersonal issues. In addition, they are very often chronic conditions. According to the American Psychiatric Association (1993), the best initial treatment results appear to be the combination of a weight restoration program combined with individual and family therapies.

Myths Surrounding Mental Illness and the Facts That Refute Them

Myth #1: *"A person who has been mentally ill can never be normal."*

Fact: Mental illness is often temporary in nature. A previously well-adjusted individual may have an episode of illness lasting weeks or months, and then they may go for years—even a lifetime—without further difficulty. To label such a recovered person abnormal is both unfair and unrealistic. Many other individuals are subject to bouts of disturbance. Between episodes, though, they may be perfectly well. People with former mental health problems deserve to be judged on their own merits.

Myth #2: *"If people who recover from other illnesses can cope on their own, persons recovering from mental illness should also be able to do so."*

Fact: Actually, most people who have been through a disabling illness need help, or rehabilitation, to return to normal functioning. As physical therapy fills this need after physical illness, social rehabilitation is usually needed after mental illness. In the case of persons with chronic mental illness, the differentness they experience makes it difficult for many of them to get back into society without help. Often, both education and social connections may have been interrupted, and self-esteem and confidence may also have been seriously damaged. People recovering from mental illnesses typically need substantial support to successfully reenter their communities.

Myth # 3: *"People with mental illnesses are dangerous. They could go berserk at any time."*

Fact: People who have come through a mental illness and have returned to the community are apt, if anything, to be anxious, timid, and passive. They rarely present a danger to the public. Most people who have been mentally ill never went "berserk" in the first place. According to experts, most relapses develop gradually, and if physicians, friends, families, or the persons themselves are alert and knowledgeable enough to recognize early symptoms, recurrences can usually be detected and dealt with before they become severe.

Myth #4: *"You can't talk to someone who has been mentally ill."*

Fact: Most people recovering from mental illness are rational and intelligent, and you may certainly be able to talk with them. Even individuals who are actively mentally ill are likely to be rational in many ways. They may suffer from certain delusions or act disturbed at times, but in their calmer moments they will probably be able to discuss many things reasonably and sensibly.

Myth #5: *"People who have experienced mental illness have a tough row to hoe, but there is not much that can be done about it."*

Fact: The way we act toward people recovering from mental illness can make a difference in their lives. Effective treatment, hard work, and good motivation are of limited value when functioning, hard-working, well-motivated individuals are refused employment, housing, or other opportunities because of false beliefs and stereotypes.

Some Things You Might Want To Do

Focus on the Individual

Learn about the person and deal with him on the basis of your knowledge. As with other people with disabilities, people with mental illnesses are the experts; they know what has worked for them and what has not. There is a tendency to assume that individuals with mental illness are not capable of expressing their own opinions or of making their own decisions. This is simply not true.

Facilitate Reintegration

Do what you can to help individuals with mental illness re-enter society. Support their efforts to obtain housing, jobs, and recreation opportunities. Because of the prejudice that often exists relative to people with mental illness, they may find difficulty in reintegrating into their own home communities. It is crucial at these early stages to provide advocacy and practical assistance.

Advocate

Do not let false statements about mental illness or people with mental illnesses go unchallenged. Many people have wrong and damaging ideas on the subject, yet they honestly believe their notions are true. Correct information may help change their minds. Spread the word; tell others what you have learned and insist that people with mental illnesses be treated fairly. Help give them what they need most: a chance. Challenge the inappropriate use of words such as crazy, schizo, psychopath, and maniac.

Implications for Recreation

In the past there has been a tendency to encourage many people with mental illnesses to take up simple, unskilled activities in segregated settings. Community inclusion is best promoted by encouraging participation in a wide range of self-determined recreation activities. Specific adaptations to equipment and programs are seldom necessary.

Leisure education has been identified as a useful approach for facilitating the leisure needs of people with mental illness (Bullock & Luken, 1994). The Reintegration Through Recreation leisure education program was developed by Bullock and Luken in response to the needs of people with severe and persistent mental illnesses. This model, which is discussed in detail in Chapter 16, is rooted within the cognitive-behavioral approach. In addition to leisure education, other recreation-based approaches to the facilitation of wellness and independence in people with mental illnesses are leisure counseling (Moon Hickman, 1994), exercise (Hall, 1994), and various therapeutic recreation-based treatment approaches (Annand, 1994). Compton and Iso-Ahola (1994) provide a very detailed overview of some contemporary leisure-based approaches to facilitating the needs of people with mental illness.

Health and Safety

Mental illnesses are treatable. When care and treatment are available, improvement and/or recovery may be expected. The health and safety of people with mental illnesses in recreation environments will generally not need to differ from that of other participants. Some individuals with mental illness take prescription drugs and may experience side effects. Depending on the medication, these may include hypersensitivity to sun exposure, fine motor tremors, weight gain, inability to eat certain foods, blurred vision, dry mouth, sedation, and stiffness of movement.

Conclusion

Mental illness is often described as the least understood of all disabling conditions. In fact, it is often thought of as less of a disability and more of a social problem that society would just as soon sweep under the rug. With the advent of deinstitutionalization in Canada and the United States, more individuals have moved back to their home communities. The transition has and continues to be a challenge for people with mental illnesses, members of their social support network, and service providers. One of the areas where this is particularly true is in recreation. People with mental illnesses often experience difficulty both in reintegrating into their communities and in reconnecting with previously enjoyed leisure pursuits.

The purpose of this chapter was to familiarize you with mental illness as a disability; to ensure that you have some understanding of the nature of this disability. In addition, we have provided you with some things that you may wish to know about the lives of people with mental illness. Most importantly, we have offered some basic strategies to help ensure that people with mental disabilities become included in their communities and are able to experience leisure and life satisfaction.

Learning Activities

1. Discuss the similarities and differences between mental illness and mental retardation. Write out how you would explain this information to a friend or relative.

2. In the following section we will discuss strategies for ensuring that people with disabilities expedience the benefits and enjoyment of recreation and leisure. As a precursor to reading this section, discuss what the implications of the dual diagnosis of mental illness and mental retardation might be for recreation participation.
3. Notwithstanding the unidentified needs of individuals with mental illness with whom you may work, how might recreation programming differ for a person with anorexia nervosa as compared to a person who exhibits signs of depression?
4. Assume that you are the program coordinator for a local recreation complex that houses a swimming pool, a gymnasium, an arts and crafts room, and a weight room. How could you structure your programs to ensure that people with mental illnesses would feel comfortable using your facility?

References

American Psychiatric Association (1993). Practical guideline for eating disorders. ***American Journal of Psychiatry, 150***, 207-228.

American Psychiatric Association (1994). ***Diagnostic and statistical manual of mental disorders: DSM-IV*** (4th ed.). Washington, D.C.: Author.

American Psychiatric Association (1998). APA online: Mental Illness (an overview). http.www.psych.org/public_info/overview.html

Annand, V.S. (1994). Therapeutic recreation treatment in psychiatry. In D.M. Compton & S..E. Iso-Ahola (Eds.), ***Leisure and Mental Health: Volume I.*** Park City, UT: Family Resources Inc.

Bandura, A. (1977). ***Social learning theory***. Englewood Cliffs, NJ: Prentice Hall.

Boorse, C. (1982). What a theory of mental health should be. In R. Edwards (Ed.), ***Psychiatry and ethics***. Buffalo, NY: Prometheus Books.

Bullock, C.C., & Luken, K. (1994). Reintegration through recreation: A community-based rehabilitation model. In D.M. Compton & S.E. Iso-Ahola (Eds.), ***Leisure and mental health: Volume I.*** Park City, UT: Family Resources Inc.

Compton, D. (1994). Leisure and mental health: Context and issues. In D.M. Compton & S.E. Iso-Ahola (eds.). ***Leisure and mental health: Volume I.*** Park City, UT: Family Resources Inc.

Compton, D.M., & Iso-Ahola, S.E. (1994). ***Leisure and mental health: Volume I.*** Park City, UT: Family Resources, Inc.

Docherty, J.P. (1993). One size fits all: Mental health care requires providers to find a good fit. ***Business Insurance, 27*** (5), 19.

Hall, E.G. (1994). Exercise and depression: Beyond physical fitness. In D. M. Compton & S.E. Iso-Ahola (Eds.), ***Leisure and mental health: Volume I.*** Park City, UT: Family Resources, Inc.

Hickey, J.S., & Baer, P.E. (1988). Psychological approaches to the assessment and treatment of anxiety and depression. ***Medical Clinics, 72***, 917-922.

Ineichen, B. (1979). ***Mental Illness***. London: Longman Group Limited.

Kalat, J. (1990). ***Introduction to psychology***. California: Wadsworth Publishing.

Mental Health Consumer Task Force. (1991). ***Mental health: Statements of rights and responsibilities***. Canberra, Australia: Australian Government Publishing Services.

Moon Hickman, C. (1994). Leisure counseling and depressed women. In D.M. Compton & S.E. Iso-Ahola (eds.), ***Leisure and Mental Health: Volume I.*** Park City, UT: Family Resources, Inc.

Nevid, J.S., Spencer, A.R., & Green, B. (1994). ***Abnormal psychology in a changing world.*** New Jersey: Prentice Hall, Inc.

Patrick, G. (1994). A role for leisure in treatment of depression. In D.M. Compton & S.E. Iso-Ahola (Eds.), ***Leisure and mental health: Volume I.*** Park City, UT: Family Resources, Inc.

Richter, D. (1984). ***Research in mental illness***. London: William Heineman Medical Books, Ltd.

Note: The authors would like to thank Karen Luken for her significant contributions to this chapter.

Other Sources of Information

National Mental Health Association
1021 Prince Street
Alexandria, VA 22314-2971
(703) 684-7722
Fax: (703) 684-5968

Mental Health Information Center 800/969-NMHA
TTY Line 800/433-5959
http://www.nmha.org/

National Mental Health Association
http://www.nmha.org/

National Consumer/Survivor
http://www.nasmhpd.org/ntac/

Related Websites

http://depression.cmhc.com/
(Disorders and Treatments—Depression)

http://www-hsl.mcmaster.ca/tomflem/depress.html
(Illness Health Care Information Resources—Depression Links)

http://www.schizophrenia.com/
(Schizophrenia.com)

http://www.well.com/user/tow/schizoph.htm
(Schizophrenia Resource Links Page)

http://www.adaa.org/
(Anxiety Disorders Association of America)

http://www.algy.com/anxiety/index.html
(The Anxiety Panic Internet Resource—Tapir)

http://www.aabainc.org./home.html
(American Anorexia Bulimia Association, Inc.)

http://www.kathy-on-the-edge.com/
(Eating Disorders Online)

http://www.nami.org/fact.htm
(National Alliance for the Mentally Ill)

http://hna.ffh.vic.gov.au/acmh/mh/mental_illnesses/stigma.htm
(What is Stigma?)

Section III

Chapter 13

Recreation Services

> Therefore as I said before, our children from the earliest years must take part in all the more lawful forms of play, for if they are not surrounded with such an atmosphere they can never grow up to be well conducted and virtuous citizens. — SOCRATES (420 B.C.)

Introduction

Recreation is a powerful force in everyone's life. It provides us pleasure. It gives us balance among the various parts of our lives. It revives and rejuvenates us. Many of our social relationships and friendships are made and maintained during our recreation involvement. No one wants that part of his life taken away. Recreation is something that most people take for granted. However, many people with disabilities do not have access to a full range of recreation opportunities. They still have the same needs, wants, and desires as anyone else, but for a number of reasons, they may not have access to recreation opportunities like everyone else. Some are denied this right because of a lack of skills or a lack of opportunities. Some do not have access to recreation because of a recent injury or psychological trauma that has left a permanent or temporary disabling condition. A lot of reasons exist for a person not to have the opportunity to enjoy a full and satisfying life, yet all people are entitled to the full benefits of citizenship, including all of its rights, privileges, opportunities, and responsibilities.

In this chapter we will look at both organizational and individual issues that encourage and inhibit access to recreation programs and services.

Statutory and Ethical Mandates

As we discussed in Chapter 6, providing recreation services for people with disabilities does not automatically mean that services provided are necessarily therapeutic recreation services. What is true is that all recreation *is* therapeutic, but that subject was dealt with in Chapter 6. To reiterate, most parks and recreation departments are mandated by their enabling legislation to provide recreation, not therapeutic recreation, services. We are not suggesting that therapeutic recreation services cannot and do not occur in public recreation services for people with disabilities; however, we want to reiterate our discussion of mandate for service.

We will start with the assumption that in public recreation departments the overriding mandate is for professionals to provide recreation services to all people, regardless of their level of disability. We will further assume that except in situations in which the mandate may be overridden or expanded by a contractual arrangement with a bona fide treatment agency, therapeutic recreation services do not occur in public recreation programs. Having established that public recreation providers must provide recreation (not therapeutic recreation) services, the question then becomes, "What kinds of recreation services must be provided and how are those services provided?"

The Americans with Disabilities Act (ADA) is very clear about the kinds of services that must be provided for people with disabilities. The ADA contains a ***most integrated setting*** concept:

> Essential to the ADA is the belief that services, programs, and activities shall be provided in the most integrated setting possible. The ADA does not oblige a parks and recreation department to guarantee successful participation, but an obligation does exist to provide equivalent opportunities. That obligation requires that the opportunity is first available in a purely integrated setting (McGovern, 1992, p. 15).

The ADA expects that inclusive services will be provided so that people with disabilities will have access to the same kinds of opportunities and choices as people without disabilities. But the ADA is equally clear that it does not prohibit or exclude segregated or specialized recreation services. It is also clear about when segregated recreation options are legitimate. A violation of the ADA occurs if an agency's segregated recreation programs and services are the only ones made available to people with disabilities (McGovern, 1992, p. 15). A local parks and recreation agency can have beginning guitar lessons for persons with severe mental retardation; however, if the agency requires that anyone with severe mental retardation who wants to take beginning guitar lessons has to do so in the segregated program and will not enroll him in a regular beginning guitar lesson, then the agency is in violation of the ADA. The thrust of the statute is that people with disabilities must have access to settings that enable interaction between people with and without disabilities to the maximum extent feasible. The ADA also clearly states that whatever supports and accommodations are needed to allow a person to successfully participate in community activities must be made. Later in this chapter we will discuss principles of adaptation and suggest ways in which accommodation might occur.

This position of most integrated or inclusive recreation opportunities for people with disabilities is reinforced by many people with disabilities, parents, and parent groups, and advocacy groups. The delegate body of the Arc (formerly the

Association of Retarded Citizens of the United States), one of the largest advocacy groups, adopted a position on inclusive recreation and leisure in 1992. Although their position relates to people with mental retardation, it is not unlike the positions of other major advocacy organizations. Their position statement is reprinted in Table 13.1.

Table 13.1
Inclusive Recreation and Leisure

Issue

People with mental retardation should have opportunities to participate in the same recreation and leisure activities that are offered to all citizens. Currently, most opportunities available are limited to segregated activities.

The presence of quality inclusive recreation and leisure activities in the community has a positive impact on all citizens in a number of ways:

1. People with disabilities have opportunities to interact with, and learn from, others who do not have disabilities. Peer interaction and modeling helps them develop appropriate social skills, self-esteem, and self-worth.
2. People with disabilities learn to use a wide array of recreation and leisure options used by other people in the community, which increases their participation in recreation activities, thus developing higher levels of physical fitness and energy.
3. Inclusive recreation options help people without disabilities learn that people, regardless of abilities, can participate if given an opportunity.
4. People with and without disabilities, interacting successfully in age-appropriate recreation and leisure activities, develop skills and attitudes needed to live harmoniously in communities.

Position

The Arc strongly supports the following:

1. Promoting recognition of the need for inclusive recreation and leisure activities as an essential component of quality of life for people with mental retardation.
2. Encouraging organizations currently providing segregated recreation and leisure activities to develop inclusive options.
3. Developing strategies and techniques to help people with mental retardation and their families make the transition to inclusive recreation and leisure activities, including competitive sports.
4. Identifying and expanding resources that facilitate inclusive recreation and leisure activities.
5. Promoting participation of people with mental retardation in organized recreation and leisure groups that are appropriate for their chronological age.

(Adopted by the delegate body of the Arc, October 1992)

On October 29, 1997, the Board of Directors of the National Therapeutic Recreation Society (NTRS) developed and subsequently approved the NTRS Position Statement on Inclusion providing principles so that recreation, park resources, and leisure services professionals and citizens can move toward inclusive lifestyles for individuals with disabilities. At the 1998 National Recreation and Park Association (NRPA) mid-year Forum in Washington D.C., the American Park and Recreation Society presented a resolution adopting the Position Statement on Inclusion. In early 1999, NTRS forwarded a resolution to the NRPA National Forum for consideration, resolving that the Position Statement on Inclusion be adopted by the entire NRPA organization. A copy of the resolution is included in Table 13.2

Table 13.2
NTRS Position Statement on Inclusion

Diversity is a cornerstone of our society and culture and thus should be celebrated. Including people with disabilities in the fabric of society strengthens the community and its individual members. The value of inclusive leisure experiences in enhancing the quality of life for all people, with and without disabilities, cannot be overstated. As we broaden our understanding and acceptance of differences among people through shared leisure experiences, we empower future generations to build a better place for all to live and thrive.

Inclusive leisure experiences encourage and enhance opportunities for people of varying abilities to participate and interact in life's activities together with dignity. It also provides an environment that promotes and fosters physical, social and psychological inclusion of people with diverse experiences and skill levels. Inclusion enhances individuals' potential for full and active participation in leisure activities and experiences. Additionally, the benefits of this participation may include:

- providing positive recreational experiences which contribute to the physical, mental, social, emotional, and spiritual growth and development of every individual;
- fostering peer and intergenerational relationships that allow one to share affection, support, companionship, and assistance; and
- developing community support and encouraging attitudinal changes to reflect dignity, self-respect, and involvement within the community.

Purpose

The purpose of the Position Statement on Inclusion is to encourage all providers of park, recreation, and leisure services to provide opportunities in settings where people of all abilities can recreate and interact together.

This document articulates a commitment to the leisure process and the desired outcomes. Accordingly, the Position Statement on Inclusion encompasses these broad concepts and beliefs:

Table 13.2 Cont.

Right to Leisure

- The pursuit of leisure is a condition necessary for human dignity and well-being.
- Leisure is a part of a healthy lifestyle and a productive life.
- Every individual is entitled to the opportunity to express unique interests and pursue, develop, and improve talents and abilities.
- People are entitled to opportunities and services in the most inclusive setting.
- The right to choose from the full array of recreation opportunities offered in diverse settings and environments and requiring different levels of competency should be provided.

Quality of Life

- People grow and develop throughout the life span.
- Through leisure an individual gains an enhanced sense of competence and self-direction.
- A healthy leisure lifestyle can prevent illness and promote wellness.
- The social connection with one's peers plays a major role in his/her life satisfaction.
- The opportunity to choose is an important component in one's quality of life; individual choices will be respected.

Support, Assistance and Accommodations

- Inclusion is most effective when support, assistance, and accommodations are provided.
- Support, assistance, and accommodations can and should be responsive to people's needs and preferences.
- Support, assistance and accommodations should create a safe and fun environment, remove real and artificial barriers to participation, and maximize not only the independence but also the interdependence of the individual. People want to be self-sufficient.
- Support, assistance, and accommodations may often vary and are typically individualized. Types of support, assistance, and accommodations include, but are not limited to: qualified staff, adaptive equipment, alternative formats for printed or audio materials, trained volunteers, or flexibility in policies and program rules.

Table 13.2 Cont.

Barrier Removal

- Environments should be designed to encourage social interaction, "risk-taking," fun, choices, and acceptance that allow for personal accomplishment in a cooperative context.
- Physical barriers should be eliminated to facilitate full participation by individuals with disabilities.
- Attitudinal barriers in all existing and future recreation services should be removed or minimized through eduction and training of personnel (staff, volunteers, students, and/or community at-large).

The National Therapeutic Recreation Society is dedicated to the four inclusion concepts of:

- Right to Leisure (for all individuals)
- Quality of Life (enhancements through leisure experiences)
- Support, Assistance, and Accommodations
- Barrier Removal

in all park, recreation and leisure services. Properly fostered, inclusion will happen naturally. Over time, inclusion will occur with little effort and with the priceless reward of an enlightened community. Encourage in the right way, inclusion is the right thing to plan for, implement, and celebrate.

Long before the ADA, there was an ethic of inclusiveness that was evident in North America. All citizens have the right to choose the ways in which they will participate in public life. The right is embedded in our law and our heritage. Providing *only* segregated recreation opportunities for people with disabilities violates this right. The responsibility of recreation service providers is to be sure that all citizens, whatever their abilities, are afforded an equal opportunity to participate in *all* recreational programs and to be as "non-special" as anyone else.

For equal opportunity to become a reality in recreation service provision, *full* physical and programmatic accessibility must be accomplished. A building cannot be the only place that is barrier free; programs must be barrier free as well. After a person gets into a recreation building, accommodations must be made in the recreation programs to allow and to encourage participation. Physical accessibility without programmatic accessibility is like letting someone in the door but not letting that person play. The situation is unthinkable, but it unintentionally happens all of the time. Programmatic accessibility without physical accessibility can mean continued separateness and exclusion even though federal legislation exists to ensure that opportunities are available in integrated settings.

Being sure that every person has equal opportunity to participate in a particular activity does not have to be a difficult, time-consuming task. The process is actually pretty simple. It is not unlike the process that any person goes through. The first step is to look at the ***particular activity*** as it is offered by a particular recreation agency and then to determine what kinds and levels of skills and capabilities are required to participate in that activity. The second step is to look at the ***specific individual*** who wants to participate and then to determine if that individual has the kinds and levels of skills and capabilities identified as necessary for participation. If the answer is yet, the program may already be accessible. If the answer is no, the activity may be made accessible through some kind of adaptation—either by the specific participant to compensate for a skill or capability deficit or by the activity itself—in a way that does not significantly affect the enjoyment and satisfaction of other participants.

Later in this chapter you will learn more about adaptation and accommodation. In the meantime, continue to think conceptually about integrated/inclusive recreation services versus special/segregated recreation services. Consider the example of the following paragraph.

Many recreation departments, as well as any other nonprofit recreation agencies, offer special (serrated) bridge programs for people with visual impairments. Yet, there is no good reason to offer a recreation program such as bridge strictly for people with visual impairments. People with visual impairments are just like other people when it comes to the game of bridge. Their capabilities in assessing their hands, bidding, figuring out what everybody else has, creating and following a strategy, and playing the game are as variable as a sighted person's. Their one disadvantage is their difficulty in identifying cards in their hands and cards played by sight. If an accommodation can be made to overcome this difficulty, such as using cards marked with Braille patterns, the game itself can be played by two people who are visually impaired and two sighted people, by three sighted people and one person who is visually impaired, and so on. Assuming physical accessibility is not a problem, the addition of Braille playing cards easily makes this bridge program programmatically accessible.

You might be thinking, "But what if people with visual impairments want to play bridge with other people with visual impairments?" The concepts of inclusion and programmatic accessibility do not ignore personal choice. In fact, they strengthen personal choice by giving people more options. Inclusion and programmatic accessibility do not preclude people with visual impairments playing bridge with people without visual impairments. In fact, it specifically allows for accommodations to be made so that people of varying abilities can participate in the same activity.

Besides being legislatively mandated, making programs accessible to people with disabilities has both social and practical benefits. It encourages the assimilation of people with disabilities into the mainstream of society and discourages their isolation and exclusion. Making programs accessible to all people may also reduce the need for dedicating resources to special, segregated programs and can increase participation (and possible revenue) in regular programs without additional expenses. In these days of fiscal austerity and increased accountability, this is indeed attractive. However, the primary reason for making recreation programs fully accessible is the basic right of all people to be judged according to their capabilities, not their disabilities—their rights to be included in all aspects of public life and to have fun like anybody else.

Before moving to segregated versus inclusive recreation services, we should look at what currently occurs in most public or quasi-public recreation services for people with disabilities. First, we will look at ways organizations are structured.

Organizational Structures

The ways organizations are structured can either encourage or discourage the provision of inclusive recreation services. The way that a department organizes its services in large measure determines the extent of inclusive or segregated services. Following are three examples of structures of parks and recreation departments (Figures 13.1, 13.2, and 13.3). These three examples represent three types of services to people with disabilities. Take a look at Figure 13.1.

Figure 13.1 provides an example of the most prevalent type of organizational structure with respect to services to people with disabilities. This particular structure provides a special section for people with disabilities. The specialized services are called different things by different agencies. In some states and provinces, this special section is called the special populations' division; in others, it may be called the adaptive services division; still others call it the therapeutic recreation division (even though we have argued that to call a public recreation program for people with disabilities that name is confusing and often inaccurate). Whatever it is called, the special section denotes a special program unit that is devoted specifically, and usually exclusively, to the provision of recreation services to people with disabilities.

When you look at Figure 13.1, what do you see? As you study it, you will see a separate section for specialized services (special pops/TR). There are two obvious concerns with this type of organizational structure:

1. The *title* of the special pops/TR specialist stands out from the other specialists. The other three are identified by activity areas while the special pops/TR specialist is identified by the people served. This emphasizes the differences and implicitly advertises, "We are the ones who provide recreation services to people with disabilities." This type of organizational structure sets up an ***us and them*** mentality among the staff. The way this organization is structured encourages separateness and discourages interaction between people with and without disabilities.
2. Although not shown on Figure 13.1, the other concern relates to ***duplication of program offerings.*** One would assume that within the special pops/TR division, there are the usual program offerings that include art and crafts, athletics, and outdoor/nature programs, among others. As you look at Figure 13.1, you will see that there are already program offerings that include arts and crafts, athletics, and outdoor/nature program. By having a specialized section that provides a similar array of services to people with disabilities, there is duplication, and potentially costly duplication.

Figure 13.1
Organized Structure - 1

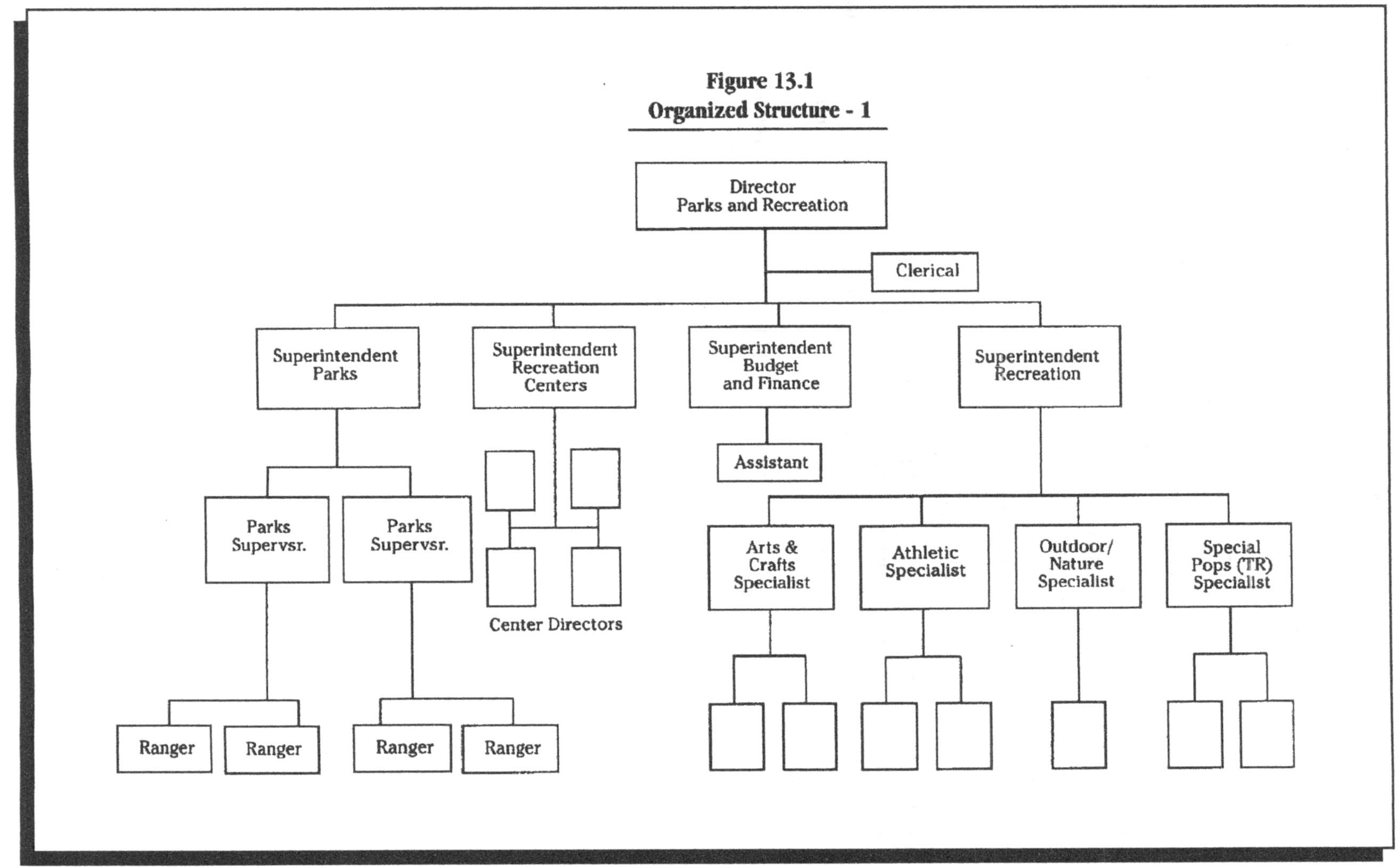

Other structures also inhibit access to regular recreation, though less than the first example (Figure 13.1). Take a look at Figure 13.2. How is it different from Figure 13.1?

Figure 13.2 represents a move from the most separate, segregated organizational structure to a structure that by design is less separate. The second example (Figure 13.2) does not organize programs for people with disabilities only with other people with disabilities. This organizational structure organizes specialized services by activity. As such, potential duplication could be avoided. Although this structure clearly has a place for special or segregated programs, an entire separate unit is not devoted to programs for people with disabilities. As such, this particular structure can fairly easily allow for segregated and inclusive services. That is, since the special program are located within activity units, it would be easy, especially for persons who are higher functioning, to be integrated and included in other levels of activities within that unit.

For example, if a person with Down syndrome was included in a special section of beginning swimming for people with mental retardation, but was found to be a good swimmer, moving that person into a regular beginning or intermediate swim class would be easy. The reason it would be easier in this structure than in the first is that the second structure is organized by activity, including people with disabilities; as discussed above, duplication and lack of articulation among units is structurally built into Figure 13.1.

One main difference in the structure in Figure 13.2 is that the ***special population staff*** report to a program/content specialist and not to a coordinator of specialized programs. Although a better alternative than the first example, some concerns about Figure 13.2 still exist. For example:

1. There is still a specialist in this model who provides services to people with disabilities. It is still easy for the "nonspecial" recreator staff in this particular unit to abdicate their responsibility to provide programs for all people. In this particular unit, it is easy for them to say, "Put them in Jackie's program; she takes all the people with disabilities."
2. As mentioned before, there are, however, more opportunities for inclusion into regular existing programs, especially for the higher functioning person. The danger is that recreation staff will start drawing lines relative to who can and who cannot be included into regular programs. In other words, regular recreation staff might say, "Josh is too disabled to be included." Typically such judgments are not based on what types of adaptations or accommodations might be able to be made; rather, they are often based on perceptions about a particular disability. This stereotyping, although often unintentional, further discourages participation into programs of choice by all people.

The third organizational structure provides more access and encourages more participation into regular recreation programs than the first two examples (Figures 13.1 and 13.2). Take a look at Figure 13.3. How is it different from 13.2?

Figure 13.3 represents the most inclusive model because it has no specialized section nor are there specialized staff devoted to specialized services within a particular unit. Figure 13.3's recreation staff, which is often specialized recreation

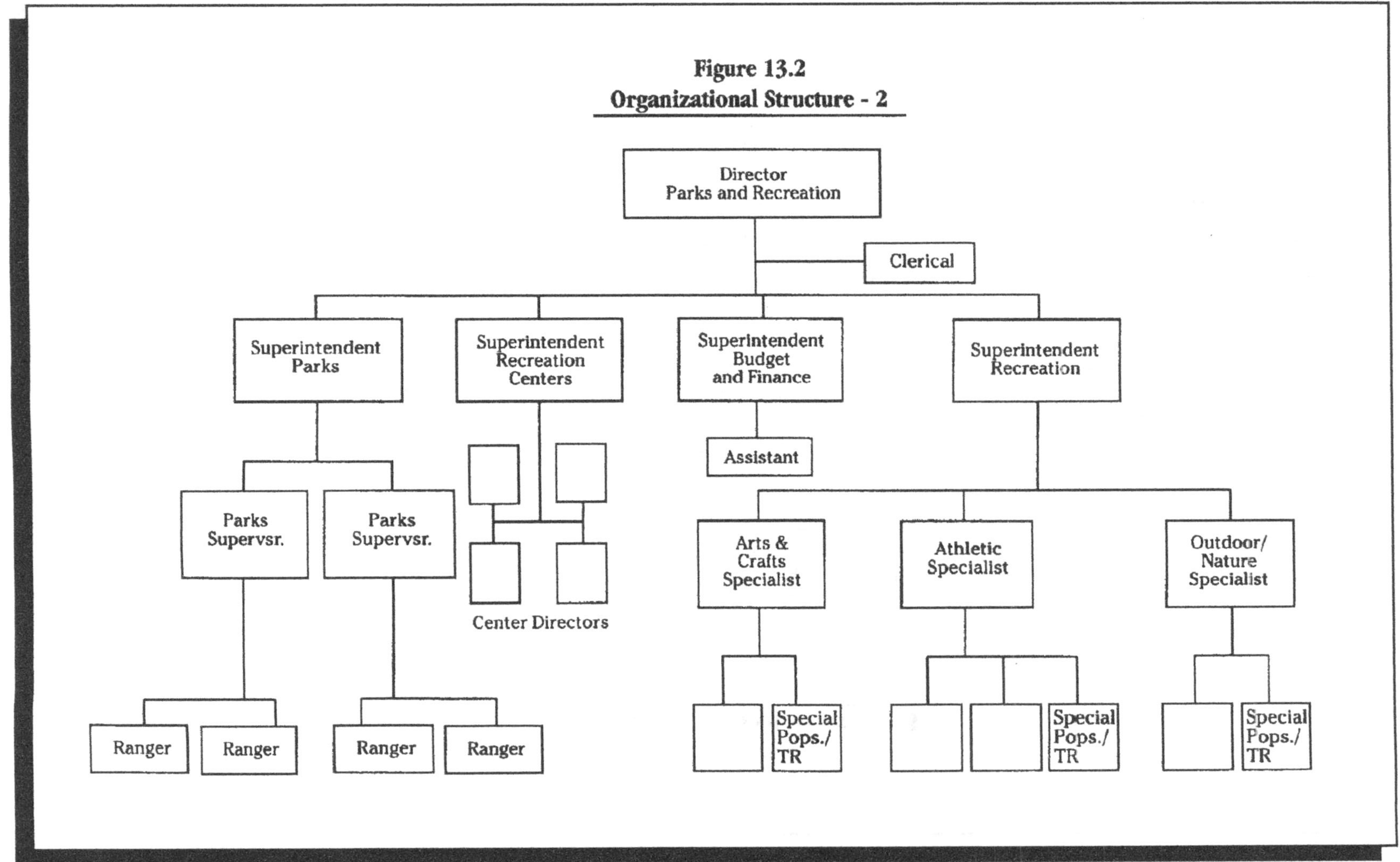

Figure 13.2
Organizational Structure - 2

Figure 13.3
Organizational Structure - 3

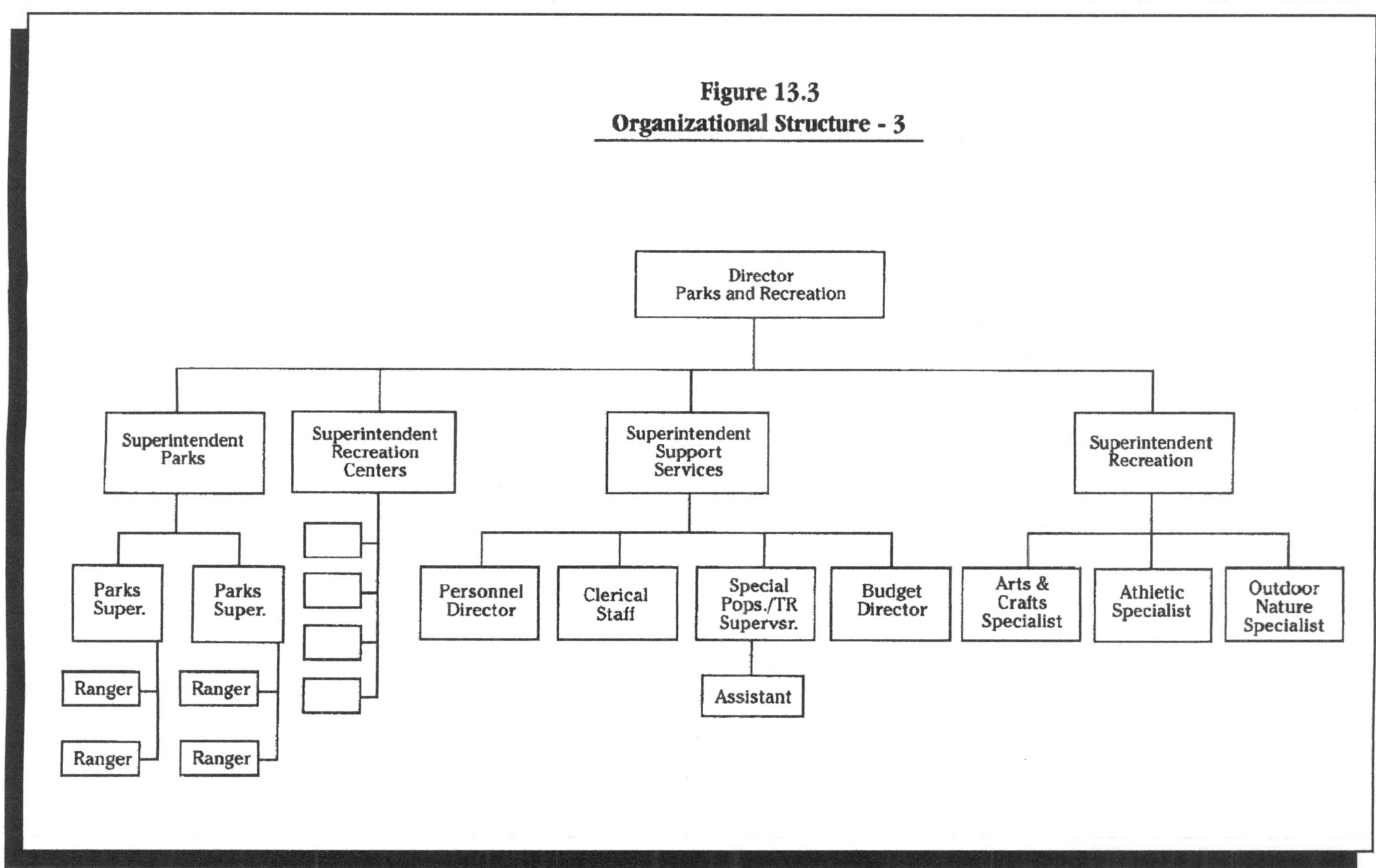

staff with therapeutic recreation training, provide support services that re needed to assist in the inclusion process. Special populations' staff are available to assist the regular recreation staff in training, consultation, or even direct service. This model assumes that the general recreation staff, not a specialized staff, are the ones responsible for providing recreation services to people with disabilities. Few recreation agencies are set up this way. This is an organizational structure that discourages segregated services and sets up a situation in which people with disabilities are not assumed to need special programs; rather, they are assumed to need possible accommodations to allow them to participate in regular programs. The special populations' staff serve more as advocates than a direct service providers. This structure can cause problems, however. For example:

1. Regular recreation staff see the specialists not providing services to people with disabilities. In that case, resentments could easily arise. Training must be provided to regular recreation staff so that they will understand that people with disabilities have the same wants and needs as people without disabilities, and that with a little creative thinking, many people with disabilities can be included into regular programs. Training must, however, be ongoing so that the best interests of people with disabilities are served.
2. Another concern is for the special populations staff, who have for many years provided services to people with disabilities. They begin to question their worth when someone says specialists are not needed. Many of these specialized staff also truly believe that people with disabilities, (especially people with severe disabilities), will not receive quality recreation services by regular staff. As such, some of the specialized staff might sabotage the change. Training for this staff is essential.
3. The other concern is a fiscal one. When there was a special unit, funding was designated to people who were provided recreation services within that unit. In a model like this one, where recreation services are provided by the activity staff (i.e., swimming is provided by aquatics staff and not by special populations' staff), fear emerges that the funds that heretofore were designated for people with disabilities will not be redistricted among the other units. Again, ongoing training and awareness are needed to ensure that not only staff but also funds are available to facilitate adaptations and/or accommodations.

With some sense of how organizations operate, we will discuss both segregated and inclusive services. Because of the ADA and the sentiment among most people with disabilities about the importance of opportunities for inclusion, we will pay more attention to ways people with disabilities can be included into regular programs. The following section will discuss the process of full program accessibility.

From Deinstitutionalization to Programmatic Access

In Chapter 2 we discussed the move toward deinstitutionalization, where people with disabilities were moved from institutional and restrictive environments to hopefully more inclusive communities. The intent was that people with disabilities would be able to achieve a standard of living commensurate with same-age peers who do not possess disabilities. Scheerenberer (1987) describes what deinstitutionalization is supposed to be. He suggests that it is about seeking greater emphasis of freedom, independence, individuality, mobility, personalized life experience, and a higher degree of interaction in a free society. Baroff (1986) reminds us however that "although for at least a decade our rhetoric has called for deinstitutionalizing persons with disabilities and the creation of community-based services, the development of these services has lagged behind this rhetoric." One area that lagged particularly far behind was recreation, even though individuals with disabilities (and particularly severe disabilities) have an excess of free time (Burke & Cohen, 1977; Stanfield, 1973; Wehman & Moon, 1985), and typically may not use time in constructive ways (Sternberg & Adams, 1982; Wehman & Schleien, 1981). As a result, a number of special recreation programs began in the 1960s and 1970s. Not surprisingly, the first programs were in large cities where there were larger population bases. Fewer offerings were found in smaller towns at first, but over time programs began in smaller towns, often with volunteers serving as leaders. The model that began with those first programs is still largely the same. Some changes have occurred; however, most programs are still mostly special programs for people with disabilities. Some offer a type of ***reverse mainstreaming***, where people without disabilities are invited to join the special programs. Some offer opportunities in regular programs, but are often only for the higher functioning people with disabilities. The process of full programmatic accessibility is a process in which recreators ask *how* a particular person with a disability can participate and not *if*. A discussion of the process and some of its inherent implications follows.

Achieving Full Programmatic Accessibility

The achievement of full programmatic accessibility in recreation and leisure services can seem to be an enormous task. The most obvious and common question is "Where do I start?" The most productive point to begin your efforts toward accessibility in recreation programming is with specific participants and the activities in which they want to participate. This is consistent with the person-centered approach that has been advocated throughout this book. This approach assures the immediate relevance of your efforts and also prevents the implementation of large-scale changes in programming that realistically may not be called for. It will encourage you and you staff to program specific activities according to the desires and capabilities of the population you serve.

The following process will help you to figure out how specific recreation opportunities can be made accessible to any individual who wants to participate in them. This process is relatively simple, but it requires a willingness to look closely at your programs and to ask people questions about what they can, cannot, and might do. An enthusiastic, imaginative, problem-solving approach towards achieving accessibility in recreation programming is an indispensable asset when attempting to achieve programmatic access. The ultimate goal is to define the form of a specific recreational activity that will be equally accessible to all those who desire to participate and that will provide all participants with the greatest possible satisfaction and enjoyment.

The three key elements of this process are the participant profile, the activity profile, and adaptation. Working on these elements can be considered as three separate and distinct tasks, each of which will provide you with valuable information in its own right. However, the key to the problem of determining how accessibility can be achieved is to consider each of these elements as a component in the larger process—a process requiring constant attention to the ways in which its components are interrelated.

This process as a whole will lead you to a description of the ideal form of any leisure activity—the form that will facilitate the inclusion of all those who wish to participate.

Participant Profile

How should the recreation provider determine how a particular individual will be able to participate in a particular activity? Not many recreation professionals are qualified to make this determination based on a thorough assessment of physiological and psychological data. Even if they were qualified, is gathering such data and performing such an assessment within the right and/or responsibility of the recreation professional? We maintain that it is not.

We do, however, feel that it is appropriate for the recreation service provider to help individuals determine how they can participate within the recreation agency environment in specific activities they choose, whether or not those individuals have disabilities.

The participant profile (Figure 13.4) is a means of encouraging the recreation professional to look at the skills and capabilities of participants with disabilities as these skills and capabilities are related to a specific activity in which they want to participate.

It consists of a number of questions related to the skills and capabilities required for participation in an activity that he has selected. As is also evident in Figure 13.4, the activity profile is an important part of the participant profile. In order for the participant to make a decision about whether he will participate in a given activity, an activity profile must be completed. This process is discussed in detail in the next section.

Activity Profile

Determining the eligibility of a person or a group for participation in a specific activity, based on competence, is a familiar practice in recreation. The general procedure is to define some criteria for the activity that must be met by any individual who seeks to participate. For example, prospective participants must be able to swim 100 yards before gaining eligibility for a beginning water skiing class.

The activity profile is a method of applying this practice to *all* activities, not only specifically defining the skills and capabilities required for participation but also pointing out several other characteristics of the activity that will help to find

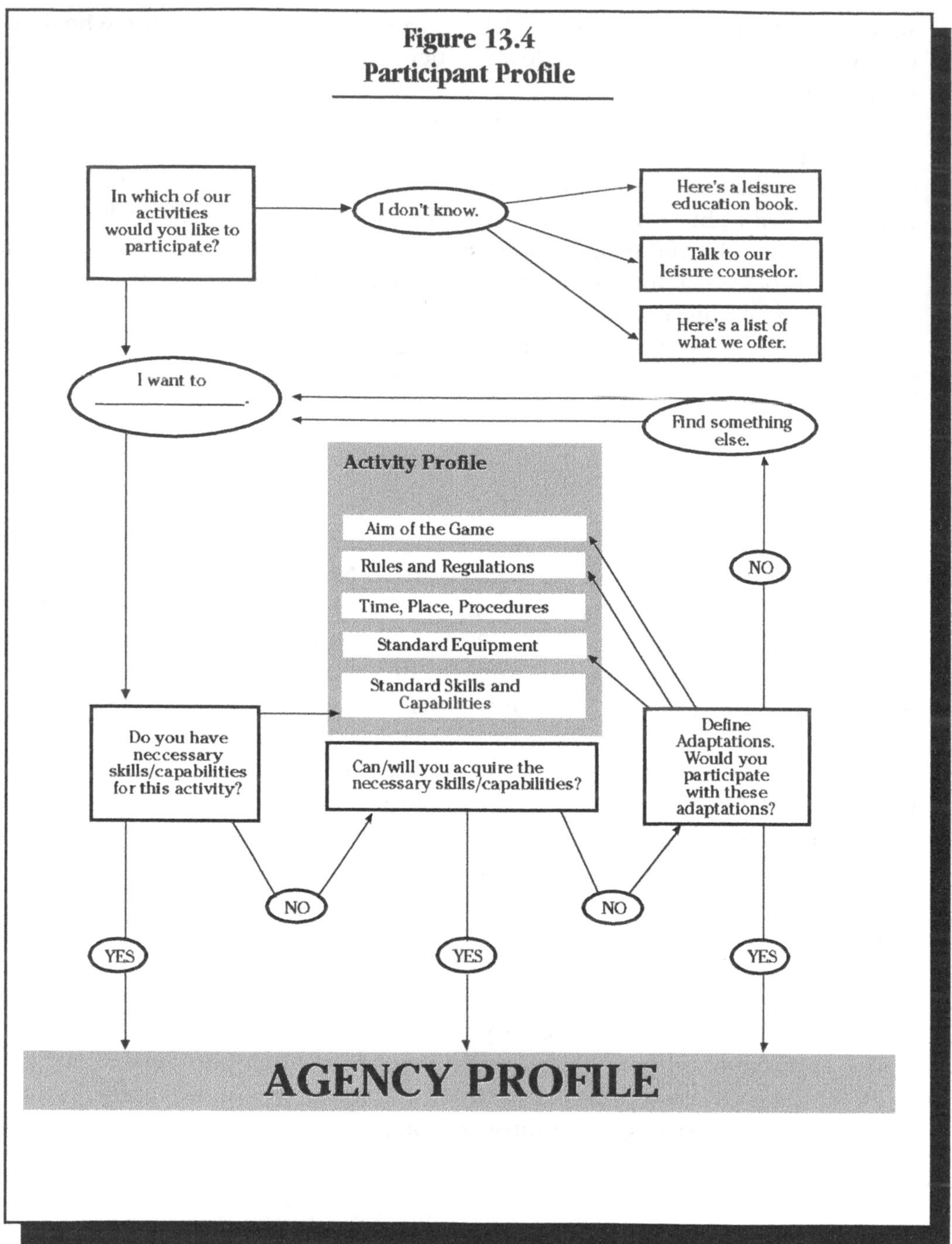

appropriate adaptations, if necessary, and to recognize subtle barriers to equal access, if and when they exist. Knowledge of all of these characteristics is essential reference material in completing a useful participant profile.

To many people, literally defining some of the more fundamental characteristics of an activity will seem an exercise in simplistic thinking. You will discover that it is not as simple as it seems, and that you will have problems deciding when

Figure 13.5
Activity Profile

 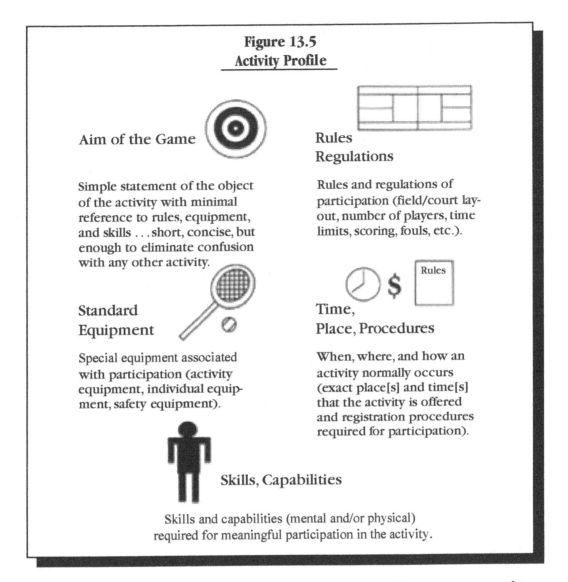

Aim of the Game

Simple statement of the object of the activity with minimal reference to rules, equipment, and skills . . . short, concise, but enough to eliminate confusion with any other activity.

Rules
Regulations

Rules and regulations of participation (field/court lay-out, number of players, time limits, scoring, fouls, etc.).

Standard
Equipment

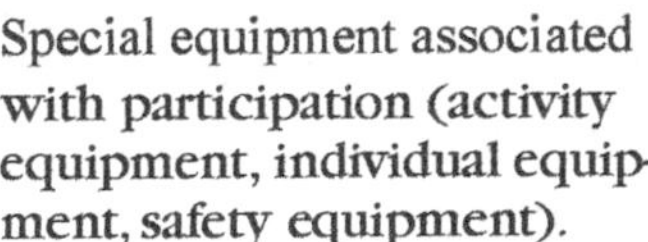

Special equipment associated with participation (activity equipment, individual equip-ment, safety equipment).

Time,
Place, Procedures

When, where, and how an activity normally occurs (exact place[s] and time[s] that the activity is offered and registration procedures required for participation).

Skills, Capabilities

Skills and capabilities (mental and/or physical) required for meaningful participation in the activity.

to stop defining. That is OK. The important aspects are to make an attempt and to be sure that the definitions you derive are based exclusively on an examination of the activity. Later, it will become clear how examining activities in the light of these characteristics will be of substantial value if some sort of adaptation is necessary to interest or include specific individuals or groups who might otherwise not have had the opportunity to participate.

You will find the six major characteristics of Figure 13.5 listed below with a short definition. Remember, when you profile a given activity, you are considering that activity as it is typically offered in a recreation agency. Now refer back to Figure 13.5.

1. *Aim of the Game* is the simplest possible statement of the object of the activity with minimal reference to rules, equipment, and skills generally used in participation. Such a statement should be as short and concise as possible, yet still be sufficiently descriptive to eliminate the possibility of confusion with any other activity.

2. ***Rules and Regulations*** are a listing of the rules and regulations, if any, that are generally associated with participation in the activity as you offer it. This may include such considerations as field/court playout, number of players, time limits, scoring, fouls, and playing procedures. If there is a readily available book or list of rules, refer to this.
3. ***Time, Place, and Procedures*** are considerations of when, where, and how the activity normally occurs in the organization. It tells the exact place or places where it will be offered, the times the activity is offered, the time frame within which it occurs, and the registration procedures required for participation.
4. ***Standard Equipment*** is a listing of the special equipment associated with participation in the activity. Such equipment can usually be classified in one of three categories: activity equipment, individual equipment, and safety equipment.
5. ***Standard Skills*** is a listing of the skills (and levels of competence, if applicable) usually required for meaningful participation in the activity. The term skills here implies physical and/or mental processes related to the accomplishment of some goal.
6. ***Standard Physical and Mental Capabilities*** are listings of the physical and/or mental capabilities not directly related to the performance of skills that are generally required by participants in the activity (e.g., stamina, strength, coordination, sight, hearing, dexterity, concentration).

Example 1
Recreational Swimming

Aim of the game:

- To propel self through the water from one point to another.

Rules and regulations:

- Pool rules
- Time factors
- No impeding others

Time, place, and procedures:

- Place: Community Center pool, downtown
- Time: Tuesdays/Thursdays, 3-7 p.m.
- Duration: Open hours
- Fee: $15 month
- Registration: In person at Center

Standard equipment:

- None

Standard skills:

- Beginning to advanced: Staying afloat for 5 minutes, stroking with arms, kicking with arms, kicking with legs, rhythmic breathing

Standard capabilities:

- Some stamina
- Some coordination

Example 2
Baseball (Adult League Play)

Aim of the game:

- To score runs by safely progressing from 1st to 2nd to 3rd and finally to home base, usually either after striking a baseball with a bat into the field of play or after a teammate has struck the ball.

Rules and regulations:

- See official Baseball Rules
- General rules: Four bases and out-of-bounds lines; 3 outs per inning; 4 balls and 3 strikes per at bat; 9 people per team; out when either batted ball caught on the fly, 3 strikes tagged with ball off base, or thrown out.

Time, place and procedure

- Place: Beal Park Athletic Field, outside of town
- Time: Saturday evenings, 6-10 p.m., in summer
- Duration: About 2 hours per game.
- Fee: $150 per team
- Registration: By mail with check

Standard equipment:

- Activity: Bats, ball, bases
- Individual: Glove
- Safety: Catcher's gear, helmets

Standard skills:

- Moderate to advanced: Running, throwing a ball, catching a ball, hitting a ball with a bat

Standard capabilities:

- Sight
- Some strength
- Understanding of rules
- Judgment (when to hit, run, stop, etc.)
- Moderate concentration

Adaptation

Sometimes in order to be able to participant in a game, sport, or activity, we must make necessary adaptations (refer back to Participant Profile, Figure 13.4). All of us use adaptations at some time and in some form to maximize success and to compensate for personal limitations. For example, choking up on a baseball bat enables us to compensate for limited strength and yet still be able to swing the bat smoothly. We may purchase a tennis racket with a smaller than normal grip to compensate for small hands. We may hit two balls off the tee and play the best ball to compensate for a weakness in our driving expertise.

Simple adaptations such as these allow us to achieve both a skill level required to take part in the activity and a feeling of success that keeps us interested and involved. Adaptation in recreation and sport to accommodate people with disabilities in particular functions is a time-honored tradition.

Consider the designated hitter in the American Baseball League. This is the addition of another player, a tenth player in a nine-player game, to accommodate for the fact that pitchers are typically not good hitters.

Consider the 3-point shot in basketball, implemented at least in part to accommodate for the fact that many players (usually under 6'5") do not have the inside moves to compete around the basket.

Consider the enlarged head of many contemporary tennis rackets, made to accommodate for the fact that, for most of us, the old size just was not big enough to hit that little tiny ball.

All of these adaptations were made for people who have deficiencies in specific skills. We adapt all the time. There is no reason to treat people with non-remediable skill deficiencies any differently if we care about their right to enjoy recreation and sport activities. The fact that such deficiencies may be the result of a physical or mental disability is inconsequential. The goal is participation. The means to get there may be adaptation—creative, resourceful adaptation.

When considering adaptation as a means to participation, it is interesting to look at the common adaptations we mentioned before in terms of their impact on the activities within which they were made. Let us look at the three previous examples:

The designated hitter required a significant change in the rules of baseball participation. Only the American League would accept those changes. The National League claimed the change perverted the game of baseball. At World Series time, when teams from one league finally play those from another, dissension and controversy always arise over the designated hitter rule.

The 3-point shot in basketball is also controversial in both the professional and college ranks. Is this adaptation good for the sport or does it so change the rules that the fundamental nature of the game is affected? The debate continues.

On the other hand, the enlarged tennis racket head does not seem to have bothered anybody very much. That is because it does not alter the game of tennis as we know it ***and*** it does not affect anybody else's game very much. All that really changes is that, maybe, the ball is coming back over the net more often.

The same two principles affirming the use of the enlarged racket head also apply in affirming the use of adaptation as a strategy for including people with disabilities in recreation activities. First, the more extensive an adaptation, the greater the chance that it will significantly affect the basic nature of the activity; the activity may then no longer provide the same kind or level of benefits to the participant. Second, the more an adaptation for one participant affects other participants, the more difficult it will be to implement.

Only adapt when necessary and only as much as necessary. Look for adaptations that apply specifically to the required skills and capabilities that the person with a disability lacks, and only adapt enough to allow participation by that person. Avoid the often-used adaptational theory known as the lowest common denominator approach, as exemplified in the following scenario:

> Today we are going to play baseball. Regular rules apply except there will be no curve balls allowed because Arnie, Beth, and Charley cannot hit them. Also there is no stealing...our catcher, Dave, has a sore arm. Hits to right field have to be on the ground because Eunice does not like fly balls. Oh, and Fred has asked that he only be tagged on the legs; he has a bad sunburn. Gloria has to bat cross-handed and run the bases blindfolded because of those four homeruns she hit last game. Because Harry argues so much, we will be flipping a coin on all close calls. Oh, and we will not be using third base because Inga and Jerry do not like being stranded there. Remember the rules and have fun!

Extensive adaptation may be necessary for some people to participate in some activities, but do not make assumptions before you look at particular person/activity combinations. Examine the skills and capabilities required by the activity, the skills and capabilities that the person possesses, and if a match is not there, look at ways you can include that person in the activity with the *least* amount of adaptation.

Three basic forms of adaptations exist, as illustrated by the three examples mentioned earlier:

1. ***Find, create, or modify equipment*** or add an assistive device that allows a person to accomplish a skill or compensate for lack of a capability (the tennis racket).
2. ***Change the method*** by which the individual accomplishes or performs a skill (the designated hitter).
3. ***Change the rules or procedures*** to allow modification of the lacking skill, elimination of that skill or capability as a necessity for participation, or the addition of an alternative skill for all participants involved in the activity (the 3-point shot).

Using adaptations for individuals and activities in the first two forms mentioned above is usually simpler than the third because the changes involved are less likely to have a significant effect on any other people who take part in the activity or on the essential nature of the activity. For example, if a person in a photography class uses a special camera mount attached to his wheelchair, this has no impact on the participation and enjoyment of other people in that class. If a person with one arm has adapted by throwing and catching well with that arm, doing so will not have an impact on the other members of a softball team. However, if a basketball goal is lowered from 10 to 8 feet to accommodate one person's disability (an example of the third form of adaptation), this will have significant impact on other players without disabilities.

Often, professionals, family, or friends can develop or modify equipment for an individual. Some examples of finding, creating, or modifying equipment include the following:

- automatic fishing reels,
- swimming flotation devices,
- hand propelled tricycles and bicycles,
- built-up handles on paint brushes, ceramic tools, etc.
- closed-captioned videotapes,
- Braille playing cards,
- bowling ramps,
- handle-grip bowling balls,
- bowling guide rails,
- outrigger snow skis,
- nerf and foam balls, and
- built-up handles on pinball and video games.

Many suppliers provide adaptive recreation equipment and assistive devices. Some of the best adapted equipment or adapted devices are homemade and not necessarily widely available. Remember, each person is unique and may need something slightly different to meet personal needs.

The second form of adaptation—changing the method by which a person accomplishes a skill—can be approached in two basic ways. First, a substitute or alternative method can be used, such as follows:

- tossing an underhand rather than an overhead tennis serve,
- painting with a brush held in the toes or teeth,
- feeling to identify the location of paints, glazes, and supplies,
- using both hands to roll a bowling ball, or
- seeing a leader demonstrate directions rather than just hearing them.

A second way of changing the method of accomplishing the skill is through additional cues or assistance provided by the leader coach, or instructor, this method might also include paring a participant with a partner, volunteer, or friend. Some examples of this kind of adaptation are as follows:

- both raising a hand and blowing a whistle as a signal by the referee, coach, or leader,
- both pointing and saying left and right,

- both demonstrating and describing movements, skills, and techniques,
- having partners give verbal cues for people who are blind when skiing or running,
- interpreting for people who are deaf at instructional classes, plays, and lectures, and/or
- having companions give assistance in arts, crafts, exercise, and dance class, and at Scout troops, clubs, and other activities.

Companions, peer tutors, or friends can enhance the opportunities for participation of people with disabilities—even those with severe disabilities. Assistants can promote the acquisition of social skills required in a recreation setting, can facilitate the learning of skills needed to participate more fully, or can provide the opportunity for partial participation by those people whose disabilities preclude involvement without assistance.

The third form of adaptation involves changing the rules or procedures to allow modification or elimination of a skill or capability, or substituting an alternative skill for all participants involved in the activity. This form of adaptation is the most likely to affect the nature of an activity and other participants but is also a powerful tool in the philosophy of inclusion. Some examples include the following:

- allowing an additional bounce (ping-pong, tennis),
- increasing or decreasing the number of players on a team,
- providing an extra turn or chance (4 strikes in baseball, first ball in for a tennis serve),
- standing closer to a dart board, horseshoe pit, or bowling pins,
- adjusting the size of the playing area or boundaries (shorten distance between bases, make court size smaller, lower the net, make the goal larger), and/or
- using a different body position (sitting rather than standing, lying down rather than sitting).

Changes in rules or procedures may also be required to allow for adaptations in the forms mentioned earlier, using adaptive equipment and assistive devices or changing the method by which a person accomplishes a skill. For example, a procedural change may need to be made to allow someone in a wheelchair to participate in a 10K run or to allow an assistant to be on a softball field with a person who is severely mentally retarded, even if the assistant does not directly participate.

The key to a successful adaptation is remembering that it may be the only means to a meaningful recreation participation by people with disabilities. Use common sense, ingenuity, flexibility, and sensitivity as you use adaptation as a tool for including everyone in recreation activities.

Other Organizational Issues

Once recreation staff know the processes described above, individual access is much less problematic. There are, however, several organizational issues other than organizational structure that are important. They include advertising, participant fees and charges, transportation, legal liability, training, and use of volunteers. All of these issues will be discussed in the following pages.

Advertising

Any organization trying to achieve full accessibility must give careful consideration to the ways in which the organization communicates with the community (e.g., information, publicity, and advertising) and the ways the community communicates with the organization (methods and procedures used by the public to contact and interact with the organization). Since theses two kinds of communication usually precede actual participation in specific programs and could preclude the participation of some citizen groups, the recreation organization should consider the nature of its communication policies and procedures a critical precondition for full access by the community to recreation programs and facilities.

Methods and Procedures

Individuals with disabilities represent important markets within the service area of your agency. Some persons with disabilities rely on alternate forms of communicating (i.e., large print, Braille, audio cassette, captioned television, sign language). Therefore, publicity and other materials must be offered in various forms:

1. **What are the various methods by which people with disabilities get information about recreation organizations?**
   - Determining the range of media by which people receive information is a standard advertising technique and is always worthwhile in designing a strategy for getting information to specific target populations. When *you* do it, however, look beyond the specific media outlets, such as WXXX radio, KYYY and KZZZ-TV, the *Daily Gazette,* etc. Examine the generic media possibilities (e.g., radio, newspapers, TV, direct mail, etc.) with reference to their accessibility to all populations, especially people with disabilities in the main disability groups discussed in section two. Make a list of primary method(s) by which people with these disabilities find out about agencies like yours and programs like the ones you offer. It is a good bet that most recreation agencies do not use the alternative forms of communicating/marketing mentioned above, to the extent that they are *not* providing true programmatic accessibility.

The Message

The methods and procedures used to advertise are important but not as important as the message. Identifying problems with the ***message*** that is contained in the publicity, advertising, and public relations' activity is essential. It is the content and tone of this message in a wide variety of forms that largely determine whether people with various kinds of disabilities will feel welcome.

As we discussed in Chapter 1, the words used to describe people often influence behavior and self-perceptions and are a reflection of general attitudes. In order to avoid perpetuation of the potential negative effects of a "self-fulfilling prophecy," efforts should be made to represent programs and the groups to be served in a positive way. Non-stigmatizing advertising and publicity will promote acceptance and positive self-images and are important elements in achieving access.

1. **What general guidelines for advertising/publicity should be followed?**
   - Use terms that will identify potential participants as capable of participating in community life as fully equal members. Avoid terms perpetuating negative stereotypes—portraying any individuals as dependent or pitied.
   - Use the symbol of accessibility and the international symbol for the deaf on all printed materials to indicate which events, activities, or facilities are accessible and the types of support services offered (i.e., sign language staff, loop systems).
   - Include a phone number (and a TDD number) to be called for more information in all publicity and advertising.
   - In advertising and registration materials, include photographs of individuals with disabilities participating on an equal basis with individuals without disabilities.
   - Use a format for registration that promotes access for all.

Registration and programs listing materials may be designed in a way that subtly discourages people with disabilities from seeking to participate in nonspecial programs. Some agencies publish information about programs for "special populations" or "the handicapped" in a separate section of the general program brochures and publicity materials. Other agencies publish separate brochures and materials for "special populations" that may be the only information that people with disabilities receive about the agency's programs.

One possibility for including information about special programs in regular publicity materials is to place it with information about programs of the same classification. For example, a roller skating program designed to teach skills to people who are mentally retarded could be placed under the "athletics" or "sports" section of publicity materials. The description of the program could indicate that it is a developmental or beginning offering for people who may need a slower pace of instruction with special assistance.

After the Publicity

Let us assume that the people you are trying to reach have somehow found out about what you have to offer and are interested in participating in one or more of your programs. Their next step is to get in touch with you, to ask questions, to get clarification and further information, and to apply and register for specific programs and activities.

This is a critical step in ensuring accessibility for people with disabilities. People with hearing impairments may not use the telephone to speak to you about program, although they can use a relay system which is available in all states and provinces. Or they may use a TDD, a telecommunication device for the deaf that has a keyboard and enables people with hearing impairments to communicate over the telephone, if the agency has a TDD available. People with visual impairments might have a problem with written registration information that is sent through the mail. People with cognitive impairments might have a problem with written registration information that is sent through the mail. People with cognitive impairments may have difficulty following directions to registering.

Participant Fees and Charges

Some people with disabilities have limited discretionary funds to spend on recreation activity participation. Low pay, lack of employment, and greater expenses for adapted or specialized equipment (i.e., hearing aids, communications boards, wheelchairs) are often contributing factors. Fees and charges for class participation and facility use may prevent some people with disabilities from taking part in opportunities offered by an agency.

Whether to reduce or eliminate fees for people with disabilities poses a dilemma for the recreation professional committed to offering access. If people with disabilities are to participate in programs with everyone else, should they be given "special" treatment? On the opposite side, without some special consideration in terms of fees and charges, participation by certain individuals with disabilities may not be possible. Consider the following questions that need to be asked and answered:

1. **Should a recreation agency develop a policy to allow people with limited financial resources to participate in programs?**
    - Check with administrative staff to find out if special funds are available for individuals who need assistance or if procedure for waiving fees exist. Some agencies that offer special or therapeutic recreation programs set lower fees for these programs than for other agency activities. Such a practice encourages those individuals with limited finances to remain in segregated programs. Perhaps the same lower fee can be set for all programs in the same category and certain individuals with disabilities can participate regular programs at the fee charged for the special program.
2. **What other actions can you take to enable people with disabilities with limited finances to have access to programs?**

- If no organization solutions have been developed, eliminate or reduce fees for your programs based on certain criteria that you establish. This could involve the design of some type of sliding fee scale for all participants. Some agencies allow people with disabilities to donate their services to the agency in exchange for program fees.
- Set up scholarship fund for people needing assistance. A fund raising project or a solicitation of community groups could raise money to begin such a fund.
- Recruit civic clubs, churches, or corporations to sponsor a specific individual(s). Sponsors could assist with activity fees and could provide volunteer assistance, if required.
- Secure donations of craft supplies and other equipment and materials to help reduce the participation fee that must be charged.

Transportation Problems

Lack of transportation will be a major factor limiting the access of people with disabilities to community recreation participation. Many public transportation systems are not physically accessible to people with disabilities. Some individuals with disabilities have not developed skills or do not have the funds to use public transit. Specialized systems that are accessible often are available on a reservation only basis or are restricted to ***life sustaining services*** (i.e., medical, social services). Many recreation agencies with transportation resources limit the transportation provided to segregated or special programs.

All of these factors may contribute to a transportation problem that you may need to help solve in order for an individual with a disability to take part in your program. Whether a recreation provider should be involved in solving a transportation problem is a legitimate question. Such a task may not be specifically included in job descriptions. However, as part of an agency committed to access, you should be ready and willing to expend the time and effort if it will lead to the participation of an otherwise excluded person. Consider the following questions that need to be asked and answered:

1. **What are the transportation resources/policies in the agency?**
    - Find out whether buses, vans, or cars are available to provide transportation for people with disabilities. Also, find out about the procedures for arranging transportation. If resources are available, learn whether transportation can be scheduled for any program or only for special programs.
2. **If transportation is limited to special programs, can policy/procedural changes be made to enable people with disabilities to attend any program?**
    - Probably the administrative and therapeutic recreation or special populations' staff will have to look for ways for present transportation resources to broaden access to general programs. Agencies that provide transportation for groups of people with disabilities to gather only for special programs may unknowingly be denying individuals with disabilities the opportunity to move into nonspecial programs.

3. **Are you knowledgeable about general transportation resources and specialized transit services for people with disabilities in your community?**
   - Contact public transportation companies (buses, trains, subways) and private agencies (taxis, limousine services) to determine what types of services are available, the accessibility, costs, scheduling of services, etc. You should consider the schedules of these public transportation services when determining the activity schedule for your facility/program in order to assure equal opportunities for participation to individuals who use public transit. Transportation brochures from these resources could be displayed in your facility.
   - To gather information about specialized transit services, check with people with disabilities or professionals who work with disabled individuals. You should get information about costs, scheduling, and whether such services will transport people to recreation programs.
4. **Do potential participants have the skills to independently use transportation services? Do they have the financial resources to afford transportation services?**
   - Some people with disabilities will not have the required skills but could learn them. Work briefly with these individuals to help them develop such skills. Special education teachers, parents, volunteers, and residential services staff may all be resources for information on how to teach this material to a specific individual or may themselves be willing to teach the individual how to use transportation resources.
   - If the financial resources of potential participants are a problem, you may want to set up a scholarship or sponsorship fund to cover transportation fees for those who need assistance in this area.
5. **What are other possible resources for transportation for people with disabilities?**
   - Arrange car pools using other program participants, volunteers, parents, etc. Also, corporations that use van pooling for employees may donate transportation services at certain times when not needed by the company.

Legal Liability Problems

Liability is a reason frequently offered by recreation professionals for not providing equal opportunities to people with disabilities. The tendency is to deny people with disabilities the opportunity to participate because it seems obvious that they are more likely to be injured and, therefore, are an increased legal risk for an individual provider or an agency to assume. However, the exclusion of a person with a disability because of an assumed increase in liability risk, due solely to that disability, seems to violate the spirit—if not the letter—of the law.

Federal legislation such as Section 504 of the Rehabilitation Act of 1973, the Individuals with Disabilities Education Act, and the Americans with Disabilities Act, *guarantees* programmatic access to people with disabilities. Antidiscrimination laws exist in most states and provinces to prevent an agency or an organization from excluding people with disabilities. These laws suggest that recreation professionals have a legal responsibility to serve *all* citizens, including any person who has disability and wants (chooses) to be in a regular recreation program.

This responsibility should focus attention on liability not as a rationalization and legal defense for ***exclusion***, but as a potential barrier to ***inclusion*** that needs to be addressed. Before accepting liability as a reason or excluding someone from a program, give attention to liability-related topics and issues. How does offering access to people with disabilities affect personal and agency liability? What action can an agency take to allow for safe access to programs and facilities?

Here are some specific questions and issues to consider and some basic information that may help to understand and to work on liability problems:

1. **Do you have a working knowledge of the concepts of legal liability and negligence?**
   - Legal liability and negligence are complex concepts that cannot be briefly explained. If you are not familiar with the meaning of these terms, review the definitions and concepts below. Another source of information is administrative staff in recreation agencies.
     i. **Legal liability** infers a responsibility between partners that the courts recognize and enforce. For the public administrator, legal liability usually refers to financial settlements or a court award of damage for personal injuries suffered on a park or recreation site or at an agency's program.
     ii. **Negligence** is the failure of a person to act as a reasonably prudent and careful person would act under similar circumstances to avoid exposing others to unreasonable risk of injury (Fifis, S.H. (1975), *Law Dictionary.* Woodbury, NY: Baron's Educational Series, Inc.) The person who is seeking remedy for damages, the plaintiff, must allege and prove four elements in order for negligence to be demonstrated: a) an applicable standard of care to which a duty is owed by the defendant; b) breach or violation of the applicable standard of care; c) causation, the logical proximity between the carelessness and the injury; d) damages, real as opposed to purely speculative injury, to the plaintiff's person or property.
2. **Are you more liable for people with disabilities who participate in your facility or in your program?**
   - The four elements described must be proven in any determination of liability, regardless of the characteristics of the plaintiff. A key point is that while the standard of a care of due care is an objective criterion based upon accepted practicing standards of a reasonably prudent person, the amount of care and kind of conduct may vary with the circumstances. A greater standard of care is required when a person with limitations (i.e., a child, an elderly person, or a person with a disability) is involved in certain activities.
3. **Realizing that you must demonstrate a greater standard of care for some people with disabilities, how can you determine what actions are required on your part?**

- Basically, your actions on the job should always be based upon the ***reasonable person*** standard. A reasonable person is one who will anticipate or foresee potential for injury or accident under the existing circumstances and will act to correct contributing factors.
- The three basic duty criteria for a reasonable professional are as follows: i) providing adequate supervision, ii) exercising good judgment, and iii) providing proper instruction.
- In many cases, the participation of people with disabilities in activities that you offer will require no greater standard of care on your part. When a person who uses a wheelchair registers for a painting class or a person with a hearing impairment is a member of a softball team, minor adaptations to the activity may be involved. No adjustments to your duties are necessary to act as a ***reasonable professional*** when these individuals take part.
- Your standard of care will be affected in some cases, dependent upon the activity in which a person chooses to participate and the capabilities and skills of that person. In some situations, participation by a person with a disability will require you to take some course of action to meet the reasonable person standard. For example, when a child with a visual impairment (total blindness) signs up for a beginner's swimming class, some safety precautions will be needed. You should ask yourself, "What are the foreseeable risks for injury and how can I get rid of them?"

  i. Determine some of the risks involved. For instance,
     - — the child could fall into the pool since he cannot see the edge,
     - — he could wander into the deep end when in the water, or
     - — she could run into the side of the pool or into another participant.

  ii. Eliminate these risks by doing some of the following:
     - — orient the child to the facility
     - — if the lip or edge of the pool is a different texture than the rest of the deck, show this to the child,
     - — pair all participants with a buddy outside and inside the pool,
     - — block off the deep end to prevent accidental movement into it,
     - — recruit a volunteer instructor to assist with the participants, and
     - — space the participants in the water with adequate area for movement without hitting someone else.

  iii. Select which precautions you will institute to eliminate the risks. You may not know which risks, if any, are posed by the participation of a person with a disability in a particular activity. If not, ask other professionals about the activity. Most importantly, meet with the people with disabilities to find out more about their abilities and limitations, what risks are posed by their participation, and what you can do to reduce the risks.

- The reasonable person standard does not make the professional recreation programmer or the agency the absolute insurer of the safety of the participants, nor does it relieve the participant of the responsibility to exercise reasonable care and to be observant.
- If the recreation programmer acted as any reasonable, prudent person would under similar circumstances and, nevertheless, a participant was injured, the staff person or agency should not be held responsible.
- It is important to realize that in a park and recreation case the recreation professional is the *expert*. In such a case, the ***reasonable person*** is not just any person, but rather an educated and experienced programmer with the knowledge and skills common to members of the profession. This standard charges the professional with the responsibility of keeping current with the development of new safety standards, programming trends, product investments, and so on. The practices and standards are common in the profession will be utilized to help determine whether an activity is appropriate and whether the individuals involved behaved in a negligent manner.

4. **What if I cannot provide the standard of care necessary for safe access?**
   - It may not be possible for every person to participate in every program or activity that is offered. However, you cannot refuse the opportunity for participation based upon your assumptions about what constitutes due care.
   - Gain knowledge about the limitations and capabilities of a specific individual who wants to participate in a particular activity. The criterion for taking part in an activity should be based solely on the ability to perform the skills and capabilities that the activity requires, not on the presence or absence of a disability.
   - Rather than excluding a particular individual, work with her to develop an adaptation that enables her to perform the skills and capabilities required for participation. You may want to refer the individual to pre-participation activities or instructional programs where skills can be developed. If you do not offer opportunities for skill development, you may want to expand your program to include these.
   - In a situation where you are reasonably certain that you cannot provide the standard of care necessary for safe access, check with the attorney of your city, county, or agency. The attorney can assist in determining in whether equal opportunity has been offered and can help assure that discrimination is not occurring.

Training

You will often find that to implement an adaptation that you and a potential participant have devised, you will need to train somebody associated with your organization to do something. Good training is not something that you can ignore and expect to come out all right. You need to take some time to analyze what kind of training is necessary, who will give it, and when it will be given. Consider the following questions that need to be asked and answered:

1. **Who needs the training and what should it include?**
    - Look carefully at the adaptation that has been devised. Determine who will be involved in implementing that adaptation and what they should be able to do. Then figure out what kinds of knowledge and skills will be required for them to do it. Next, find out which skills and what knowledge those people already have. The difference is what needs to be provided through a training program.
    - Assess attitudes and provide training activities involving attitude change if you perceive this to be a problem among those staff involved in implementing adaptations or among the staff in general.
2. **Who should do the training?**
    - Find someone who has an expertise in the knowledge and/or skills that you have determined should be included in a training program. This is your subject matter expert. Do not settle for less than the best you can find. The quality of the knowledge and skills this person possesses will be directly reflected in the performance of the staff that receives the training. Tell this person well ahead of time exactly what you want your trainees to be able to do with respect to the subject/skill are involved. This will help them to focus their presentation. You should also inform him what the time constraints of your training experience are and find out what tools, props, or other assistance you can provide. In many cases, the trainer will be you, the recreational professional, who has had a course like this one, where you learn a lot about people with disabilities and about ways to provide full access.
3. **When should you do the training?**
    - The schedule for training sessions has to be determined at the local level since only you know the realities of your organizational time frames. However, it is important not to overload staff with training that is too intensive. When feasible, space your training activities over several one to two-hour sessions.
    - Also, do not do your training during "off" hours or squeeze it into otherwise unoccupied time slots. The importance that your trainees assign to the training will be a reflection of the importance that you assign it. If it is something to be done in "spare" time, they will assume that it must follow everything else in priority.

Human Resources—Use of Volunteers

Sometimes, a specific activity adaptation or an environmental adaptation will require an increase in staff. The first response to this kind of problem is generally to ask for more money to hire and pay the additional people needed, on either a full- or part-time basis. Sometimes it works. Most of the time it does not. A negative response by the agency to a request for money to fund additional staff should not be a justification for exclusion of the participant or abandonment of the adaptation. Other alternatives exist.

Volunteers can be a very important resource to an agency committed to providing access to all people. They can help with adaptations in at least two ways. First, they can handle routine tasks ordinarily performed by paid staff, thereby allowing paid staff members to help people who require some sort of assistance in order to participate in recreation activities. Volunteers can also provide such assistance themselves if the proper level of training is provided. An enhanced recreational experience for both the participant and the volunteer and the avoidance of liability can be achieved through a good volunteer training program.

Secondly, volunteers can enhance an agency's image in the community. A well-run volunteer program is extremely cost-effective. It can help you expand your services to all people in the community at little or no cost to your agency and also involves the community itself more heavily in the number, nature, and quality of the recreation services it receives. Consider the following questions that need to be asked and answered:

1. **What kind of assistance can volunteers provide to people with special needs in recreation participation?**
   - Specific tasks of a volunteer involved in providing access to individuals with disabilities might include the following:
     i. assisting the participant during registration,
     ii. explaining to able-bodied peers the nature of the participant's disability, if this is necessary and he is not able to do so himself,
     iii. managing problem behaviors if they occur,
     iv. facilitating interpersonal relationships with other participants,
     v. physically prompting the participant to perform a task (e.g., helping a person with poor balance to bend over to touch her toes in an exercise class or identifying colors of glazes for a person with a visual impairment),
     vi. task analyzing and teaching leisure skills to a participant,
     vii. evaluating participating involvement in the recreation program,
     viii. providing transportation assistance to and from the recreation program site,
     ix. assisting during toileting, lifting, dressing, grooming, etc.,
     x. assisting with mobility throughout the program length (e.g., pushing wheelchairs, walking beside and providing support, if needed), and
     xi. assisting in areas as determined by people with disabilities and the instructor and/or leader.

   Note: Perhaps the most significant volunteer role to ensure access for a person with a severe disability is to serve as a companion, special friend, peer tutor, or buddy. This type of volunteer accompanies the individual with a disability to provide support and eliminate barriers.

- The volunteer has the opportunity to act as an advocate to highlight the individual's abilities, to emphasize similarities to peers, to diffuse subtle attitudinal barriers, and to help develop a climate of acceptance. The volunteer can help to break down the participant's intrinsic attitudinal barrier and replace them with healthier, more open attitudes. The companion provides one-on-one assistance so that regular recreation staff are not monopolized by attending to a single participant. This extra assistance allows the normal rhythms of the program to remain largely undisturbed.

2. **Where can you recruit volunteers?**
   - Your organization may have a volunteer coordinator or some other staff person responsible for recruiting volunteers. If so, make him aware of your specific volunteer needs. If there is no one else to recruit volunteers, you must do it yourself. Parents, siblings, friend, school classmates, and neighbors of people with a disabilities should be contacted as possible volunteers. Also, youth-serving agencies (e.g., Boy and Girl Scouts, 4-H Clubs, YM/YWCA's, churches, schools) often look for service projects for their members. Colleges and universities may require students to participate in fieldwork or internships. Corporations sometimes provide volunteer resources for recreational programs and special events where people with disabilities will participate.

3. **How do you recruit and retain volunteers?**
   - There are three key steps you can take to recruit and retain volunteers:

     i. Develop a volunteer job description format that outlines specific responsibilities and expectations. This description might include the following:

     — title (e.g., volunteer advocate, special friend),

     — job description (duties to be performed),

     — days needed,

     — hours needed, length of program, location of program,

     — immediate supervisor

     — special skills needed (e.g., sign language),

     — description of the participants to be assisted and their needs, and/or

     — other considerations (e.g., transportation needs, self-care).

     ii. Recruit potential volunteers from the community at large, local schools, youth-serving agencies, businesses, etc. Appropriate methods to solicit volunteers include some of the following:

     — advertising in municipal parks and recreation program brochures,

     — disseminating news releases to media sources (e.g., newspapers college publications, church newsletters),

     — writing public service announcements for local audio, TV broadcast, and cable stations,

— creating a speakers' bureau made up of parents, consumers, and advocates to speak to various agencies and organizations (e.g., schools, parent groups, senior centers), and

— registering the municipal parks and recreation department and/or individual community centers with the local volunteer clearinghouse.

iii. Provide orientation and training for volunteers once they have been recruited, interviewed, and selected. Basically, your volunteers will need to understand the overall goals and polices of your program and be able to effectively perform tasks that you assign to them. Well-planned orientation and training sessions will help volunteers feel comfortable, competent, and confident. It is important to make plans for orientation and training before volunteers are actually selected and matched with job assignments. If you wait until you have recruited volunteers, you may not have enough time to prepare effective sessions. It is best to make tentative plans early, such as determining broad topics that should be covered, about how many sessions will be needed, who will conduct them, how often they will occur, and where they will take place. Then adapt the sessions to meet the specific needs of the volunteers you recruit.

4. **What should be included in the orientation?**

- The purpose of orientation is to provide volunteers with a general understanding of your agency and how your volunteer program "fits in" to the overall picture. It should give volunteers a firm idea of the policies, procedures, and facilities of your agency as well as broad knowledge about its background, structure, purposes, and goals. You might want to brainstorm a list of things you want volunteers to know about your agency and its activities. The following is a brief list to get you started:

i Procedures:

— where to park,

— where to put coats and hats,

— how to sign in and out,

— who to contact if they are unable to work at regularly scheduled times,

— how to handle discipline problems,

— what to do in emergency situations (accidents/illnesses),

— how to follow fire dill procedures,

— how to follow first aid regulations and safety rules, how to obtain needed supplies, and how to register for programs.

ii. Policies:

— rules about clothing, eating, smoking,

— center hours and holidays,

— what is expected (caliber of work, hours, etc.)

— what is required (e.g., health forms, insurance),

— rules about phone use,

— participant eligibility, and

— registration requirements.

iii. Facilities:

— location of bathrooms, lounges, cafeteria and/or snack services, safe storage places for valuables, exits, and

— location of administrative offices.

iv. General information:

— organizational structure,

— background/history of agency,

— purpose,

— philosophy, and

— goals and objectives.

- A good idea is to distribute a handbook that outlines major orientation topics. That way, volunteers will have something to take home to remind them of the information they receive in an orientation session. The handbook should contain a map of the building(s), copies of public transportation schedules, a calendar of agency holidays and upcoming events, important agency phone number and addresses, and other practical information.

5. **What should be included in training programs?**

- Volunteers will need training to help them in the specific tasks they will perform for your agency. In addition, they will benefit from a knowledge of how the tasks they will perform fit into the overall service goals of the agency. The first step is to examine the volunteer job descriptions and to look at what the volunteers are expected to do. Determine what skills at that level are required by the job. Then determine the present level of competence in these skills that your volunteers must acquire to bridge the gap between their present capabilities and the capabilities required by the job they will perform. Training can occur in three phases: pre-service, on-the-job, and in-service.

- Pre-service training provides a volunteer with the information and skills required to do the job that they have been assigned. It is usually defined as formal training and takes place before the volunteer actually begins work. This is the kind of training that we most often think of when we consider a training program. On-the-job training provides opportunities for volunteers to practice newly-acquired skills on the job in order to reinforce what has been learned in the training program. It should always be considered as an informal type of training that compliments, but does not substitute for, pre-service training. If this is the only type of training that is done, confidence and competence are usually the casualties.

- In-service training provides an opportunity to review previously learned knowledge and skills, to share concerns, discuss problems, improve knowledge and skills and learn new techniques. It is formal training that can be very beneficial to volunteers who have been performing a job for a period of time. You should be sure that the persons you select to do training are thoroughly knowledgeable and accomplished in the area they will cover. The quality of the training your volunteers receive will be reflected in the quality of the work they do. Never assign training duties to whomever is "available." Choose the person who does the best work in that area to train others, and you then perpetuate the best work.

Conclusion

For people with disabilities to be encouraged and supported to achieve their full potential and to be able to live, learn, work, and play in environments of their choice, recreation services must do the following:

1. Be provided in as normal an environment as possible.
2. Employ or develop specialized services only when those used by the general public cannot reasonably accommodate the needs and choices of individuals with disabilities.
3. Be fully accessible and culturally sensitive and empower people with disabilities to be primary decision makers.
4. Be directed by and towards the enhancement of quality of life and the achievement of self determination, independence, interdependence, and inclusion into the community.

Learning Activities

1. Think of two examples of segregated recreation programs that would not be violations of the ADA. Explain to a classmate why they are appropriate segregated programs.
2. Get an organizational chart from your local parks and recreation department or some other public or quasi-public recreation agency. Examine it. How does the structure of the organization promote inclusive or segregated services? Give specific examples.
3. Collect examples of advertising from a local recreation agency. Review it for terminology, inclusion, accessibility statement, etc.
4. Interview a special recreation and a regular recreation staff person. What are their similarities/differences in perception, interests, etc.?
5. Write an essay on the pros and cons of providing segregated versus inclusive recreation services.
6. Pick something you enjoy. Do an activity profile, paying particular attention to the skills and capabilities needed to participate.

7. Use the AADAG standards to conduct an accessibility survey of a recreation facility.
8. Design a training program for a recreation agency that wants to move away from segregated recreation services and move toward inclusive opportunities.

References

The ARC of the U.S. (1994). *Position statement on inclusive recreation and leisure*. Arlington, TX: Author.

Baroff, G.S. (1986). *Mental retardation: Nature, cause and management (2nd ed.)*. Washington, D.C.: Hemisphere.

Burke, D., & Cohen, M. (1977). The quest for competence in serving the severely/profoundly handicapped: A critical analysis of personnel preparation programs. In E. Sontag, J. Smith, & N. Certo (eds.), *Educational programming for the severely and profoundly handicapped* (pp. 445-465). Reston, VA: Council for Exceptional Children.

McGovern, J. (1992). *The ADA self-evaluation: A handbook for compliance with the Americans with Disabilities Act by parks and recreation agencies*. Arlington, VA: National Recreation and Park Association.

Rankin, J. (1977, July). Legal risks and bold programming. *Parks and Recreation*, 47+.

Scheerenberger, R.C. (1987). *A history of mental retardation: A quarter century of promise*. Baltimore, MD: Paul H. Brookes Publishing Co.

Stanfield, J.S. (1973). Graduation: What happens to the retarded child when he grows up? *Exceptional Children, 39*, 548-553.

Sternberg, L., & Adams, G. (1982) *Educating severely and profoundly handicapped students*. Rockville, MD: Aspen.

Teague, M., & Mobily, K. (1986, First Quarter). Litigation: A growing threat to community centers. *Therapeutic Recreation Journal, XX*, 18-31.

Wehman, P., & Moon, M.S. (1985). Designing and implementing leisure programs for individuals with severe handicaps. In M.P. Brady & P.L. Gunter (Eds.), *Integrating moderately and severely handicapped learners: Strategies that work* (pp. 214-237). Springfield, IL: Charles C. Thomas, Publishing.

Wehman, P., Schleien, S. (1981). *Leisure programs for handicapped persons: Adaptations, techniques, and curriculum*. Baltimore: University Park Press.

NOTE: Significant portions of this chapter are adapted from Bullock, C.C., McCann, C.A. & Palmer, R.I. (1994). *LIFE resources: The LIFE resources manual* (2nd ed.). Published by the Center for Recreation and Disability Studies, Curriculum in Leisure Studies and Recreation Adm., University of North Carolina at Chapel Hill. The authors would also like to thank Carrie McCann for her significant contributions to this chapter.

Related Websites

http://www.activelivingalliance.mb.ca/
(Active Living Alliance for Canadians with a Disability—Manitoba Chapter)

http://activeliving.ca/activeliving/alliance/alliance.html
(Active Living Alliance for Canadians with a Disability)

http://www.corecom.net/ATA/recreat.html#top
(Assistive Technologies of Alaska's Guide to Adaptive Recreation)

http://www.ddrcco.com/recreate.htm
(Developmental Disabilities Resource Center — Recreation Services)

http://www.users.interport.net/~sprout/index.html
(Sprout—Travel and Recreation for People with Special Needs)

http://www.activeliving.ca/activeliving/cpra/open_r.html
(Candadian Parks/Recreation Association—Opening Doors: Keys to Inclusive Recreation Policy for Persons with a Disability)

http://www.gwrhn.com/camplotsoffun.html
(Camp Lotsafun)

http://www.users.bigpond.com/achievable_concepts/
(Achievable Concepts Adapted Recreation and Sporting Equipment)

http://www.infinitec.org/sports_orgs.html
(Infinitec — Adapted sports organizations)

http://www.gorp.com/gorp/eclectic/disabled.htm
(GORP—Great Outdoor Recreation Pages — Disabled Access)

CHAPTER 14

INTRODUCTION TO THERAPEUTIC RECREATION: AN EVOLVING PROFESSION

CO-AUTHORED BY LAURIE SELZ

INTRODUCTION

What is therapeutic recreation? What makes a recreation activity therapeutic? Is all recreation therapeutic? If recreation is therapeutic, then why would a person with a disability need ***therapeutic recreation*** rather than, simply, recreation experiences? What does therapeutic recreation offer that is unique among health care of therapeutic disciplines? If recreation is all about freedom and self-determination, how can it still be recreation if a therapist is directing it? Does this not violate the principle of choice? Does therapeutic recreation imply segregated recreation for people with disabilities? If so, does this not violate the principle of inclusion?

These questions are very understandable for the student of recreation and/or therapeutic recreation. In fact, they are not only understandable questions, but crucial topics for reflection as each student begins to develop her own professional identity and niche. These very same questions have been tackled by many of the pioneers in the field of therapeutic recreation and have challenged recreation therapists to become increasingly clear and articulate about the philosophy and practice of therapeutic recreation.

Therapeutic recreation as a discipline is still relatively young. The profession has evolved in response to many factors, including the following:

1. Advances in research regarding the process of therapy and rehabilitation.
2. Advances in research regarding the therapeutic benefits of recreation, the specific elements of the recreation experience which yield positive outcomes, and the importance of leisure in promoting ongoing health and wellness.
3. Changes in the contexts or settings in which health care is provided, to include greater emphasis upon community-based services.
4. Changes in the standards and mandates guiding the practice of health care, with an increased emphasis upon measurable and functional outcomes, accountability, standardization of service, cost-effectiveness, and preventive care.

In this chapter the student will be invited to reflect upon the therapeutic nature of recreation; to develop a working definition of therapeutic recreation; to explore various models describing the therapeutic recreation services; and to synthesize principles of person-centeredness, inclusion, and self-determination, as they relate to models and practice of therapeutic recreation.

The Therapeutic Value of Recreation

Strictly speaking, *therapeutic* refers to "having the power to heal or cure" (Websters II, 1984), and is a term that, historically, has been largely associated with medical cures for disease and illness. Recently, however, the term has been used more broadly to describe a variety of activities or experiences—for example, exercise, meditation, listening to music, and interpersonal relationships—that yield positive health outcomes.

This use of the term *therapeutic* typically implies that the experience to which an individual is exposed has made an impact upon the quality of his life. In some cases, the therapeutic value of the experience may be short-term, as may happen when listening to a sonata by Bach. In other situations, the experience may have a more lasting impact upon the quality of the person's life, as may happen when a person with a mental illness joins a writing class an is able to widen her network of social support, learn possible employment-related skills, and creatively express her experience of stigma within the mental health system.

The field of therapeutic recreation has, since its inception, claimed that recreation has therapeutic benefits for people with disabilities. In fact, therapeutic recreation is founded upon the basic premise that recreation has therapeutic value. But, what exactly is it about the recreation or leisure experience that is therapeutic? Subjective descriptions of leisure have been characterized by such experiences a competence, mastery, and control; involvement and focus; relaxed alertness; optimal levels of challenge; and freedom and absence of constraints (Csikszentmihalyi, 1990; Gunter, 1987; Iso-Ahola, 1980, 1984; Neulinger, 1974). Various researchers have found that these types of experiences can assist people to manage and reduce the impact of stressors in their lives (Reich & Zautra, 1988; Wheeler & Frank, 1988); to cope with the transitions of aging (Kelly, Steinkamp, & Kelly, 1986); and to maintain overall physical and psychological health (Kobasa, 1979). In addition, Shank & Kinney (1987) have asserted that the experience of leisure, as described above, may assist individuals with disabilities to cope positively with change, to increase their levels of comfort, and to try out new behavior and to receive immediate feedback.

These very questions regarding the therapeutic value of recreation experiences, and of therapeutic recreation interventions, prompted a major conference designed to facilitate in-depth study and discussion. In the fall of 1991, Temple University, though the support of a three-year grant from the National Institute on disability and Rehabilitation Research (NIDRR), conducted the National Consensus Conference on the Benefits ofTherapeutic Recreation in Rehabilitation. Panels of expert practitioners and educators were convened, representing skill in treating a wide spectrum of people with disabilities. Each panel compiled the results of existing research related to its particular disability, relevant recreation and therapeutic interventions, and resulting health outcomes.

The findings of this conference indicated recreation and therapeutic recreation have value for individuals in many areas of functioning. These benefits were organized according to the following categories: 1) Physical health and health maintenance; 2) Cognitive functioning; 3) Psychosocial health; 4) Growth and personal development; 5) Personal and life satisfaction; and 6) Societal and health care system outcomes (Coyle, Kinney, Riley, & shank, 1991, p. 353). Based upon the work of the expert panels, Coyle et al. identified specific health outcomes within each of the six categories resulting from therapeutic recreation and related interventions. In addition, the work of the expert panels enabled the authors to identify promising areas for further research regarding the therapeutic benefits of recreation. Table 14.1 provides a summary of the health benefits identified for each of the six categories.

Table 14.1
An Empirically Derived List of the Benefits of Involvement in Therapeutic Recreation Programs

Category	Benefits
A. Physical Health Health Maintenance	1. Reduction in cardiovascular and respiratory risk. 2. Reduction in the risk of physical complications secondary to disability 3. Improvement in general physical and perceptual motor functioning in individuals with disabilities.
B. Cognitive Functioning	1. Improved general cognitive functioning. 2. Improved short- and long-term memory. 3. Decreased confusion and disorientation.
C. Psychosocial Health	1. Reduced depression. 2. Reduced anxiety. 3. Improved coping skills. 4. Reduced stress level. 5. Improved self-control. 6. Improved self-concept, self-esteem, and adjustment to disability. 7. Improved general psychological health.

Table 14.1 Cont.

	8. Improved social skills, socialization, cooperation, and interpersonal interactions. 9. Reduced self-abusive and inappropriate behaviors.
D. Growth and Personal Development	1. Improved communication and language skills. 2. Reduced inappropriate behavior and increased age-appropriate behavior. 3. Increased acquisition of developmental milestones.
E. Personal and Life Satisfaction	1. Increased life and leisure satisfaction and perceived quality of life. 2. Increased social support. 3. Increased community integration, community satisfaction, and community self-efficacy. 4. Increased family unity and communication.
F. Societal and Health Care System Outcomes	1. Reduced complications secondary to disability. 2. Improved follow-through with rehabilitation regimes, satisfaction with treatment, and dedication to treatment. 3. Increased outpatient involvement and post-discharge follow-through with treatment plans.

This list of the benefits of therapeutic recreation compiled by Coyle et al. (1991) lend credence to the argument that recreation can, in fact, have therapeutic benefits.

The Need for Therapeutic Recreation Intervention

What would indicate that a person with a disability would benefit from therapeutic recreation intervention, as opposed to freely chosen, intrinsically satisfying, recreation experiences? One way to think about this question is to consider some philosophical thoughts about freedom. In his essay on leisure and freedom, Hemingway (1987) discusses the difference between freedom from constraints and obstacles and freedom to pursue what one chooses. Hemingway states that:

> full liberty...is not simply removal of barriers, but giving persons the power to carry themselves beyond these barriers; to remove a barrier without also providing the means of moving beyond the point at which one finds oneself, is empty (p. 5).

In other words, for the person with a disability, it may be that, while she is *free from* anyone telling her what to do or organizing her life, she may not be *free* to pursue what she desires and hopes for in her recreation due to limited awareness, ability, resources, or opportunities. So, in this way, the individual with a disabling condition is often not truly *free*.

Restoring *freedom* to has been advanced as one philosophical rationale for the existence and use of therapeutic recreation intervention. However, intervention requires a provider and a recipient, or therapist and a client. Often, the therapist may assume, temporarily, some of the control in choosing and structuring the individual's recreation experience. Thus, while the ultimate goal of therapeutic recreation intervention may be freedom, the means of reaching that goal may involve the client temporarily giving up some of her freedoms to the therapist.

This process of asking that someone relinquish her freedom to an expert is called *paternalism*, and is described as "the practice of overriding an individual's self-determination in the name of his/her best interest" (Lahey, 1987, p. 19). Paternalism is one characteristic of many health care relationships, and it raises extremely important ethical questions, including the following:

1. Who decides what is in the *best interest* of the individual? The individual himself? The family? The health care provider?
2. What is the dividing line between *competence* to make one's own choices, and *incompetence* to do so? Who defines that line?
3. How much freedom is appropriate to take away from an individual in the name of her own best interest? Who defines this?

These questions move into the area of ethics in therapeutic recreation practice and are beyond the scope of an introductory text. However, even the beginning therapist needs to being grappling with these questions and formulating some personal answers.

Toward a Definition of Therapeutic Recreation

Given the philosophical dilemmas surrounding recreation and therapeutic recreation it comes as no surprise that the development of a definition statement that can accurately and comprehensively reflect the dynamic nature of therapeutic recreation has presented many challenges to both the academic community and to practitioners working in the field. Definition statements are important for many reasons. On a most practical level, the practicing recreation therapist must have an adequate way to describe her services to her clients or participants, to other professionals, and to various funding sources who control reimbursement or payment for services.

Acknowledging that—as the profession evolves, so the definition of therapeutic recreation will also evolve—is it possible to construct a viable working definition of therapeutic recreation that can be useful to the student? Several recent texts have advanced the following definitions:

- Therapeutic recreation is a means, first, to restore oneself or regain stability or equilibrium following a threat to health (health protection), and second, to develop oneself through leisure as a means to self-actualization (health promotion) (Austin, 1991, p. 13).
- Therapeutic recreation is the purposive use of recreation...to promote independent functioning and to enhance optimal health and well-being in persons with illnesses or disabling conditions (Bullock, 1987, p. 203).
- Therapeutic recreation refers to the specialized application of recreation and experiential activities or interventions that assist in maintaining or improving the health status, functional capacities, and ultimately—the quality of life of persons with special needs (Carter, VanAndel, & Robb, 1995, p. 10).
- Therapeutic recreation is a planned process of intervention directed toward specific environmental or individual change. The goals of the change process are to maximize the quality of life, enhance the leisure functioning of the individual, and promote acceptance of persons with disabilities within the community (Howe-Murphy & Charboneau, 1987, pp. 9-10.

Each definition listed above seems to highlight a particular aspect of therapeutic recreation. Austin's definition stresses a continuum of health and recreation's role in both restoring ***equilibrium*** and promoting long-term wellness. Bullock's definition stresses independence of functioning as one element of optimal health. Carter, Van Andel, and Robb stress the link between planned activity-based intervention and functional outcomes. Howe-Murphy and Charboneau highlight the importance of considering the individual in his context or environment and role of the recreation therapist in promoting social as well as individual change.

Other definitions of therapeutic recreation have been advanced by a variety of researchers and by numerous state and national professional organizations; for the sake of simplicity, let us examine the four definitions proposed above to identify the "threads" that seem to run through each of these definitions, and to thereby identify what seem to be the core components of therapeutic recreation. Some of the "threads" that emerge are as follows:

1. **Purpose and Direction.** Each definition emphasizes the purposeful nature of therapeutic recreation intervention—in other words, to be considered ***therapeutic,*** recreation activities must be purposely selected to address specific, health-related, functional , or quality-of-life related outcomes. For example, wheelchair basketball might be used as therapeutic recreation intervention for a person with a spinal cord injury if the individual has needs in the area of fitness and/or

social interaction. Similarly, ceramics might be a therapeutic recreation intervention for a person who has experienced a stroke if that individual has a need to increase hand strength. Finally, puppet play might be used as therapeutic recreation intervention for a young child who is facing major surgery and needs to learn about the procedure to reduce anxiety.

2. **Enhancement of Functioning.** Each definition states or implies that one aim of therapeutic recreation intervention is the enhanced mastery of a variety of life tasks or improved functioning in the world. While the definitions differ in their focus upon leisure-related functioning vs. broader life-skill functioning, therapeutic recreation appears clearly focused upon this domain of concerns. For example, interventions that address transportation, money management, or using the telephone are all relevant to improving an individual's ability to function in recreation pursuits; these skills are also relevant to improved functioning in a wide variety of other life pursuits as well. Often, life-skill teaching in the context of recreation can be more enjoyable than in other contexts, and thus, can assist an individual with a disability to maintain motivation and interest in change and growth.

3. **Quality of Life, Wellness, and Optimal Health as Core Concerns.** Each definition stresses that one role of therapeutic recreation intervention is to assist people with disabilities not only to ameliorate symptoms or deficits but also to make lifestyle changes resulting in improved long-term health and in an enhanced sense of satisfaction, fulfillment, and quality regarding life. For example, stress management and relaxation instruction, which are a part of many programs and therapeutic recreation intervention, are designed to be useful not only in the short-term, in terms of relieving immediate symptoms, but also in the long-term, in terms of preventing stress from reaching unmanageable levels.

4. **The Individual in Her Context.** While only the Howe-Murphy and Charboneau definition refers specifically to the individual's context (her interpersonal and physical environment), the importance of the environment is implied in each of the definitions. In order to function effectively and independently, the individual must not only have her own skills well-developed, but, in addition, must have working supports and resources within her work. Many recreation therapists work effectively with the individual's environment as a form of therapeutic recreation intervention. For example, the therapist may teach a simple leisure planning process to the parents of a child with mental retardation so that they can use this process with their child when planning family recreation; the therapist is intervening in the child's interpersonal environment to increase its supportiveness. In another example, the therapist might work with an art teacher at a local park and recreation department and assist her to improve the accessibility of her classroom to students in wheelchairs. In this intervention, the therapist is increasing the resources available to her client.

With the above threads in mind, the beginning student could viably think about therapeutic recreation as a purposeful intervention directed at the individual and his environment that aims to enhance health and to impact functioning in many crucial life domains. The student's next task will be trying to describe a model, or ***map***, for the way that therapeutic recreation interventions are actually organized and conceptualized.

Models of Therapeutic Recreation Services and Interventions

Any profession where people intervene in the lives of others must have a ***model*** that guides those interventions. A model is important because it provides a framework for selecting, sequencing, and organizing interventions. It guides the therapist in the process of decision making and assists her in answering such questions as "How do I make a choice regarding what direction to take with this person?"; "What is the range of intervention options that I have?"; "How are these options connect or sequenced?"; and finally, "What am I ultimately aiming for when I use my therapeutic techniques to intervene with this person?"

Usually, a model is based on certain assumptions or beliefs that, in turn, influence people's behavior and choices. For example, the teacher who believes that students' brains are like "blank slates" that need to be "written on" or "filled" with knowledge will probably choose such instructional techniques as reading and memorization, lecture, and objective testing. In contrast, the teacher who believes that students learn through directly experiencing a phenomenon, and who bring their own way of looking at the world to the act of learning, would be more likely to choose direct experience, reflection assignments, and group or individual projects as her teaching methods.

To provide another example, the recreation therapist who believes that the aging process is basically a slow decline or deterioration of abilities will likely choose interventions that help people to adjust to their limitations, such as simple table games, reminiscing, and outings to local coffee shops. In contrast, the therapist who sees the aging process as a transition in which there are, perhaps, some losses, but also some new and exciting freedoms and ways of thinking and feeling, will likely choose interventions that foster physical, intellectual, social, and emotional stimulation; that invite participation in new recreational pursuits; and that encourage active involvement in the process of choosing, planning, and pursing personally-chosen recreation.

As health care has evolved over the years, several different models, or sets of assumptions and beliefs, have emerged regarding the nature of development and growth, the definition of health and illness, and the process and goals of therapy. For example, the ***medical model*** of health care services is based upon the assumption that growth and development are biological processes that occur in a predictable fashion; that there is a "normal" and an "abnormal" way to grow and develop; that health represents an absence of illness or of symptoms; that illness represents a breakdown of biological processes; that the goal of therapy is the removal of symptoms of illness; and that the health care provider possesses the knowledge, expertise, and ability to restore the individual to a state of health.

Working within this model, the recreation therapist would tend to take the role of the expert who determines the problems to be addressed, the desired outcomes of treatment, and the specifics of the how the intervention will occur. The goal of the recreation therapist's interventions would be to remove or to reduce the symptoms of the illness. The client's role would simply be to comply as closely as possible to the therapist's instructions and recommendations.

In contrast, a more ***wellness-oriented model*** of health care is based upon the assumption that growth and development are unique to each individual and occur in response to both internal biology and a supportive and nourishing environment; that ***health*** represents a full and optimal expression of the individual's capacities and uniqueness; that illness occurs in response to an interaction between internal and environmental conditions and represents a restricted or limited expression of the self; that the goal of therapy is to enable to individual to fully experience his own uniqueness and health; and that the health care provider cannot control the process of healing, she can only support it.

The recreation therapist working within this model would tend to take the role of a facilitator and supporter. She would collaborate with the client in defining the problem, the desired outcome, and the means of achieving that outcome, and would then do her part to assist the client along his own path. The client, rather than being asked to comply, would essentially be asked to be an expert on his own health and would be asked to join actively with the therapist in their common pursuit.

As with the definition statements discussed above, the models guiding therapeutic recreation intervention have evolved over time in response to advances in research, social change, and changes in health care. Several models of therapeutic recreation intervention that have been advanced over the past 20 years will be summarized; we will then examine the contrast as well as the "threads," or similarities, among the models, with the hope of arriving at some basic component that appear central to each of them.

The Leisurability Model

The first attempt to "model" the design and practice of therapeutic recreation was presented by Peterson & Gunn in 1984. This model is based on the belief that ***leisure*** is an optimal state of mind, and that ***recreation is*** inherently therapeutic because it evokes that leisure state. The authors state, "Individuals with disabling conditions are entitled to a meaningful existence that includes satisfying recreation and leisure experience" (Peterson & Funn, P. 4). The Leisureability Model focuses, therefore, on the individual's ***ability to*** choose, take part in, and to fully experience ***leisure*** (hence, ***Leisurability***), and holds "the development, maintenance, and expression of an appropriate leisure lifestyle" (Peterson & Gunn, G. 3) as the ultimate goal of therapeutic recreation intervention. According to the model, intervention may occur in a wide range of settings and addresses individuals with "physical, mental, social, or emotional limitations" (Peterson & Gunn, p. 4). The intervention model is conceptually divided into three phases along a continuum of client functioning and restrictiveness. The graphic representation of this model is pictured in Figure 14.1.

Figure 14.1
Therapeutic Recreation Service Model

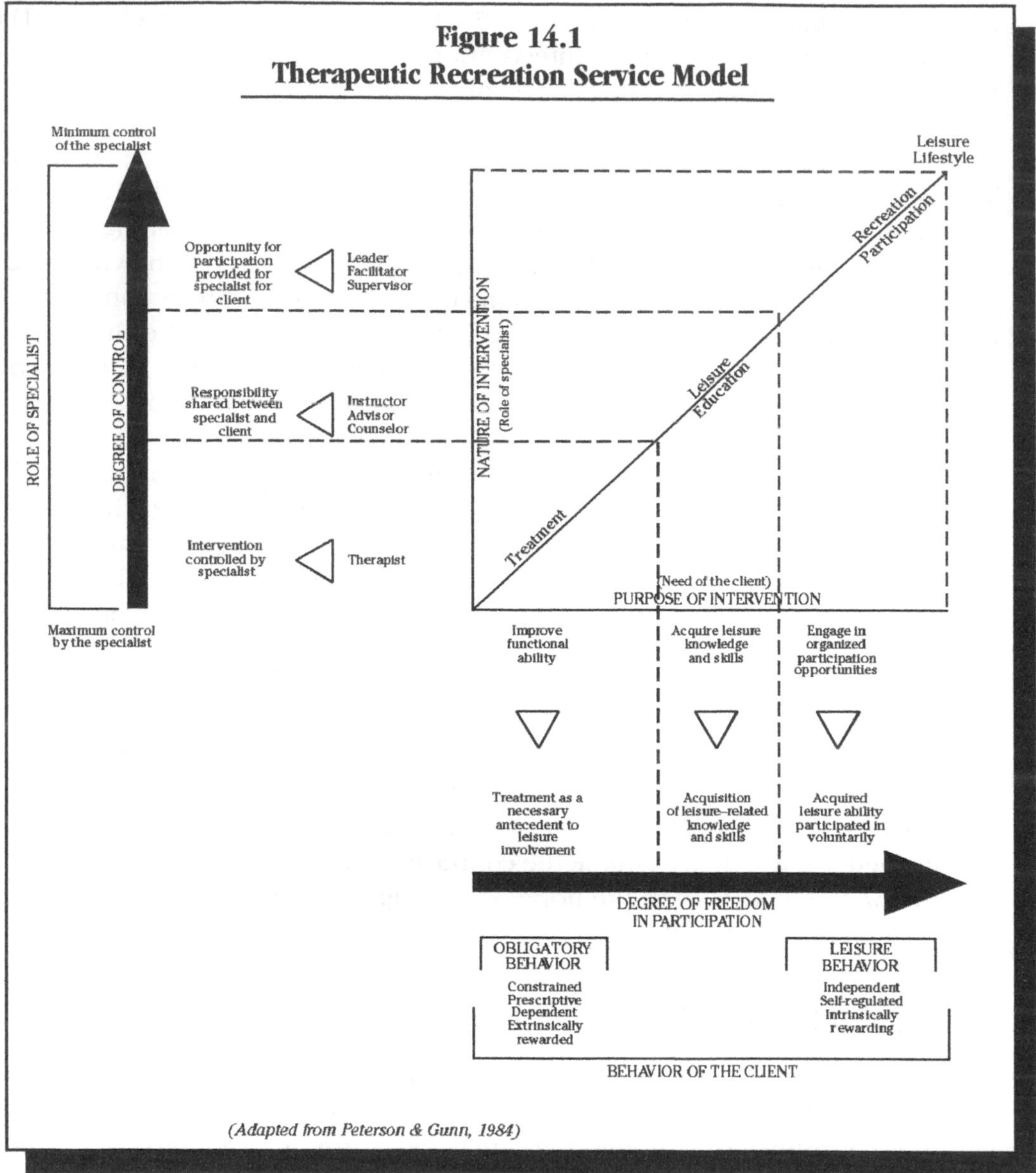

(Adapted from Peterson & Gunn, 1984)

As is represented in the model, the first phase of intervention is ***treatment.*** Treatment refers to activities that are specifically meant to ***improve functional skills*** in a given domain. For example, an activity using clay to mold a simple pot might be used to increase hand and arm strength in an adult woman who has experienced a stroke, thereby improving functioning in the physical domain. Similarly, a ***trust fall*** activity might be used to increase trust and cooperation in a residential treatment center for adolescents, thereby improving functioning in the social and/or emotional domain. A memory game might be used to improve short-term memory in people who have experience head injuries, thereby improving functioning in the cognitive domain.

The second phase of intervention is ***leisure education,*** which addresses the "development and acquisition of skills, attitudes, and knowledge related to leisure participation and leisure lifestyle development" (Peterson & Funn, 1984, p. 6). In other words, in this phase, the client is assumed to have the basic functional skills to participate in leisure pursuits but may not have the skills, attitudes, and/or knowledge to successfully do so. Leisure education may address leisure awareness, social interaction, leisure resources, and/or leisure activity skills.

The third phase of the continuum of intervention is ***recreation participation,*** where the client receives activity-based programs and services that "provide the opportunity...to engage in structured, group recreation experiences for enjoyment or self-expression" (Peterson & Gunn, 1984, p. 7). While these programs focus more on the process of participating than on specific functional outcomes, they are thought to be an important component of the leisureability continuum, as they provide opportunities for practice, for choice, and for interaction.

The three phases of therapeutic recreation intervention are arranged in a sequence, from greater therapist control to lesser therapist control, and from lesser client independence to greater client independence. This arrangement is purposeful and is meant to convey that the ultimate aim of the ***appropriate leisure lifestyle*** is that it be engaged in dependently and freely.

The Health Promotion Model

As knowledge and expertise in the practice of therapeutic recreation have evolved over the years, and as the mandate of health care organizations have called for greater emphasis on functional outcomes and accountable services, considerable thought has been given to alternate models of service. The assumption that the attainment of an ***appropriate leisure lifestyle*** is an adequate and comprehensive aim of therapeutic recreation intervention has come into question. As a result of this questioning, a series of models have been proposed that conceptualize therapeutic recreation intervention in the boarder context of ***health promotion,*** including the restoration and/or maintenance of health, the prevention of health dysfunction, and the achievement of optimal states of wellness. One such model proposed by Austin and Crawford (1996) is the Health Promotion Model. This model is graphically depicted in Figure 14.2.

As stated by Austin and Crawford, therapeutic recreation within the Health Promotion Model serves to help clients to strive for both health protection (illness aspects) and health promotion (wellness aspects) (Austin & Crawford, 1996). As with the Leisureability Model, the student will note that, within the Health Promotion Model, individual travels from left to right along a continuum of functioning. Unlike the Leisureability Model, however, which maps a continuum of ***leisure functioning***, the Health Promotion Model maps a continuum of ***optimal health***, in which the individual moves through a state of ***illness***, to a state of ***stabilization*** (or freedom from symptoms), and then beyond to a state of ***actualization,*** where she reaches the fullness of her potential for health and healthy functioning.

Therapeutic recreation intervention is conceptualized within this model as a contributor in each phase of the individual's journey toward maximal health. Within the ***illness*** phase, therapeutic recreation in implemented as ***prescriptive activity***, not unlike the ***treatment*** phase of the leisurability continuum. The purpose of prescriptive activity is to assist the individual to begin to regain the control over her life that she lost as a result of her illness or disability. As stated by Austin & Crawford:

> For (persons with disabilities),...activity becomes a necessary prerequisite to health restoration. They must being actively to engage in life to order to overcome feelings of helplessness and depression. They need to become energized so that they are not passive victims of their circumstances but can take action to restore their health" (Austin, 1996, p. 8).

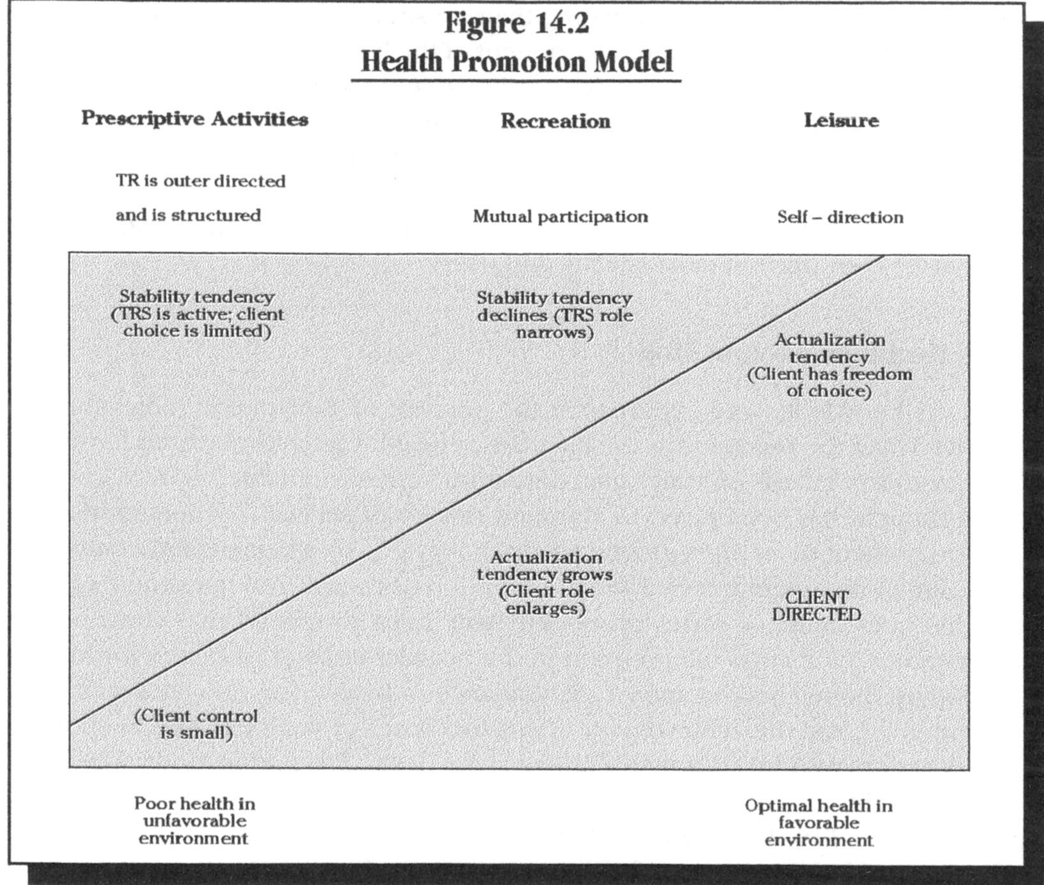

Within the ***prescriptive activity*** phase of the Health Promotion continuum, therefore, therapists design and implement therapeutic activities focused specifically upon engaging individuals and assisting them to exercise choice and control.

Within the ***stabilization*** phase, therapeutic recreation interventions become more focused upon the recreation experience itself as an aspect of health protection. The overall purpose of this phase is to assist the individual, through recreation, in "adapting so as to keep the level of stress in a manageable range in order to protect...from possible biophysical or psychosocial harm" (Austin & Crawford, 1996, p. 7). The focus of the recreation interventions is upon creating experiences of mastery and success, self-confidence, and rewarding interaction.

Finally, in the ***actualization*** phase of the health promotion continuum, therapeutic recreation interventions focus upon assisting the individual to attain ***optimal health,*** or the kind of freedom, self-determination, self-expression, and deep satisfaction that can be experienced through ***leisure***. As in the ***recreation participation*** phase in the Leisureability Model, the therapist working with an individual in the ***actualization*** phase serves as a facilitator and supporter, encouraging independent and self-determined participation.

The Therapeutic Recreation Outcome Model and Service Delivery Model

Carter, Van Andel, & Robb (1995) propose two models that contain elements of both the Leisurability and the Health Promotion Models. The Therapeutic Recreation Outcome Model (Figure 14.3) is a graphic depiction of overall ***quality of life*** as being related to ***both*** health status and functional capacities.

Figure 14.3
The Therapeutic Recreation Outcome Model

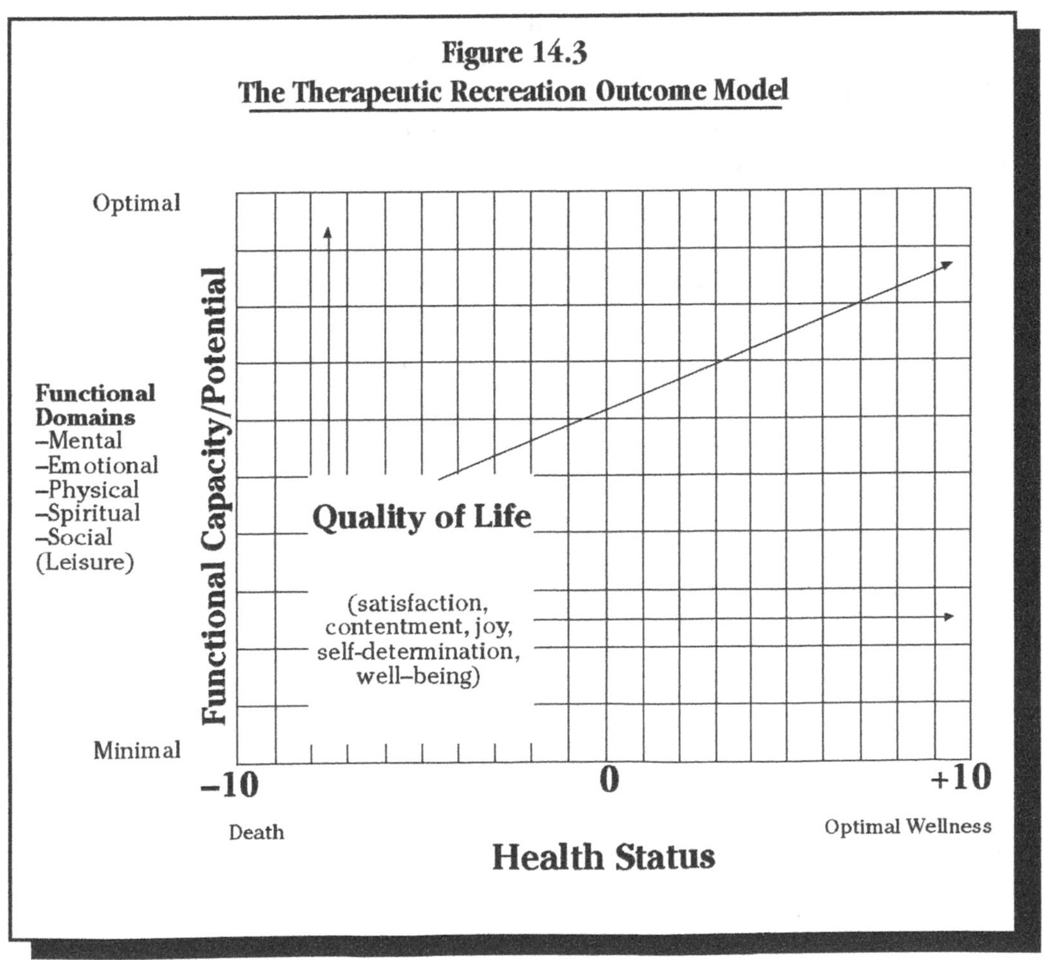

As can be seen in Figure 14.3, quality of life does not relate solely to the presence of absence of illness, but also to the individual's ability to function within her world. This is an important argument for therapeutic recreation's focus upon ***both*** functional capacity and symptom reduction in assisting a client to improve the quality of life.

As in the outer models, the Outcome Model is organized in a continuum, or sequence, whereby the individual might, theoretically, progress in health status and functional capacity at approximately the same rate. However, this is not always the case, and is, in fact, an important consideration for therapeutic recreation interventions. For example, a young woman with schizophrenia might be receiving psychiatric medications and therapy to minimize her hallucinations and delusions (the symptoms of the illness). However, even with her symptoms stabilized, she may lack the exposure, experience, or skills to successfully interact with other people in a way that allows her to participate in daily activities that are truly satisfying or enjoyable to her. Therefore, in assisting her to improve her quality of life, the therapist would need to address both the symptoms of the illness and her capacity to function in social situations.

In the Therapeutic Recreation Service Delivery Model (Figure 14.4), Carter et al. (1995) explore the continuum by which health status, functional capacities, and quality of life can be addressed by the recreation therapist. The student will notice some similarities between this model and the others.

Figure 14.4
Therapeutic Recreation Service Delivery Model

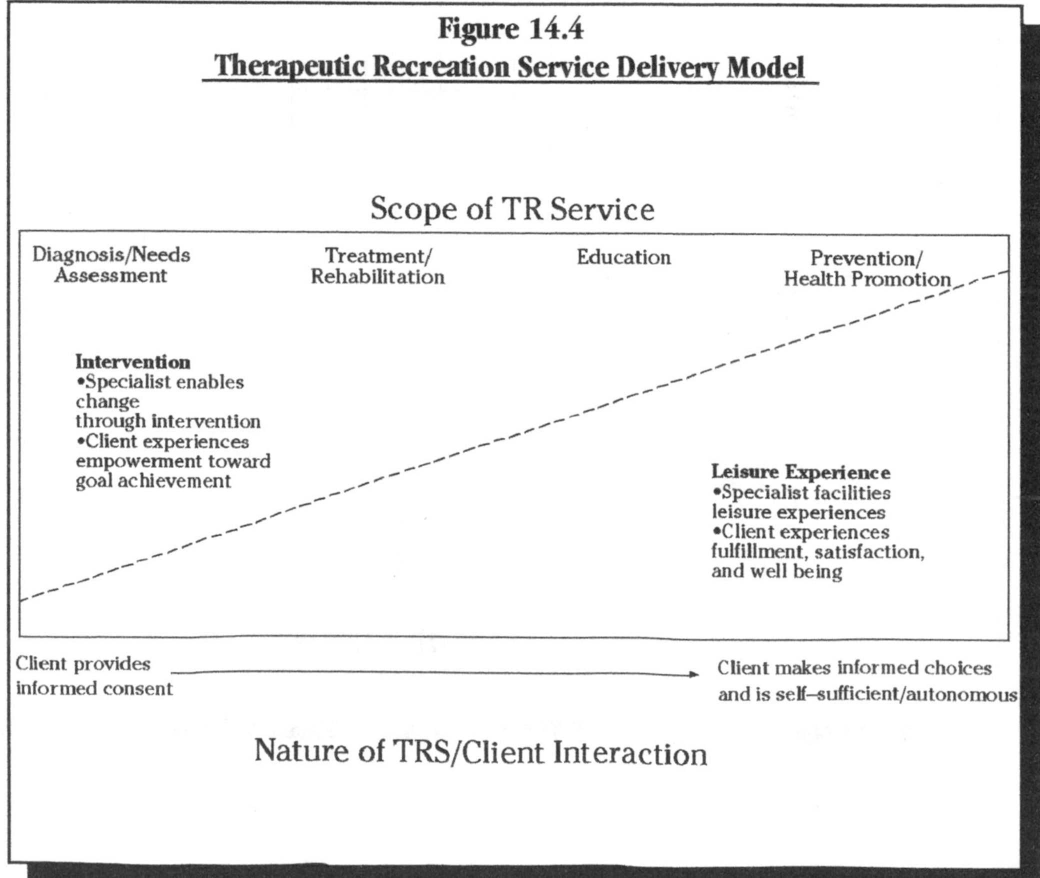

In the *treatment/rehabilitation* phase of this continuum, the focus is upon "interventions that have a direct or indirect objective of restoring or ameliorating the primary or secondary effects of a disease process or injury" (Carter et al., 1995, p. 21). In the education phase, the emphasis is upon health maintenance and upon specific skill development activities related to leisure as well as other life pursuits, for example, stress management, planning skills, or social interaction. In the *prevention and health promotion* phase, the focus is upon "promot(ing) and reinforc(ing) healthy lifestyle behaviors..." (Carter et al., p. 21)

Self-Determination and Enjoyment Enhancement: A Psychologically-Based Service Delivery Model for Therapeutic Recreation

The first edition of this text included only three models. In the second edition, we have added the conceptual model presented by Dattilo, Kleiber, and Williams (1998) as a fourth model. This fourth model did not exist as a service delivery model at the time of the writing of the first edition. Dattilo and Kleiber has proposed a conceptual model (1993), however it was not until 1998 that Dattilo, Kleiber, and Williams expanded that conceptual model into a service delivery model. As such, it is added to the service delivery models in this chapter.

The components of the psychological model previously (Dattilo and Kleiber, 1993), demonstrated the dynamics of the relationship between self-determination and enjoyment. The components included, self-determination, intrinsic motivation, perception of manageable challenge, investment of attention, enjoyments, and functional improvements (see Figure 14.5).

The authors (Dattilo and Kleiber, 1993), used extant psychological theories to posit the components of their model. They explicitly linked self-determination

Figure 14.5
The Relationship and Enjoyment

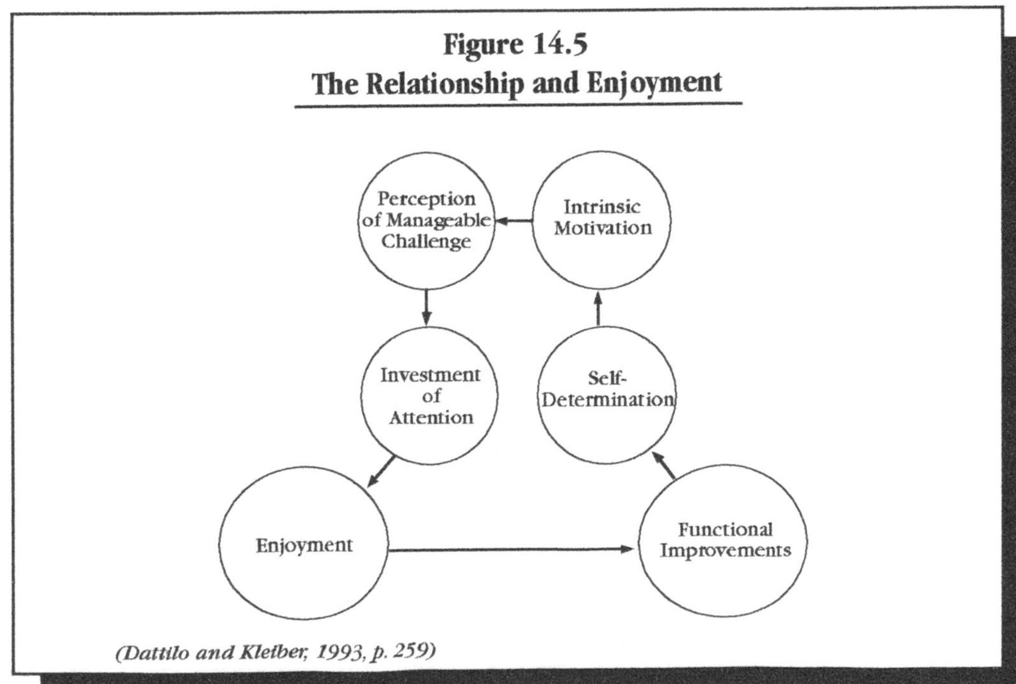

(Dattilo and Kleiber, 1993, p. 259)

and intrinsic motivation as had been done in the literature. They said, "intrinsically motivated activity energizes behavior and results in feelings of self-determination." They continued, "[p]eople who are intrinsically motivated are generally seeking challenges that are commensurate with their competencies...Fortunately, intrinsic motivation does not depend on a particular level of ability; therefore, interest, excitement, and relaxation can arise with anyone" (Dattilo, Kleiber, and Williams, 1998, p. 261).

Another component of the model is the perception of manageable challenge. The belief is that it is, "important that people [with disabilities] learn about the availability of challenging opportunities, be given the chance to engage in challenging activities, and be encouraged to overcome their fears and try." (Dattilo, Kleiber, and Williams, 1998, p. 261). Another component of their model is investment of attention. They recognize the importance of challenge in maintaining a person's attention and therefore closely tie the management of challenge to the ever-changing skill level so that attention will be maintained and enjoyment can be achieved. The authors then logically state that, "enjoyment is the experience derived from investing one's attention inaction patterns that are intrinsically motivating" (Dattilo, Kleiber, and Williams, 1998, p. 261). The final component of the model (see Figure 14.5) recognizes the importance of functional improvement for people with disabilities. They cite literature that suggests that enjoyment leads to functional improvements. For a review of the originally proposed model and its components, see Dattilo, J., Kleiber, D., and Williams R., (1998).

To render their psychological model a service delivery model, (Dattilo, Kleiber, and Williams, 1998) expanded the original model (see Figure 14.6). They showed

Figure 14.6
The Relationship and Enjoyment

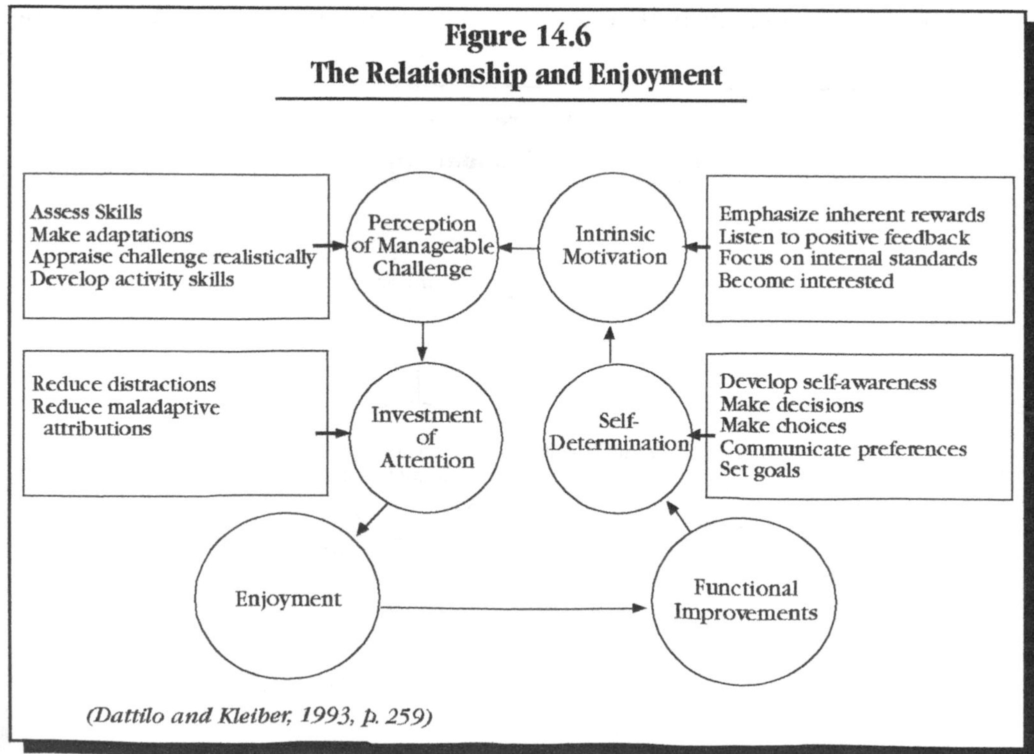

(Dattilo and Kleiber, 1993, p. 259)

how each component of their model fit into a programming model that includes assessment, planning, implementation, and evaluation.

As depicted in Figure 14.6:

> Self-determination can be enhanced when people are encouraged and supported to become aware of themselves in leisure contexts, make decisions and choices, communicate their preferences, and set goals. Intrinsic motivation is enhanced when people focus on internal standards, emphasize inherent rewards, listen to informative feedback, and become aware of their interests. These patterns can be facilitated (or disrupted) by service providers. To increase the chance that participants consider the challenge of an activity to be manageable, they can be encouraged to assess their skills, make adaptations, make realistic appraisals of challenges, and develop activity skills. Practitioners can recognize and avoid sending messages that undermine self-determination and creating conditions that are distracting. Teaching participants to make accurate attributions relative to their success and failures encourages investment of attention and enjoyment. In turn, generating enjoyment can help facilitate functional improvements (Dattilo, J., Kleiber, D., and Williams, R., 1998, p. 262).

For a review of the service delivery model and its components, see Dattilo, J., Kleiber, D., and Williams R., (1998).

Toward a Unified Model of Therapeutic Recreation Services and Interventions

Each of the models mentioned before takes a slightly different perspective on the focus and scope of therapeutic recreation services and interventions. However, as was demonstrated in the discussion of the definition of therapeutic recreation, we can draw out a set of core "threads" or themes that seem to appear in some form in each of the models. What are these themes, and what do they convey about the core beliefs and philosophical perspectives that form the foundations of therapeutic recreation practice?

1. **A Continuum of Growth and Intervention.** Each model is structured along a *continuum* of functioning, health, and intervention; in other words, each model rests upon the assumption that growth and change occur in a way that is not random, but systematic, and, therefore, to be effective, the therapist's interventions must also be systematic and must "match" the individual's particular strengths and needs. There is less explicit discussion of a continuum in the Dattilo, Kleiber, and Williams model.
2. **A Belief in the Strengths and Abilities of the Individual.** Each model presented proposes that individuals move in a direction of increasing expression of personal strengths and abilities; this notion rests upon the assumption that individuals, in fact, have the capacity to develop and express strengths and abilities. This crucial belief will be discussed later in this chapter as one truly unique element of therapeutic recreation intervention.

3. **Increasing Freedom and Self-determination.** A core foundation of each *continuum* is the individual's progression from a state of relative constriction and dependence upon others (not only in functional skills and knowledge, but also in opportunities, resources, and supports), to a state of relative autonomy, self-responsibility, and interdependence regarding, creating, choosing, and following through with valued life pursuits. For example, the Leisurability Model culminates in freely-chosen and independently implemented leisure pursuits; the Health Promotion Model culminates in actualization and wellness; the Outcome Model culminates in optimal quality of life, health status, and functional capacity; and the Psychologically-Based Therapeutic Recreation Model culminates in functional improvements, as well as the "promotion of participants' self-determination associated with leisure participation, creation of leisure environments conducive to the development of intrinsic motivation, cultivation of perceptions of manageable leisure challenges, and fostering the investment of attention so that optimal experience and enjoyment will be abundant..." (Dattilo, J., Kleiber, D., and Williams, R., 1998, p. 268). It seems that values of self-determination and self-responsibility are central not only to the philosophy of recreation for all individuals (including those with disabilities), but also to the practice of therapeutic intervention as well.
4. **Decreasing Therapist "Control."** Related to the above "thread," each model highlights the shifting role of the therapist as the individual moves along the continuum of growth and change. While the therapist intervenes in the more acute stages of illness or disability with considerable directiveness and structuring, central to each model is the notion that, as growth occurs, the individual increasingly "takes over" responsibility for his own life and chosen activities. In fact, many of the educational interventions that are described within each model are conceptualized specifically to assist the individual to develop the skills, supports, and resources to function independently of therapist intervention. Self-awareness, decision making and problem-solving, resource education, and coping skills are all examples of therapeutic recreation interventions that address those skills that are crucial to successful independent functioning. In this way, the therapist's "job" is to "work herself out of a job"; in other words, the sign of an effective therapeutic intervention often comes when the client no longer needs the therapist in the same was as before.
5. **Increasing Involvement and Participation in the "Natural" Community, or Inclusion.** Finally, each model rests upon a belief in and focus upon true inclusion as an ultimate goal; that is, a part of the continuum of growth is that the individual becomes increasingly able to participate fully in activities, settings, and social groups of her own choosing, and that these choices are based upon abilities and preferences, rather than upon disability grouping or other labeling process. While not explicitly stated in the models that were summarized before, this endpoint implies that the person within his environment is a key consideration of therapeutic recreation intervention. This point is crucial and will be discussed further in the sections addressing assessment and intervention plans.

During 1998, the *Therapeutic Recreation Journal* ran a special series on Therapuetic Recreation Practice Models. Each of the four models presented in this edition were presented by their author(s). Each model was then critiqued by two reviewers. One review addressed the ability of the model to advance the practice of therapeutic recreation. The other review focused on the conceptual and theoretical strengths of the model related to research. The purpose of the special series was to stimulate dialogue and the exchange of ideas among therapeutic recreation specialists. You are encouraged to read the presentation of the models and critiques in volumes 2, 3, and 4 of the 1998 *Therapeutic Recreation Journal*.

The Contexts of Therapeutic Recreation Intervention

Models of therapeutic recreation services and interventions only make sense within contexts in which they are practiced. In other words, different contexts as well as different agency mandates will demand that the therapist function within different parts of a model. This introductory text is into the place to go into detail about all the intricacies and subtleties of models and contexts; however, you need to remember that the type of service and intervention provided must fit within the context in which it is provided and within the skills of the recreation therapist.

One of the biggest mistakes a recreation therapist can make is to assume that his service is a "one-size-fits-all setting." Shortly, we will discuss the major contexts (sometimes referred to as settings or environments) where therapeutic recreation is delivered. Even within similar settings, we find it impossible to say which models or which portions of a particular model fit best. Such a determination can only be made as it fits into the philosophy and expectations of particular agencies and their staffs.

Remember our discussion in Chapter 5 about the importance of mandate for service? You should remember that it is not the setting but rather the mandate that legitimizes therapeutic recreation as a clinical service. As such, we will briefly review the various settings or contexts in which recreation therapists might work.

Historically, most recreation therapists have worked either in hospitals or long-term care settings. More specifically, most have worked in psychiatric services, physical medicine services, or nursing homes. Today, however, recreation therapists working a broader range of environments, including inpatient health are (hospital) settings in many service areas; outpatient health care settings, also in many service areas; schools; and, increasingly, in community- or home-based contexts. Theses have been described by Kraus and Shank (1992) and are summarized next.

Inpatient settings include such places as acute care hospitals as well as long-term rehabilitation centers. The length of stay is determined by the type and condition of the patients it serves. In some settings, patients are admitted for acute care and stay only until they are stabilized. In other settings, such as long-term rehabilitation facilities, people who are past the acute phase but still need 24-hour care and rehabilitation may have extended stays of many months in which they receive varied forms of physical, psychological, vocational, and recreational rehabilitation to facilitate their return to their families and to community life. Inpatient clinical settings operate under various sponsorships such as Veterans' Administration, military, universities, public health, state, county, municipal, voluntary, sectarian, and proprietary entities. They serve many types of patients: general medical and surgical, psychiatric, pediatric, chronic disease, geriatric, burn, and others.

Outpatient health care settings have become much more prevalent in the past decade. As an alternative to rising health care costs, many people who may previously have been treated or served in inpatient settings are increasingly being treated in outpatient settings. That is, rather than being admitted to an inpatient setting, the care of treatment occurs often in the same or at least similar facilities, yet, on a daily basis or occasional basis. Such settings are less expensive than traditional inpatient settings because they are daily rather than 24-hour care. Initially, the only outpatient settings, often called partial hospitalization, were for psychiatric care, yet as health care costs have continued to skyrocket, examples of outpatient services are in virtually every area of health care. In addition, as health care costs rise, average lengths of stays in inpatient settings are becoming shorter and shorter. Therefore, much follow-up and aftercare occur in an outpatient setting, whereas before it was often accomplished by readmissions. Although there are not a lot of recreation therapists in outpatient settings now, a strong case can be made of increasing numbers of recreation therapists in those settings.

Another context or setting which recreation therapists work is long-term care. Institutions are one type of long-term care setting. As we discussed earlier in this book, as a result of deinstitutionalization, there are far fewer institutions in North American now than 20 years ago; however, in most states, state institutions exist for people who are profoundly mentally retarded as well as for people with severe and persistent mental illness. Though far fewer residents reside in these state institutions, this remains a setting where some recreation therapists work.

Another type of long-term care setting is the nursing home. Nursing homes are facilities that provide extended care for people who can no longer function in their homes or with their own families. Nursing homes are generally thought of as facilities for older adults; however, many younger people—who because of mental retardation, mental illness, head injury, stroke, or other trauma, cannot live independently—are sometimes residents of nursing homes. In the past, many of these younger residents of nursing homes lived in state institutions, but as a result of deinstitutionalization, nursing homes are often the only alternative for many people.

A number of people cannot live independently or with their families, but do not need intensive nursing or medical care. Such people can meet some of their needs independently. As a result, a number of large and small group homes exist for different types of people. These are aggregate living situations where residents are taught and encouraged to do as much as possible for themselves. The most well-known group homes are those for people who are mentally retarded or who are mentally ill; these became very popular during and following deinstitutionalization.

Another type of setting in which a recreation therapist might work is adult day care, which is a nonresidential program for seniors who may need some level of medical or nursing care, but who are able to live with their families outside of nursing homes. As the population ages and with increased incidence of physical disability and dementia associated with aging in some people, adult day care settings have become more and more of an option for some families.

Schools are another setting where recreation therapists work. For many years, there have been thousands of state or segregated schools throughout North America. Although many of these schools for people who were mentally retarded or who were mentally ill no longer operate because of deinstitutionalization, many of these schools for children who are blind, deaf, or blind/deaf still function. The focus of such schools has changed in recent years. Previously, they functioned more like state institutions—where someone lived for life rather than attending for just specialized schooling. Currently, such schools are more like specialized residential schools where a resident learns not only academic skills but also skills needed for independent community living.

Since the advent of Public Law 94-142 and through its most current reauthorizations, other schools have emerged as viable settings for recreation therapists, as discussed in Chapter 4. Now therapeutic recreation is a legitimate ***related service*** of special education. Students in public and private schools can expect to learn community living skills along with academic skills.

One of the most exciting new contexts in which recreation therapists work is in community and/or home-based treatment programs. These psychosocial rehabilitation programs are highly individual and provide intervention within the context of the person's life. It is a type of intervention that is more costly initially; however, research is beginning to show that it is more cost effective in the long run because the changes that occur within a person's real environment do not have to be transferred from a hospital, they change ***in context***. For the entrepreneurs of the future and for the forward-thinking health care providers, this type of context will provide a ripe ground for recreation therapists.

Additional components of *context* are important to the delivery of therapeutic recreation services as well. In addition to the place where intervention occurs, other people play a role in intervention. Again, there is no way to say exactly who becomes part of the context in particular situations. It is clear, however, that the more people who are intimately involved in the intervention, the better chance that the intervention will have not only short-term, positive gains but also meaningful and sustained change.

In most health care settings teams of professionals become integral parts of the intervention context. These professional *teams* are composed of individuals with various types of professional training and expertise who work together as a unit to assist an individual seeking health and maximum functioning (Howe-Murphy & Charboneau, 1987, p. 225). The composition of the team varies based on the specific setting and philosophy of that setting. In general, teams include such professionals as physicians, nurses, physical therapists, occupational therapists, and social workers. These professional teams are organized as multidisciplinary, interdisciplinary, or transdisciplinary.

The multidisciplinary model utilizes the efforts of appropriate disciplines but without a great deal of skill sharing among professionals. Each professional maintains a more of less traditional role consistent with her training. The working of an interdisciplinary team, on the other hand, is based upon the assumption that the client is a dynamic organism who functions within an integrated environment; therefore, treatment must be dynamic and integrated as well. In the interdisciplinary model, problems cannot be treated in isolation. All members of the team share information in an effort to develop an integrated intervention for each person. The transdisciplinary team goes even further toward integrated and holistic intervention. The transdisciplinary team functions much like an interdisciplinary team, yet recognizes the inevitable overlaps among related professions. Rather than never crossing perceived or real disciplinary practices, the transdisciplinary team encourages blurring of disciplinary practices in an effort to provide the most effective and appropriate interventions for each client.

As you begin to learn more about the process of therapeutic recreation intervention, keep in mind that the service is delivered within various settings and contexts. Also, remember that at the center of the service is the ***person*** (often called the client in treatment/clinical settings), and not the settings or the professionals!

The Process of Therapeutic Recreation Intervention

Clearly, the practice of therapeutic recreation encompasses a wide and varied spectrum of individuals, interventions, activities, and contexts. Are there, then, any consistent processes that guide practice? Clinical process in therapeutic recreation provides this consistency—that is, regardless of the context or content of the intervention, recreation therapists follow a systematic sequence of ***assessment, planning the intervention, implementing the intervention, planning for transition, evaluation, and systematically documenting the outcomes of their interventions.*** These processes and activities maximize the likelihood that the services provided by the recreation therapist are individualized, purposeful, outcome-focused, and, ultimately, effective. Each phase of the therapeutic recreation process will be discussed in the following pages.

Assessing the Individual and His World

Assessment must be the first step undertaken by recreation therapists because it sets the direction for the ***purposeful intervention*** by enabling them to focus specifically upon the strengths, needs, and health concerns of the individual being serviced. ***Assessment*** may be defined as a systematic process of gathering and synthesizing information about an individual and his world in order to determine the most effective course of intervention. An effective assessment will provide information about the individual's functioning at the beginning of the intervention, his desires and goals for intervention, and some possible ways to structure the intervention. It provides a ***baseline*** against which to measure progress and outcomes.

Each setting or agency has priorities regarding the type of information to be sought in the assessment process, as well as regarding the methods of assessment and sources of information. The choice of assessment instrument often directly reflects the philosophy and values of the agency. For example, a traditional ***medical model*** psychiatric setting may have an assessment process in which the patient is administered formal psychological tests and is observed in the unit by a staff member, who then writes a diagnostic report that focuses on the major psychiatric symptoms that appear to be the most evident.

By contrast, a community-based ***psychosocial rehabilitation*** program may have an assessment processing which the individual himself is asked to state what he sees as his greatest strengths and areas of need and is asked to define his own priorities and needs. In addition, he may be encouraged to have a family member or friend with him to provide additional information. In the staff member's write-up of this assessment, the issue of the particular diagnosis or psychiatric problem may never appear, except if it is identified as a troublesome barrier by the individual and something for which he would like help.

A vast amount of information may be collected from any one individual. Generally, the therapist focuses her efforts on those areas in which the individual is likely to have the greatest need. This is determined from the therapist's general knowledge of the disability area being addressed. Some of the basic information about strengths and needs that the recreation therapist may wish to gather in the assessment process includes the following:

1. **Physical Functioning.** For example—mobility, flexibility, balance, dexterity, coordination, endurance, strength.
2. **Cognitive Functioning.** For example—attention, memory, problem solving, decision making, following steps or directions, abstract thinking.
3. **Social Functioning.** For example—formal and informal conversational skills, assertion, conflict resolution, cooperative and/or competitive interaction.
4. **Emotional Functioning.** For example—the experience and ability to cope with anxiety, depression, anger, stress, and/or the ability to experience enjoyment.

In addition to these basic functional skills, the recreation therapist will also assess functioning in the areas of recreation and leisure. Again, depending upon the setting in which services are offered and the general group of individuals being served, any of the following areas of leisure functioning may be assessed:

- **Leisure Interests and Preferences.** For example—past, present, and future possibilities.
- **Access to and Successful Use of Leisure Resources.**
- **Barriers to Satisfying Recreation Experiences.** For example, *external* barriers, such as finances & transportation; *internal* barriers, such as physical and/or mental health concerns; *interpersonal* barriers, such as limited friendships and/or friendship skills; and *system* barriers, such as limited or noninclusive recreation options, social stigma, and discrimination.
- **Ability to Successfully Choose, Plan, and Implement Leisure Pursuits.**

The therapist has a wide a variety of assessment tools from which to choose. Some assessment tools are meant to be used only with those receiving treatment, while others are meant to be used with family members or significant support people in the individual's life. Some assessments are specific to leisure functioning, while others may be borrowed from other disciplines (i.e., psychology, education, or physical medicine) and used by the recreation therapist.

Some assessments are ***standardized,*** which means that they have been developed and tested to ensure that they reliably measure a given set of characteristics, and that they are always administered in the same way. Some assessments are more ***flexible***, allowing the therapist more latitude in how and when to administer them. Some assessments are based upon the individual's answers to specific ***questions***, either written or verbal; others are based upon more open-ended ***conversations*** and ***discussions***; still others are based upon ***observations*** of the individuals actually doing something in a given environment or upon a ***shared activity*** between the therapist and client; and some assessment instruments require that the therapist extract information from another written document, such as a medical chart or an Individualized Education Plan (IEP). Generally, professionals recommend that more than one method or instrument be used in order to gain the most accurate and complete "sense" of the individual. For example, the young adult with a spinal cord injury who ***says*** that he is having an easy time relating to other people may be ***observed*** to be alone and to shy away from conversation with others.

The choice of assessment may be determined by the individual therapist or by the facility or agency. Regardless of the specific assessment instrument used, however, the values of person-centeredness, inclusion, and self-determination should be attended to by any recreation therapist. These values translate into the following guidelines regarding assessments:

1. **Seek as much input as possible from the individual.** This includes asking informal as well as formal questions, which often involves taking some extra time to develop a comfortable rapport. In addition, it is advisable that the individual be encouraged to state his own desires and goals in his own words and that these be preserved in original form to the greatest degree possible.
2. **Assess the physical and human environment as well as the individual's skills and needs.** A person's ability to function effectively is often as much a reflection of his environment and supports as it is a reflection of his specific skills and deficits. Are there people on whom he can rely? Is he able to share in enjoyable activities with others? Does his environment promote mobility and assess? Assessing these factors may necessitate some additional effort on the part of the therapist but will result in a more comprehensive understanding of the challenges and supports that are part of the client's life. As will be discussed in the next section, we are able to intervene on the level of the environment as well as the individual, so therefore, assessing the quality of the environment is crucial.
3. **Remain focused upon the individual's goals and how he would like them to function in his life.** While many assessment tools focus accurately upon the person's performance in certain specific skill areas (i.e., ***memory, balance, impulse control***), it is crucial for the recreation therapist to develop learning strategies that are contextual. That is, strategies that are relevant and meaningful to the individual. For example, the therapist may assess a teenager with a head injury and find that he has lost some ability to follow multistep directions. However, if the therapist also knows that this teenage had been very involved with bicycle racing, and had worked in a bike repair shop after school, then the ***point*** of enhancing his ability to follow multistep directions becomes much more

clear and meaningful. In addition (as will be discussed in the next section), the therapist can now use this knowledge to design individual and ***contextual*** interventions that will be more likely to succeed with this particular individual—for example, she might find a bicycle, adapt some directions in a repair and maintenance manual, and encourage her client to begin to work through the directions in maintaining the bike.

4. **Assess strengths, abilities, and desires as well as deficits and needs.** At the core of the recreation experience is a celebration of the individual's strengths and abilities and an expression of his unique choices. Crucial, therefore, is for the therapist to gain an accurate sense of these in order to develop high quality and successful interventions. It is interesting that strengths, abilities, and desires are often not attended to by service providers or health care professionals, especially those in highly symptom-focused, medical model settings in which payment or reimbursement is based upon the presence of problems or deficits. Especially challenging for the recreation therapist working in such a context is to remember that assessment of the ***positives*** is just as important as assessment of the ***negatives***, and that these positives may provide clues to as to the most powerful and effective interventions. In fact, the recreation therapist is often in a position to offer new and unique information to other members of the team, as it may be that she is the only person who has specifically assessed strengths, abilities, and desires.

Planning the Intervention

The planning phase (sometimes called ***treatment planning, individualized program planning***, or ***care planning***, depending upon the setting) is one in which the strengths, needs, and goals of the individual, and the expertise and contributions of the therapist, are organized into a coherent plan that maximizes the chance that the individual will reach his desired outcomes. This phase of the therapeutic recreation process is often as much an ***art*** as a ***science***, as it involves creatively and sensitively combining many elements of skill, timing, and relationship to achieve a positive and meaningful goal.

Many settings have particular guidelines or requirements for the development and formatting of intervention plans. In some settings, the recreation therapist will develop specific ***recreation goals***. For example, "the patient will be able to fish independently" is a possible recreation-based goal for an individual who has experienced a stroke and needs to master the use of adaptive equipment in order to continue his most valued recreation pursuit—fishing. In others, the recreation therapist will develop goals pertaining to aspects of functioning that are more generalized and that are attainable through participation in recreation pursuits. For example, "the client will reduce perceived levels of stress through increased physical activity" is a possible goal for an individual who is experiencing symptoms of anxiety disorder.

Regardless of the particular format or context, certain crucial phases and components compose the design of a complete intervention plan. These include the following:

1. **Stating the Desired Outcome.** The therapist must clearly state what the goal of the intervention will be. The goal must clearly answer the question, "What will the client be able to do differently at the end of the intervention?" As discussed above, the greater the direct involvement of the client in determining the intervention goal (i.e., the more person-centered it is), the more likely the goal will be personally relevant to him and he will remain engaged and motivated throughout the course of the intervention. While a detailed discussion is beyond the scope of this chapter, there are several elements of intervention goals, including the desired behavior (stated in observable and measurable terms), the conditions under which it will be manifested, and the time frame in which it will occur.

   Intervention goals are most often followed by specific objectives, which are the distinct behaviors or activities that, when added together, indicate that the overall goal has been accomplished. Intervention planning is addressed in great detail in more advanced therapeutic recreation texts and courses. Some examples of a typical treatment or intervention goal, with related objectives, include the following:

An Adolescent with Mental Retardation

Goal: "The client will demonstrate improved personal safety behaviors in public settings."

Objective #1: When waiting at the bus stop, the client will refrain from approaching and conversing with people whom she does not know.

Objective #2: When walking in public, the client will store her money in a pocket or a purse rather than carrying it in plain view.

An Older Adult with Depression

Goal: "The resident will demonstrate increased engagement and improved affecting family activities."

Objective #1: By the end of July, the resident will increase his weekly activity attendance from two activities per week to a minimum of six activities per week.

Objective #2: By the end of August, the resident will demonstrate the ability to engage verbally with another resident a minimum of two times per activity group, in four out of six groups per week.

Objective #3: By the end of August, the resident will report increased satisfaction with and enjoyment of program activities, as demonstrated by his scores on the monthly Program Satisfaction and Enjoyment Evaluation Form.

2. **Developing the Intervention Strategy.** In this phase of intervention planning, the therapist carefully considers the area of need or skill deficit that has been identified during the assessment process. She determines whether intervention will involve learning or enhancing a new skill, adapting an old skill to a new situation or constraint (as often happens in the case of a traumatic or sudden illness or disability), or maintaining current levels of functioning to minimize decline (as may happen, for example, with an older adult with a progressive

cognitive impairment). The therapist takes into account the client's strength, dreams, and abilities; his resources; his supports; then she designs an intervention plan in which personal strengths and supports can be used to address areas of need or skill deficit.

As discussed above, this phase is where much of the art of being a clinician comes into play. Some examples of strategies combining strengths, supports, and skills with needs and deficits include the following:

- Scott is a 24 year-old man in a wheelchair from a recent spinal cord injury that he sustained in a skiing accident. His overall goals include wanting to be able to continue to participate in skiing and to remain connected to his skiing-related friends. His strengths, supports, and resources include a highly supportive group of friends, extensive knowledge of local ski schools and resorts, and past experience as a ski instructor. His needs include education regarding adaptive ski equipment and continued strength and endurance training to support his skiing. The recreation therapist works with Scott to use his resources to identify and link up with an adaptive ski program at a ski resort that he and his friends have enjoyed visiting and to arrange a visit there with five of his friends. After he has been trained in adaptive ski techniques, the therapist supports him to put together a proposal at his favorite ski resort to begin a small adaptive ski class that Scott volunteers to lead.
- Ronny is an 8-year-old boy with autism who spends two hours per day in an inclusive classroom and the remaining hours in a special education classroom. His strengths and supports include parents who are very involved with him, a friend named Annie from his inclusive classroom who has taken a liking to him, a love of music and rhythm, and considerable drawing ability. His needs include increased opportunities for structured recreation on the weekends. The recreation therapist uses her own community resources to identify a Parents-&-Kids-Together Art Class, and contacts the instructor to determine that the nature of the class would be appropriate for Ronny in terms of level of stimulation and structure. Ronny's mom and dad are able to contact Annie's parents, and they all express an interest in attending the class together. In this way, Ronnie is able to successfully take part in recreation opportunities in his community, to enjoy his art, and to have multiple social supports around him.

3. **Sequencing and Structuring the Intervention.** Finally, the therapist develops a specific plan for what activities will be undertaken in implementing the intervention. She considers such issues a the client's preferred learning style, the complexity of skills to be learned, and the components, or steps, into which the skills can be broken. She develops a plan for how frequently the intervention will occur, where it will occur, and how it will be organized to allow for time to practice and master the skills. She develops a monitoring plan and strategy so that, together, she and the client can monitor progress and growth.

The following is an example of how an intervention might be sequenced:

- Sarah is a 35-year-old woman diagnosed with paranoid schizophrenia. For the past five years she has resided in a residential group home in the community. However, she has remained quite isolated because she tends to become extremely frightened and overwhelmed in crowds or when there is lots of noise, and, when frightened, her hallucinations tend to become more pronounced. She has recently started taking medications that help her to keep her hallucinations fairly well under control, and she feels that she would like to try to get out of the house more. Sarah has few social supports, except for one older woman from the group home who she "doesn't mind too much—she is real kind and patient with me." Her strengths include a love of nature and her ability to persevere and to try things even though they are sometimes hard. The therapist works with Sarah to identify a local park with some open areas for walking and some benches under a tree. Sarah feels that this is a place that she would like to try to visit. The therapist sees Sarah two times per week and sequences her intervention in the following way so that they do one new step each week. First, they drive by the park, as Sarah feels fairly safe in the therapist's car. Then, they walk to the edge of the park and look around and then return. The next week, they walk into the park and stay for 15 minutes, walking and sitting on the benches. The next week, they take sandwiches there and stay for 30 minutes and have lunch. The next week, Sarah invites her friend to come along, and the three of them visit together. The next week, the therapist accompanies Sarah and her friend to the park, and, as planned, leaves them alone for 10 minutes before joining them to walk back. The next week, the therapist meets Sarah and her friend at the park, stays for 10 minutes, then leaves them to walk home together. Finally, the therapist assists Sarah to schedule two weekly visits to the park with her friend, and to plan for various enjoyable activities there, such as having lunch, feeding the birds, doing needlepoint, and making leaf rubbings. All throughout the intervention, the therapist has been working with Sarah to take three deep breaths when she feels afraid, to say positive things to herself, and to record her successes in a journal.

4. **Documenting the Intervention Plan.** Finally, the therapist must document the client's plan in a manner that communicates clearly to members of the health care or service team and that accurately represents the outcomes, activities, and time frames that characterize the interventions. Documentation concerns are discussed further below.

Implementing the Intervention

The next phase of the therapeutic recreation process is implementation, or the actual delivery of services. Fortunately, the recreation therapist has a wide spectrum of options for her interventions, allowing her to tailor them to the needs of the individuals being served. A significant portion of the recreation therapist's training is devoted to studying and mastering these intervention options. For the purposes of this chapter, we will summarize some of the major types of interventions in order to give the beginning student a sense of the richness of choices open to individuals who practice therapeutic recreation.

Interventions may be conducted *one-on-one* or in *groups*. Ideally, the needs and preferences of the client and the professional judgment of the therapist should drive the decision about how services are offered, and many times, a recreation therapist will have the opportunity to work with a client in both one-on-one and group contexts, as needed. Each modality has advantages and appropriate uses. One-on-one services allow for maximum flexibility in individualizing and contextualizing interventions and in truly moving at the client's own pace. They allow the therapist to devote all of her attention to the individual client, which may be important when a great deal of hands-on assistance is needed. Group interventions, on the other hand, allow for the development of interpersonal relationships and for the reinforcement and encouragement that arise from working together with a group of peers on a common goal or concern.

Services may be provided in a relatively segregated setting, as in a classroom or treatment center, or in an inclusive setting, as in a restaurant or movie theater. Common practice in therapeutic recreation interventions is to deliver them in both settings, in a sequenced manner, so that the client may receive instruction and rehearsal opportunities in the safety of the classroom but then will have the opportunity to master those skills in his natural environment, at first with support, and then with increasing independence.

Interventions may be implemented using a variety of different teaching and learning modalities. Interventions may be *verbal*, involving discussion, instruction, and/or feedback, or *nonverbal*. Nonverbal interventions may include various types of physical activity, and/or artistic or creative expression.

A brief listing of some of the commonly utilized therapeutic recreation intervention modalities follows. You will notice that many of the interventions involve sequenced skill training. Students in therapeutic recreation receive extensive training in the sequence of interventions so that the client is gradually able to successfully master the skill in increasingly challenging and natural environments and is able to choose and participate in recreation activities in an increasingly self-determined manner. The interventions provided are certainly not the only ones available to the therapist; however, they will give you a broad picture of the different choices and options available to both therapists and clients:

1. **Cognitive-Behavioral Training.** These interventions assist the client in becoming aware of the internal thoughts and beliefs that are influencing his actions and in helping to systematically practice altering those thoughts and beliefs to develop new patterns of behavior. The individual participate in careful monitoring of his actions, thoughts, and feelings in order to perceive patterns to make changes. Cognitive-behavioral interventions are particularly useful in learning to manage anxiety, stress, fear, anger, and other "unmanageable" feelings.
2. **Relaxation Training.** These interventions assist the client in effectively managing the physiological indicators of stress, and often result in reduced levels of

psychological or emotional stress as well. Some examples of relaxation, yoga, guided imagery, and meditation.

3. **Adventure/Risk Recreation.** These interventions use challenging high-risk or adventure situations to promote personal growth and self-awareness and to foster trust, self-confidence, and cooperation. They are often used with adolescents or adults experiencing difficulties in functioning because of emotional, behavioral, or social challenges, including addiction, behavioral/emotional disorders, and stress disorders. Some examples of risk or adventure recreation include ropes courses and extended wilderness adventures.
4. **Social Skills and Relationship Training.** These interventions are designed to promote improvements in the quality of an individuals' social interaction. Social skills training is often a component of intervention programs for individuals with a wide range of disabilities, including developmental disabilities, mental illness, addiction, and childhood or adolescent behavioral problems. Most social skills training interventions involve skill demonstration and learning, discussion, and active practice both in and out of group settings. Examples of social skills training topics include conversation skills, nonverbal communication, and listening skills.
5. **Community Resource Education.** These interventions are designed to assist individuals to seek out, identify, and practice using various community resources that support recreation involvement. As above, these interventions often involve a classroom-based component and an active practice component.
6. **Community Integration Interventions.** These interventions are designed to be implemented with a wide range of individuals, including those with physical disabilities, psychiatric disabilities, and developmental disabilities. They are developed as a carefully sequenced series of recreation experiences that assist individuals to be both successful and comfortable in a variety of community settings. Interventions are sequenced from less challenging to more challenging, and from more therapist-directed to less therapist-directed.
7. **Assertiveness Training.** Closely related to social skills training, assertiveness skills are often taught on their own, as the ability to clearly express one's needs and desires is so important to successful participation in recreation and leisure pursuits. Individuals with developmental disabilities, psychiatric disabilities, and addictions are often targeted for assertiveness training. Assertiveness training topics may include expressing one's needs, expressing anger, and resolving conflicts.
8. **Cognitive Training.** These interventions are designed to assist people with cognitive impairments due to aging or injury to restore or to maintain cognitive abilities, especially in the areas of attention, memory, following directions, reasoning, and problem solving. Games and activities that foster these skills are often utilized, as is sequenced practice in natural settings.
9. **Fitness and Health Education.** Health improvement and ongoing health maintenance are the concern of individuals with many disabilities. The therapist seeks

to creatively choose enjoyable and attainable activities that will foster improvement in levels of fitness and health.

10. **Adapted Activity Skills.** For many individuals with disabilities related to aging, illness, or injury, familiar activities may need to be adapted, or altered, so as to allow continued participation. The therapist combines technology, ingenuity, and available resources to successfully adapt enjoyable and valued activities.

Planning for Transition

This phase of the therapeutic recreation process is sometimes called ***discharge planning*** (in inpatient, residential, or medical model outpatient facilities) or ***transition planning*** (in educational contexts). It is a crucial part of the process that provides continuity, as it is the phase in which the individual and the therapist have the chance to look at what has been accomplished, what challenges will emerge in the future, and what supports are needed as the individual moves on to a more independent setting.

Ideally, transition planning should begin during, rather than at the end of, treatment, so that clients will have the opportunity to plan for, and preferably visit or experience, some of the settings that they will encounter in the next phase of life. Comprehensive transition planning involves exploration of the places, people, opportunities, and resources that will be part of the individual's life, exploration of the supports available to him; and identification of "next steps" for his development. An example of transition planning follows:

- Maria is a 68-year-old woman who has experience a stroke and has been on a rehabilitation unit for one month. She is preparing to go home, where she lives with her 70-year-old husband. Maria enjoys the company of friends and has loved card playing, gourmet cooking and dinner parties, and swimming. She is still experiencing some left side weakness in her extremities, making such activities as cooking, dressing, and needlework difficult for her. The therapist meets with Maria and her husband and joins with an occupational therapist to consider some simple adaptations to the kitchen and cooking equipment that will allow Maria to successfully and safely continue to create her gourmet meals for her family and friends. The therapist links her with a peer support group for women who are recovering from strokes and meets with Maria and one of her female friends who has volunteered to drive her to the group and stay there with her until she becomes comfortable. She locates a therapeutic swim class at a local community college where Maria can continue her strengthening exercises, socialize with other people, and eventually, return to her lap swimming in a nonspecialized program.

Evaluating the Intervention

The final phase of the therapeutic recreation process is the evaluation of the effectiveness of the intervention. As discussed in the *planning* phase, the therapist does not wait until the end of the intervention to evaluate its effectiveness; rather, she has already built-in mechanisms for evaluation, or monitoring, along the way. Evaluation of an intervention has become increasingly important in health care and human service settings, as issues of cost effectiveness and scarce resources become more pressing and urgent. The recreation therapist must be skilled in evaluation so that she can successfully advocate for the profession.

Various aspects of the intervention may be evaluated, depending upon the requirements and needs of the setting. These include the following:

1. **Attainment of Identified Goals.** Evaluation of outcomes provides crucial information to the therapist, the client, and administrative or reimbursing bodies. This type of evaluation answers the question: "To what extent did the intervention achieve what it was intended to achieve?" The development of measurable, observable intervention objectives makes evaluation of outcomes much more precise and accurate.
2. **Effectiveness of the Intervention Over Time.** This type of evaluation answers the question: "What happened to the effectiveness of the intervention over time? Was the individual able to maintain the progress that she had made during the intervention? Or, was there some decline in progress due, perhaps, to change in support systems or environments?" Maintaining the positive results of an intervention over time is an important and continual challenge in the provision of quality services to people with disabilities.
3. **Satisfaction with Services: Clients and Families.** Increasingly, the satisfaction of service recipients is becoming an important indicator of the quality of services. In the past, the medical expert was the primary source of evaluative data; currently, however, with increasing competition within health care and human services, the consumer's opinions regarding the effectiveness of services, as well as the process or manner in which services are delivered, is becoming a priority. In addition, such evaluation is especially critical to looking at therapeutic recreation interventions, since, at the core of the recreation interventions, is the individual's response to and way of perceiving that experience. For all of these reasons, evaluation of services by clients and families is critical.
4. **Cost Effectiveness of Services.** This type of evaluation answers the question: "How much service was provided, resulting in what outcomes, and at what cost?" In other words, this type of evaluation balances the ***benefits*** of intervention in terms of positive client outcomes with the costs of intervention in terms of staff time and resources. Often, this type of evaluation will take place at the administrative, rather than individual therapist, level; however, therapists are commonly asked to track their use of time and to report ***units of service*** in terms of hours of service to clients.

Finally, it is important for the beginning student to consider, when thinking about evaluation, that in current health care and human service climates, ***after-the-fact*** evaluation has largely been replaced by ***quality improvement*** activities, in which selected indicators of quality are tracked over time, so that improving services may occur on an ongoing basis. In many ways, this is a highly effective form of evaluation because needed changes can occur as they are identified, protecting the best interests of the clients and service recipients.

A Note on Documentation of Services

While it may seem like busywork, documentation is critical to effective work in a health care or human service setting. While this text does not address rules or processes of documentation, the beginning student should be aware that it is a vital component of providing services as a recreation therapist. Documentation is often the primary means of communication among staff members who work at different times and on different days, and who comes from different disciplines. The student of therapeutic recreation learns methods of documentation that are clear, accurate, understandable, and as free as possible of personal opinion or bias.

In addition, accurate documentation of services and outcomes often forms the basis for reimbursement or funding reports; it is imperative that such data are tracked and conveyed accurately. Finally, documentation is a part of providing ethical services; an effective documentation system will provide a complete and accurate record of what was done in the context of intervention, where it was done, when it was done, who did it, and perhaps, why a given course of action was chosen. This information is critical to maintaining accountable, high quality services.

Conclusion

What does therapeutic recreation have to offer to the individual and to health care and human service systems that is unique and of most value? This question is very important as the profession, as well as health care and human service settings, continue to evolve and grow. You are invited to consider some of the contributions that we have discussed in this chapter that are unique to therapeutic recreation. A focus has been on the following: 1) strengths and abilities, 2) enjoyment, 3) self-determination, and 4) individualized, person-centered service.

Learning Activities

1. Answer the questions: "Do you believe that recreation is therapeutic? If so, in what way? What is it that makes a recreation experience therapeutic?" Now, interview five people and ask them the same questions.

   What therapeutic aspects of recreation did your respondents mention? What kind of variation did you see in the range of responses that you received from others? How did these compare to your own experience of recreation? What does this tell you about the *therapeutic* nature of recreation?

2. Think about someone you know who has a disability or a long-term illness. Divide a piece of paper into two columns, labeled "Strength and Abilities" and "Deficits and Disabilities."

   Describe a therapeutic recreation intervention for the person, basing your ideas *only* on the "Deficits and Disabilities" list. Then, describe an intervention basing your ideas only on "Strengths and Abilities" list. Finally, design an intervention based upon information on *both* lists.

How would you evaluate the relative merits of each intervention? What happens when we look only at disability? What happens when we fail to consider the impact of the disability? What happens when we take into account both simultaneously?

3. Interview someone who has gone through treatment or rehabilitation for an illness or a disability. What changes came about as a result of the disability? How did life change?

   Ask your respondent to discuss how he was treated by health care providers and to talk about how this felt. Finally, ask your respondent to identify the most helpful and the least helpful aspect of his treatment. What did you learn from your interview?

4. Interview professionals from several different health care disciplines, for example—physical therapy, nursing, occupational therapy, psychology, speech therapy, physical medicine, psychiatry, creative arts therapy, or social work.

   Ask your respondents, "How do you understand therapeutic recreation?" Ask them to discuss what they know about therapeutic recreation, if it is practiced in the setting in which they work, and how it fits into the total rehabilitation picture.

   What do you observe about how people from other health care disciplines view therapeutic recreation? Do you believe that their perceptions are accurate?

   How might a recreation therapist go about educating other staff members about therapeutic recreation?

References

Austin, D.R., & Crawford, M.E. (1996). *Therapeutic recreation: An introduction*. Needham Heights, MA: Allyn and Bacon.

Bullock, C.C. (1987). Recreation and special populations. In A. Graefe & S. Parker (eds.), *Recreation and leisure: An introductory handbook* (pp. 203-207). State College, PA: Venture Publishing.

Carter, M.J., VanAndel, G.E., Robb, G.M. (1995). *Therapeutic recreation: A practical approach* (2nd ed). Prospect Heights: Waveland Press.

Coyle, C.P., Kinney, W.B., Riley, B., & Shank, J.W. (1991). *The benefits of therapeutic recreation: A consensus view.* Ravensdale: Idyll Arbor, Inc.

Csikszentmihalyi, M. (1990). *Flow: The psychology of optimal experience*. New York: Harper and Row.

Dattilo, J. & Kleiber, D.A., (1993). Psychological perspectives for therapeutic recreation research: The psychology of enjoyment. In M. J. Malkinm & C. Z. Howe (eds.), *Research in therapeutic recreation: Concepts and methods* (pp. 57-76). State College, PA: Venture.

Dattilo, J., Kleiber, D., & Williams R. , (1998). Self-Determination and Enjoyment Enhancement: A Psychologically-Based Service Delivery Model for Therapeutic Recreation. *Therapeutic Recreation Journal, 32*(4), 258-271.

Gunter, B.G., (1987). The leisure experience: Suggested properties. *Journal of Leisure Research, 19* (2), 115-130.

Hemingway, J. (1987). Building a philosophical defense of therapeutic recreation. The case of distribution justice. In C. Sylvester, J. Hemingway, R. Murphy, K. Mobily, and P. Shank. (eds.), *Philosophy of therapeutic recreation: Ideas and issues* (Vol. 1, pp. 1-16). Alexandria, VA: National Recreation and Park Association.

Howe-Murphy, R., & Charboneau, B.G. (1987). *Therapeutic recreation intervention: An ecological perspective.* Englewood Cliffs: Prentice Hall, Inc.

Iso-Ahola, S. (1980). Toward a dialectical social psychology of leisure and recreation. In S. Iso-Ahola, (ed.), *The social psychology of leisure and recreation* (pp. 19-38). Dubuque: Wm. C. Brown, Publishers.

Iso-Ahola, S. (1984). Social psychological foundations of leisure and resultant implications for leisure counseling. In E.T. Dowd, (Ed.). *Leisure counseling* (pp. 97-128). Springfield: Charles C.Thomas, Publisher.

Kelly, J.R., Steinkamp, M.W., & Kelly, J.R. (1986). How they play in Peoria. *The Gerontologist, 26* (5), 531-537.

Kobasa, S.C. (1979). Stressful life events, personality, and health: An inquiry into hardiness. *Personality and Social Psychology, 37*, 1-11.

Kraus, R. & Shank, J. (1992). *Therapeutic recreation service: principles and practices*. Dubuque: Wm. C. Brown, Publishers.

Lahey, M. (1987). The ethics of intervention in therapeutic recreation. In C. Sylvester, J. Hemingway, R. Murphy, K. Mobily, and P. Shank. (eds.), *Philosophy of therapeutic recreation: Ideas and issues* (Vol. 1, pp. 17-26). Alexandria, VA: National Recreation and Park Association.

Neulinger, J. (1974). *The psychology of leisure*. Springfield: Charles C.Thomas, Publisher.

Peterson, C.A., & Gunn, S.L. (1984). *Therapeutic recreation program design: Principles & procedures* (2nd ed.). Englewood Cliffs: Prentice-Hall, Inc.

Reich, J.W., & Zautra, A.J. (1988). Direct and stress moderating effects of positive life experiences. In L. Cohen (ed.), *Life events and psychological functioning*. Newbury Park: Sage Publications.

Shank, J., & Kinney, W. (1987). On the neglect of clinical practice. In C. Sylvester, J. Hemingway, R. Murphy, K. Mobily, and P. Shank (eds.), *Philosophy of therapeutic recreation: Ideas and issues* (Vol. 1, pp. 65-75). Alexandria, VA: National Recreation and Park Association.

Websters II: New Riverside Dictionary. (1984). New York, NY: Houghton Mifflin Co.

Wheeler, R.J., & Frank, M.A. (1988). Identification of stress buffers. *Behavioral Medicine, 14* (2), 78-79.

Related Websites

HYPERLINK http://www.nrpa.org/branches/ntrs.htm http://www.nrpa.org/branches/ntrs.htm
(National Therapeutic Recreation Society)

HYPERLINK http://www.recreationtherapy.com/rt.htm http://www.recreationtherapy.com/rt.htm
(Therapeutic Recreation Directiory)

HYPERLINK http://www.atra-tr.org/ http://www.atra-tr.org/
(American Therapeutic Recreation Association)

HYPERLINK http://www.nystra.org/ http://www.nystra.org/
(New York State Therapeutic Recreation Association)

HYPERLINK http://www.alberta-tr.org/index.html http://www.alberta-tr.org/index.html
(Alberta Therapeutic Recreation Association)

HYPERLINK http://www.prontario.org/branches/therptc.htm http://www.prontario.org/branches/therptc.htm
(Therapeutic Recreation Branch - Ontario)

HYPERLINK http://perth.uwlax.edu/hper/RM-TR/TRAIN.html http://perth.uwlax.edu/hper/RM-TR/TRAIN.html
(Project TRAIN — Therapeutic Recreation Access to the INternet)

HYPERLINK http://perth.uwlax.edu/hper/RM-TR/TRschooh.htm http://perth.uwlax.edu/hper/RM-TR/TRschooh.htm
(Project TRIPS — Therapeutic Recreation in Public Schools)

HYPERLINK http://perth.uwlax.edu/hper/RM-TR/wintr.htm http://perth.uwlax.edu/hper/RM-TR/wintr.htm
(WINTR — Wisconsin Network of Therapeutic Recreators)

Chapter 15

Sport and People with Disabilities

Introduction

North Americans place great value on sport and people associated with sport. To confirm this, one has only to look at the growth of professional sports during the past few decades. Professional baseball, football, basketball, and hockey players as well as golfers and tennis players provide a plethora of heroes for both our youth and adults. The value placed on sport can be measured not only in terms of the number of heroes but also by the resources contributed to professional sports in terms of salaries and advertising.

Sport has been a part of human kind for centuries. The roots of sport can be traced all the way back to the Early Dynastic period of the Sumerian civilization (3000-1500 B.C.). Since its inception, some form of sport has become a part of cultures around the world. In contrast, sport for people with disabilities has much shorter, but no less important place in the development of sport. Starting in the late 1800s with people with hearing impairments, sport for people with disabilities has developed into a very significant aspect of the delivery system that facilitates the leisure and recreation needs of people with disabilities (Sherrill, 1993). This chapter will provide an overview of the topic of sport for people with disabilities. Specifically, the following areas will be discussed within this chapter: 1) this history of sport for people with disabilities; 2) benefits of sport participation; 3) the delivery system of sport for people with disabilities; and 4) sport issues for people with disabilities.

The History of Sport for People with Disabilities

In the introduction we highlighted that the disabled sport movement first began within the deaf community. In fact, according to Winneck (1990), in the 1870s the state school for the deaf in Ohio became the first school for the deaf to offer baseball; football and basketball were introduced in the ensuing 30 years. The roots of organized disabled sport can be traced to 1924 with the establishment of the Comite International des Sport des Sourds (CISS), an organization for deaf athletes. In North America the American Athletic Association for the Deaf (AAAD) was the first organization for disabled athletes to be established. It began in 1945 to facilitate sanctioned competitive sport opportunities to athletes with hearing impairments. Clearly, the disabled sport movement began within the deaf community.

With the exception of the initiatives within the community of people with hearing impairments, the remainder of the history of sport for people with disabilities is very recent, having occurred during the past 30 years. Table 15.1 provides an overview of key dates within this history.

The Stoke Mandeville Games are typically described as the catalyst for the disabled sport movement within modern times. Sir Ludwig Guttman, a neurosurgeon of Stoke, Mandeville, England, is credited with introducing competitive sports as an integral part of rehabilitation of disabled veterans following World War II. According to Labanowich (1988), Dr. Ludwig Guttman's decision in 1948 to restrict participation in hospital sports programs to those with spinal cord impairments resulted in the adoption of a fundamental premise for organizing sports programs for individuals with disabilities—that sport competition should be organized according to etiology. Labanowich explains that Guttman defended his actions by advocating for the formation of other disability-specific international sport organizations, which eventually resulted in the creation of the International Sports Organization for the Disabled (ISOD), the International Blind Sports Association (IBSA), and the Cerebral Palsy International Sports and Recreation Association (CP-ISRA).

At the same time Guttman was establishing competitive opportunities for individuals with disabilities in England and Europe, wheelchair basketball was developing in the United States. The first tournament was held at the University of Illinois in 1949, with the NWBA established that same year. Six years later, Ben Lipton established the National Wheelchair Athletic Association to increase sport opportunities for people with physical disabilities (Winnick, 1990).

In 1960, the International Stoke Mandeville Games were held in conjunction with the Olympic Games in Rome. Since that time, the Paralympic Games have been held in the host city of the Olympics each year the Olympics have been held. The relationship between the modern day Olympic games and the Paralympic Games became formalized in 1981 (the Year of the Disabled) with the establishment of the International Coordinating Committee (ICC). This committee brought under one umbrella CP-ISRA, IBSA, ISMWSF, and ISOD. One of the principal objectives of this committee is: "To be the representative organization of sport for the disabled; to negotiate with such bodies as the International Olympic Committee and the United Nations" (ICC, 1985, p. 2, as cited in Labanowich, 1988). Since the committee was first established, two other organizations have come under its umbrella—in 1986, the International Committee for Silent Sports (CISS) and the International Federation for Sports for the Mentally Handicapped (INAS-FMH). According to Labanowich (p. 270), the ICC "represents a convenient, uncomplicated medium for participation with the IOC for the six member organizations." In addi-

Table 15.1
Chronology of Sport for People with Disabilities

1870s	Participation of schools for the deaf in team sport competitions.
1907	Track meet held between the Overbrook and Baltimore schools for the blind—the earliest recorded sporting event in the U.S. for people with visual impairments.
1924	Comite International des Sports des Sourdes (CISS) was established; the first International Silent Games competition is held at Pershing Stadium, Paris, France.
1945	American Athletic Association for the Deaf (AAAD) is formed.
1949	National Wheelchair Basketball Association (NWBA) is established.
1948	First Stoke Mandeville Games for the Paralyzed opened with 16 ex-members of the British Forces—14 men and 2 women.
1952	First International Stoke Mandeville Games took place with Holland competing against England.
1957	International Stoke Mandeville Wheelchair Sports Federation (ISMWSF) is created.
1956	National Wheelchair Athletic Association is formed.
1960	International Stoke Mandeville Games, called the Paralympic Games, are held in conjunction with the Olympic Games in Rome.
1963	International Sports Organization for the Disabled (ISOD) is formed.
1967	National Handicapped Sports and Recreation Association (NHSRA) is established.
1968	The Kennedy Foundation, with the help of the Chicago Park District, organized the First International Special Olympic Games at Chicago's Soldier Field.
1969	Canadian Special Olympic Games held in Toronto, Canada.
1974	Canadian Special Olympics, Inc. is incorporated; Harry "Red" Foster is the founding president.
1976	The U.S. Association for Blind Athletes (USABA) is established.
1978	The *Amateur Sports Act*, PL 95-606, facilitates the establishment of the Committee on Sports for the Disabled (COSA) within the U.S. Olympic Committee (USOC); the Cerebral Palsy International Sports and Recreation Association (CP-ISRA) is created; the National Association of Sports for Cerebral Palsy (NASCP) is formed.
1981	International Blind Sports Association (IBSA) and the United States Amputee Athletic Association (USAAA) are created; the Cooperative Committee is formed—renamed the International Coordinating Committee (ICC) in 1983.
1983	The Federation of Sports Organizations for the Disabled is formed in Canada.
1986	The U.S. Les Autres Sports Association and the Dwarf Athletic Association of America are both formed.
1986	The International Sports Federation for Persons with Mental Handicaps (INAS-FMH) is formed.
1994	First participation of athletes with disabilities in the Commonwealth Games in Victoria, Canada.
1998	Amendments to PL 95-606 are passed by the United States Congress to create the Olympic and Amateur Sports Act which fully incorporates the Paralympics, clearly reflecting equal status for athletes with disabilities.

(Adapted from the works of Labanowich, 1988; Sherrill, 1993; Steadward & Walsh, 1986; Winnick, 1990)

tion to the facilitation of the Paralympic Games each two years (winter and summer) by the ICC, each of the six member organizations also hold international world championships.

In 1968, an altogether different sport movement began for individuals with mental retardation. Dr. Frank Hayden, a professor from Toronto, and the Kennedy Foundation both initiated the first International Special Olympic Games at Soldier Field in Chicago for approximately 1,000 athletes with mental retardation from the United States and Canada. Since that time, Special Olympics International has developed into a worldwide program involving more than 60 countries; international winter and summer games rotate every two years. The first Special Olympic games in Canada were held in Toronto in 1969. Canadian Special Olympics, Inc. was incorporated in 1974.

Unfortunately, sport for people with disabilities has been misunderstood by the general population, service providers, the media, and even family members. Stories about athletes with disabilities were presented as human interest stories in the media. Individuals with disabilities were not often perceived as "athletes." However, the rapid growth of sport organizations and opportunities for individuals with disabilities in the late seventies and eighties helped to change many of those images. One of the most significant things that has served to reshape the image of sport for people with disabilities has been the development of integrated or parallel competitive opportunities in generic sporting events. In the United States, two wheelchair races were held at the Los Angeles Olympic Games in 1984, and in Canada, exhibition alpine and Nordic events were held at the Calgary Olympics in 1988; in 1994, the Commonwealth Games in Victoria, British Columbia, included track and swimming events for athletes with disabilities. In addition to this, many more such opportunities were held at various national, state and provincial, and local events throughout the United States and Canada. Wheelchair events also became common place at most competitive road races throughout the United States and Canada, including the New York and Boston marathons.

On October 21, 1998, Congress passed amendments to PL 95-606, to create the Olympic and Amateur Sports Act. This legislation, proposed by Senator Ted Stevens (R-AK), fully entrenches the rights of United States athletes with disabilities in national and international competition. According to Beaver (1998, p. 6):

> ... the most important aspect of the amendments of 1998 lies in those sections recognizing sport for athletes with disabilities; on their parity with other athletes, and programs provided under the aegis of the United States Olympic Committee; in the recognition of the International Paralympic Committee, the Paralympic Games, as well as the acknowledgment of the USOC as the National Paralympic Committee for the United States.

This new bill reflects the growth in sport competition by athletes with disabilities which began more than a century ago, and continues today. In many ways, it marks the arrival of athletes with disabilities into the sporting world.

Benefits of Sport Participation

The rapid growth of sport opportunities for individuals with disabilities can be traced back to the efforts of Sir Guttman. He believed that sport could play an integral role in the rehabilitation of veterans injured during World War II. The result of Guttman's belief in the benefits of sport in the process of rehabilitation led to many exciting initiatives. Over 40 years later, looking back on this rapid development of sport opportunities for people with disabilities, an obvious question that comes to mind is: "What are the benefits of sport for people with disabilities?" A growing body of literature exists to address this question. We will highlight a few key areas found.

Exercise Outcomes

According to Depauw (1988), the benefits of exercise derived from sport participation by people with disabilities are similar to those of people without disabilities. That is, participation in sports that include a regular fitness component facilitates enhanced fitness and physical health (including muscular strength and endurance, cardiovascular endurance, and flexibility). Research has demonstrated fitness games for people with physical disabilities in such areas as muscular strength (Coutts, 1986; Davis, Tupling & Shephard, 1986), body fat (Coutts, 1986) and cardiovascular endurance (Coutts, 1990).

A number of studies have also investigated the impact of participation in Special Olympics and other sport opportunities on the fitness levels of athletes with mental retardation. For the most part, research has demonstrated that people with mental disabilities are on average less fit than non-mentally disabled peers (Fernhall & Tymeson, 1987; Reid, Montgomery, & Seidl, 1985), but that engagement in physical activity can result in improved levels of cardiovascular fitness (Tomporowski & Jameson, 1985). However, there is some controversy as to whether participation in Special Olympic programs facilitates the intensity of activity necessary to increase fitness levels. Petetti, Jackson, Stubbs, Campbell, and Battar (1989) found that male participants in the Special Olympics had comparative fitness levels to non-trained individuals without disabilities, but were less fit that trained individuals without disabilities; meanwhile, female Special Olympic participants were found to be less fit that both trained and non-trained women without disabilities. This study also found limited to nonexistent gains for a small group of Special Olympic participants tested over the course of one year. However, this group was so small the results may be questioned. This study was based in the United States. In contrast, a Canadian-based study by Dahlgren, Boreski, Dowds, Mactaish, and Watkinson (1991) found that Special Olympic athletes who participated in a yearlong training program showed significant gains in fitness, particularly in relation to cardiovascular fitness. Quite likely, these differences are the result of those in training programs. In general, we can safely say that people with mental disabilities can receive health and fitness benefits from participating in well-structured sport programs.

Skill Enhancement

Most agree that active participation in a sport can serve to enhance skills in that sport. The literature clearly indicates that individuals with disabilities can improve their performance in specific sport skills through participation in sport programs and in particular through participation in programs that incorporate instructional methods based on the most current knowledge relative to teaching practices (Reid, 1993; Steadward & Walsh, 1986). One of the greatest contributions to improvements in the area of sport skills has been the dramatic changes in wheelchair design (Steadward & Walsh, 1986). Today, athletes are able to use wheelchairs designed for their specific sport. A track athlete uses a distinctly different chair than a wheelchair basketball athlete. Advances in engineering have enabled manufacturers to create chairs that are both lightweight and extremely strong. In addition the biomechanics discipline has increased our knowledge of the appropriate techniques in a variety of sports for people with disabilities, thereby enhancing the ability of athletes to improve their own skills (Alexander, 1984; Gorton & Gavron, 1987; Pope, Sherrill, Wilkerson, & Pyfer, 1993; Walsh, 1986).

Advances in the area of skill and technique are much more closely related to improvements in teaching/coaching practices among people with mental retardation. The use of behavioral and self-control techniques have enabled coaches and athletes to benefit from the increased ability of the coach to teach athletes with mental retardation such complex tasks/sports as the high jump, basketball, and alpine and Nordic skiing through the use of such methods as skill and activity analysis. The Canadian Special Olympics has developed a two level coaches' training program within the Coaching Association of Canada's National Coaching Certification Program that teaches coaches how to teach athletes with varying ability levels of a variety of different sport skills.

Psychological and Social Benefits

Expressions such as "sport builds character" and "being part of the team" are based on the long-held belief that if one participates in sport, one will experience benefits beyond learning, refining a new skill, or becoming more fit. There is little question that, indeed, any such benefits from participating in sport do exist. As with sport for people without disabilities, there has been much discussion within the field of disability related to the relative social and psychological benefits of participation in sport by people with disabilities. We will briefly discuss some of the benefits that have been identified.

The majority of work focused on psychological benefits has looked at the impact of sport participation on different psychological constructs representative of what is often described as psychological well-being. For example, Gibbons and Bushakra (1989) studied the impact on participation in a Special Olympic event on perceived competence. Perceived competence is a psychological construct often used as an indicator of psychological well-being. They found that children who participated in Special Olympic events had higher levels of perceived competence than children who were not Special Olympic participants. A more recent study conducted by Dykens (1994) of Yale University also found that individuals with mental disabilities who participated in the International Special Olympic games had greater self-esteem than either the noninternational Special Olympic participants or the individuals with mental retardation who had not participated in Special Olympics at all.

Similar studies have been conducted with participants in wheelchair tennis participants and nonparticipants. They found that the participants were more positive in their moods and were more confident about their wheelchair tennis skills and general wheelchair mobility skills. Hedrick (1985) found similar positive results among adolescent participants in wheelchair tennis. His study demonstrated participation in wheelchair tennis to have a positive impact on perceptions of competence. As cited by Hedrick (1985) and Greenwood, Dzewaltowski, and French (1990), studies by Campbell and Jones (1994), Patrick (1986), and Sherrill and Rainbolt (1988) support the positive effects of sport on the psychological well-being of athletes with physical disabilities.

Based on the research cited above that people with disabilities can experience enhanced psychological well-being from participating in sport, the growing popularity of participation is quite evident. A complementary area within the research literature relates to the impact of sport participation from a social perspective. Williams (1994) conducted a thorough review of the literature related to sport socialization and identity construction in athletes with disabilities. He indicates that the literature on sport socialization has uncovered some key areas of consensus. First, it appears that sport socialization is different for athletes with and without disabilities. For example, the literature suggests that friends and peers are the most important initial socializing agents in wheelchair sports, followed closely by other people in the community (e.g., recreation personnel). Family and schools appear to be least important. This is in marked contrast to the literature on sport socialization in the case of athletes without disabilities, where the family and schools play a much more vital role. The second important finding within this literature is that sport socialization is markedly different for people with congenital disabilities, versus those with acquired disabilities. People with congenital disabilities are exposed to a long-term socialization process, which is both general and sport specific in nature. In contrast, the socialization process for people with acquired disabilities will vary depending upon the age of onset of the disability. Williams (1994, p. 19) indicated that:

> Individuals with acquired impairments, however, will have been subjected to different socialization influences for varying lengths of time depending upon the age of acquiring the impairment. In the case of individuals with spinal cord injuries, for example, many have been subjected to nondisabled socialization prior to their injuries and subsequent disability socialization. Disability socialization, then, is conceptualized as autobiographical discontinuity for individuals with noncongenital impairments.

A third key finding identified by Williams (1994) with respect to sport socialization is that sport socialization for people with disabilities is the product of a variety of influences, that vary for each individual. Some of these influences are age, gender, type of disability, and setting. So, though training principles for athletes with and without disabilities may be very similar, the nature of a person's disability and the culture of that particular disability may result in entirely different training program structures.

In addition to focusing on the nature of sport socialization, considerable attention has been given to the impact of athletes with disabilities, and disabled sport in general, on attitudes of people without disabilities toward people with disabilities. For example, Kisabeth and Richardson (1985) studied the affect of having one person with a disability in an undergraduate raquetball class on the attitudes students towards the individual with a disability. They found significant differences in attitude between a class of students who had a classmate with a disability and one that did not.

Together, the literature of the psychological and social benefits of participation in sport by people with disabilities provide convincing evidence of the value of sport. When combined with the evidence related to physical fitness, health, and skill enhancement, it becomes very clear that sport is indeed an important leisure and recreation option for people with disabilities. Given this, we need to develop an understanding of the delivery system that exists for facilitating opportunities in sport for people with disabilities.

The Delivery System of Sport for People with Disabilities

In an earlier section we discussed the emergence of sport for people with disabilities in modern times. What is evident from looking at the history of sport for people with disabilities in North America is that since about the mid-1900s there have been many organizations that have been established in both North America and internationally to provide sport training and competitive opportunities for athletes with disabilities. Two of the most widely known international programs to be developed have been the Paralympic Games and Special Olympics International. The Paralympic sport movement consists of training and competition outlets for people with disabilities who are under the auspices of one of the following organizations: Cerebral Palsy International Sports and Recreation Association (CP-ISRA), International Blind Sports Association (IBSA), International Stoke Mandeville Wheelchair Sports Federation (ISMWSF), International Sports Organizations for the Disabled (ISOD), Comite International des Sport des Sourds (CISS), and International Sports Federation for Persons with Mental Handicaps (INAS-FMH). Together, these groups provide competitive outlets for individuals with varying types of disabilities, both physical and mental in nature, under the auspices of the International Paralympic Committee. Until recently, the one group who was not represented in the United States or Canada was INAS (International Sports Federation for Persons with Mental Handicaps). However, Canada recently formed the Canadian Association for Athletes with Intellectual Disabilities (CAMH), which is affiliated with INAS.

Within the United States there are numerous organizations that facilitate training and competition for athletes with disabilities from a grass-roots level all the way to international competition. The Committee (USOC), represents the following eight different multisport organizations who provide opportunities for athletes with disabilities:

- American Athletic Association for the Deaf (AAAD),
- Dwarf Athletic Association of American (DAAA),
- National Handicap Sports (NHS)
- National Wheelchair Athletic Association (NWAA),
- Special Olympics, Inc.,
- United States Association for Blind Athletes (USABA),
- United States Les Autres Sports Association (USLASA),
- U.S. Cerebral Palsy Athletic Association (USCPAA).

In Canada, all sport organizations for people with disabilities who have affiliation with both a national and international organization are a part of Sport Canada, which is the body that funds and monitors amateur sport in Canada. The ***majority*** of these organizations are associated with the Canadian Paralympic Committee (CPC), formerly the Canadian Federation of Sport Organizations for the Disabled (CFSOD). This organization is a member of the International Coordinating Committee which supports the Paralympic Games. Members of this group include the following:

- Canadian Amputee Sports Association (CASA),
- Canadian Association for Athletes with Mental Retardation (CAAMH),
- Canadian Association for Disabled Skiing (CADS),
- Canadian Blind Sports Association (CBSA),
- Canadian Cerebral Palsy Sports Association (CCPSA),
- Canadian Therapeutic Riding Association (CANTRA),
- Canadian Deaf Sports Association (CDSA),
- Canadian Wheelchair Sport Association,
- Canadian Wheelchair Basketball Association (CWBA).

In addition, in 1994 the Canadian Yachting Association, Federation of Canadian Archers, Racquetball Canada, and the Shooting Federation of Canada were accepted as Paralympic sport members. The mandate of these organizations is to facilitate sport training and competition for all athletes, including those with disabilities. Their application for membership illustrates the connection between disabled and nondisabled sport, which has become much more prominent.

Consistent with the international scene and the United States, the Canadian Special Olympics is not associated with the Canadian Paralympic Committee. Canadian Special Olympics is affiliated with Special Olympics International, of which the U.S. is a part.

It is important to note that though each of the organizations responsible for facilitating different sport opportunities for athletes may differ in terms of such things as rules, administrative framework, and types of athletic competitions offered, they hold a number of things in common. Kennedy, Smith, and Austin (1991) have highlighted a number of common goals of sport organizations for athletes with disabilities. These are highlighted in Table 15.2.

The breadth of the delivery system for sport for individuals with disabilities precludes us from describing in detail each of the organizations cited above. Rather, to give you some examples of the structure of organizations that facilitate sport opportunities for people with disabilities, we will provide an overview of Special Olympics and Wheelchair Sports, the latter being a part of the Paralympic system.

Table 15.2
Common Goals of Sport Organization for Athletes with Disabilities

1. Provide a method of informing the public about the unique abilities that participants possess.
2. Promote independence, sports skill development, and increased physical fitness among participants.
3. Promote maximum participation by offering local and regional events but also provide for recognition of outstanding performances though national and international competition.
4. Have some system of classification, such as degree of disability, to make the competition in events as fair as possible.
5. Use the classification system as a method of increasing participation opportunities among individuals with severe disabilities.
6. Offer some unique competitive events, or modified activities that provide the participant with a chance to display special skills not usually associated with nondisabled competition.

(Adapted from Kennedy, Smith, & Austin, 1991, p. 239)

Special Olympics

Special Olympics was the brainchild of Dr. Frank Hayden, who became the first executive director of Special Olympics, Inc. In the early sixties, research indicated that children with mental retardation were only half as fit as their nondisabled peers. People assumed this was due to their cognitive disability. Dr. Hayden, a researcher and professor at the University of Toronto, challenged this long held assumption. As a result of a rigorously controlled experimental research design, he determined that individuals with mental retardation could become physically fit and develop sport skills (Canadian Special Olympics, 1994). Spurred on by this discovery, Dr. Hayden worked to establish a national sport organization for athletes with mental retardation. His work came to the attention of the Kennedy Foundation in Washington, D.C. This led to the creation of Special Olympics and the first Special Olympic games held at Soldier Field in Chicago on July of 1968. Dr. Hayden, ever conscious of his Canadian roots, contacted Harry "Red" Foster, a well-known

Canadian broadcaster, businessman, and humanitarian, to solicit his support to bring a Canadian contingent to Chicago. Foster, who had a brother with a mental disability, accompanied a team of floor hockey players to Chicago. Thus, from the beginning, Special Olympics has been international in scope. Soon after the Chicago games, Special Olympics Inc. was created. The first Canadian Special Olympics were held the following summer, 1969, in Toronto, and Canadian Special Olympics was incorporated in 1974. Today, Special Olympics, Inc. (SOI) is the largest program of sport training and competition for athletes with mental retardation, involving over a million athletes from well over 60 countries in training and competition.

According to Songster (1986, p. 74), "the mission of Special Olympics is to provide year-round training and competition in a variety of Olympic-type sports for all mentally retarded children and adults." Individuals with mental retardation who are eight years of age or older are eligible for participation in Special Olympics. SOI uses the American Association on Mental Retardation definition of mental retardation (described earlier in this text) as a criterion for accepting athletes. However, because coaches and administrators are volunteers and probably do not have access to information related to IQ and adaptive skills, other criterion such as whether the individual receives services from an agency geared to the needs of individuals with mental retardation (such as special education and supported employment) are often used.

We indicated earlier that one of the common goals of sports organization for athletes with disabilities is that they most often offer a "classification system as a method of increasing participation opportunities among individuals with severe disabilities." This is indeed one of the cornerstones of Special Olympics. The three criterion used to classify athletes are: 1) age, 2) gender, and 3) previous sport performance. Through these three criterion, Special Olympics works to establish equal ability groups for competition. Songster (1986, p. 75) indicates that these equal ability groups help to accomplish several goals, including:

> ...it promotes the true spirit of Special Olympics by providing sport training and competition for all mentally retarded people (sic); it provides fair and equitable conditions for competition; it protects the physical well-being of the athletes; and it promotes uniformity so that no competitor can obtain an unfair advantage over another.

To facilitate the creation of ability groups for an event, actual scores, times, or distances recorded during prior meets or practice sessions are used. To avoid any competitive imbalance, Special Olympics uses the 10% rule. This simply means that an athlete should be matched in competition with athletes who performed within 10% of her own performance. For example, if an athlete's recent high jumps have been 3'6" or 42", she must compete with athletes who typically high jump approximately 4" (10%) higher or lower than she. In this case, she should compete against athletes who typically jump between 3'2" and 3'10". This way the competition is more fair.

Athletes with a physical disability who are mentally retarded are also eligible to compete in Special Olympics. Athletes with a physical disability are classified using the same criterion as is used for other Special Olympians. Thus, an athlete with a physical disability who uses a wheelchair may compete against athletes who do not use a wheelchair; however, their previous performances would have been within 10% of each other.

Organizational Structure

Special Olympics has grown to become a year-round program of training and competition in both winter and summer sports. The official winter and summer sports for SOI are listed in Table 15.3.

Special Olympics, in a sense, started as an international event with the first games in Chicago because of Canadian participation. This fact has been both a help and a hindrance to Special Olympics. While helping to facilitate the development of an international organization from the very beginning, SOI did start as an event, and so for many years was criticized for providing little or no training for athletes—just providing the "big event." In addition, SOI has sometimes been criticized for calling itself an international organization while focusing most of its energies on the United States. More recently, Special Olympics International has worked hard to develop an organization that facilitates the development of Special Olympics in the United States and around the world.

Special Olympics is organized at an international, national, and local level. The offices of Special Olympics International are located in Washington, D.C., but SOI also has offices around the world. In addition, there are a vast number of national Special Olympic organizations around the world. SOI describes each of the national organizations as chapters of SOI. To take Canada as an example, Canadian

Table 15.3
Official Winter, Summer, and Demonstration Sports for Special Olympics

Winter Sports	Summer Sports	Demonstration Sports
Alpine skiing	Swimming	Canoeing
Nordic skiing	Diving	Cycling
Figure skating	Track and Field	Table tennis
Speed skating	Basketball	Team handball
Floor hockey	Bowling	Tennis
	Equestrian	
	Football (Soccer)	
	Gymnastics	
	Roller skating	
	Softball	
	Volleyball	

Special Olympics (CSO) is located in Toronto, Ontario. CSO has 11 of its own chapters representing all of the provinces of Canada, plus the Yukon Territory in northern Canada. Each of the chapters in Canada then have local Special Olympic organizations that may represent a city, town, or area of a province. This same structure exists in the United States. Local Special Olympic organizations are sanctioned by the chapter, just as countries are sanctioned by SOI.

During the past decade, SOI has worked to create ongoing training in all of its chapters. This effort has been in response to the criticism cited earlier—that Special Olympic athletes receive minimal training. All of Special Olympic training programs around the world are run by volunteers. Volunteers come from all walks of life. A recent study conducted by Mahon (1994) of the Manitoba Special Olympic program delivery system identified the reasons that people volunteer for Special Olympics. These reasons are highlighted in Table 15.4. As is evident from the results of this study, the two most significant reasons that people volunteer are that they have a desire to work with people with mental retardation and that they want to volunteer with a sport organization. Also interesting to note is that the third most popular choice relates to the fact that volunteering with Special Olympics provides the students the opportunity to gain experience that will ultimately help them with their careers.

Competitions parallel the levels of organizational development within Special Olympics. Competitive events are offered at local, chapter, national, and international levels. Each of the competitions is bound by the rules of SOI. SOI hosts international games every two years, alternating winter and summer sports at each games. For the first two decades these games always took place in the United

Table 15.4
Why People Volunteer for Special Olympics

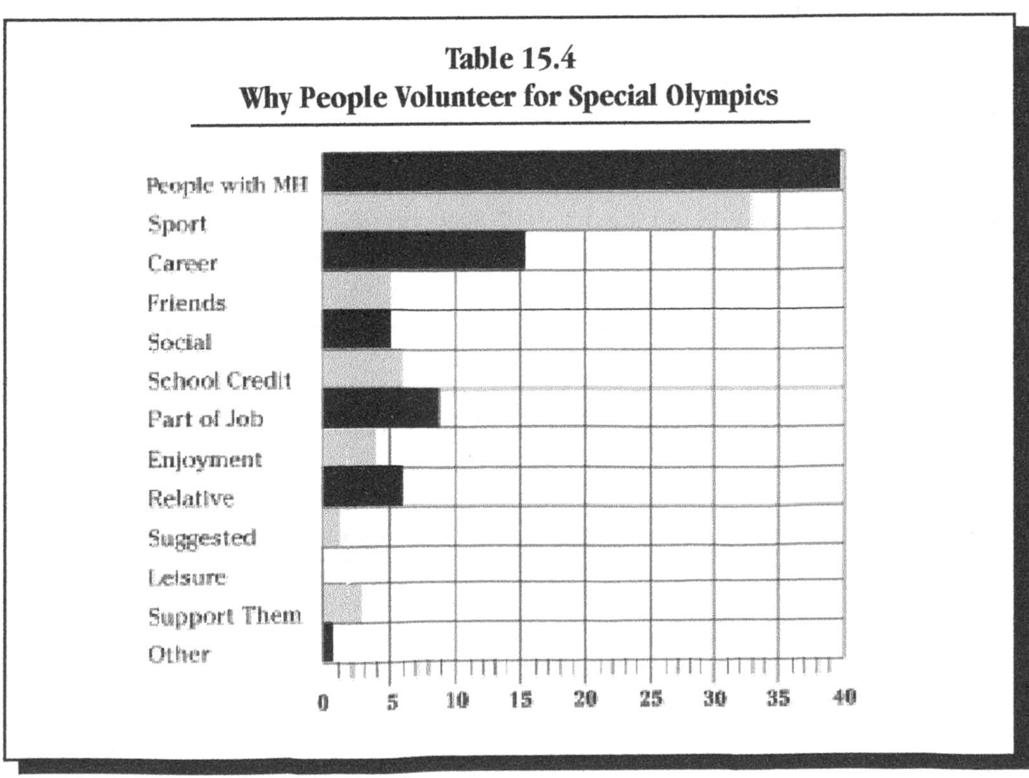

States. However, in 1993, the first games were held outside of the United States, hosted by Salzburg and Shladming, Austria. This movement to hold games outside the United States represents a continued effort on the part of SOI to be international in scope. Countries host many of their own local events and then a national event, which precedes the international hosting.

What is evident from this overview of Special Olympics is that it is a growing, variable organization. However, it is not without its controversies. We will highlight some of these controversies in the final section of this chapter.

Wheelchair Sports

The history of wheelchair sports dates back to World War II. Unlike any previous war, there was a much larger percentage of veterans who survived very serious combat related injuries. Many returned to their home communities or veterans hospitals with spinal cord injuries and amputations. As part of the process of rehabilitation, or in many cases to counteract the negative experiences of rehabilitation, many became involved in sports. Dr. Ludwig Guttman of the Stoke Mandeville Hospital in England held the first organized competition for young veterans (Labanowich, 1987). According to Allen (1981), Dr. Guttman believed that sport could provide newly disabled veterans with enjoyment, but at the same time could help them reintegrate into their home communities and establish self-respect and self-discipline. Initially, Guttman concentrated on people in wheelchairs, but he eventually expanded his vision of ***disabled sport*** to include people with other types of disabilities (Labanowich, 1987).

In the United States, Benjamin H. Lipton and Tim Nugent were responsible for the first wheelchair sports. Nugent, who was from the University of Illinois, organized the first college wheelchair basketball team in 1948 and the first National Wheelchair Basketball Tournament in 1949. Lipton initiated the first United States Wheelchair Games in 1957. The birth of wheelchair sports in the United States resulted from the development of two separate organizations. The first wheelchair sport activity in Canada took place at a field day on the front lawn of Deer Lodge Hospital in Winnipeg, Manitoba, in 1947. Five years later, two wheelchair basketball teams began practicing. The official organization of the Canadian Wheelchair Sports Association took place in Manitoba when Canada hosted the Pan-American Games. Dr. Robert W. Jackson, an orthopedic surgeon, was the first chairperson.

Philosophy and Classification System

From a philosophical standpoint, the National Wheelchair Basketball Association (NWBA), the National Wheelchair Athletic Association (NWAA), and the Canadian Wheelchair Sports Association (CWSA) believe that all sports, with the exception of swimming, should be played in wheelchairs. They believe that it is the wheelchair, almost more than the fact that a person has a physical disability, that defines the sport. Because of this, people without disabilities in many countries participate in local wheelchair basketball leagues. However, both the NWBA and the NWAA serve only people with permanent physical disabilities. Other sports organizations for people with physical disabilities are not guided by those same philosophical principles. For example, the National Sports for Cerebral Palsy believes that athletes who are able to be ambulatory should be able to compete through their own ambulation, even if this means that they must move more slowly.

As with other types of disabled sport, wheelchair sports has a classification system that is designed to both guide programming and equalize competition. In the United States, a medically-based classification system was adopted in the 1840s. The system developed then and used by the National Wheelchair Athletic Association is depicted in Figure 15.1. As depicted in the figure, the system consists of three classes for people with quadriplegia (IA, IB, IC) and four for people with paraplegia (II, IV, V, VI). In contrast to this, the system developed for the National Wheelchair Basketball Association, which is also depicted in Figure 15.1, involves three classes. Both of these medically-based classification systems have come under fire in recent years. The international community has adopted a more functional approach to classifying athletes. In the functional approach, classifiers observe the athlete to determine what their abilities are in a specific sport. Athletes are then classified based upon a functional profile. Classifications are tested to determine whether they are statistically different from one to another. Many have argued that this system is much more objective than the older approach. However, it is unclear whether the U.S. associations will move from their traditional classification approaches to a functional approach.

Scope of Opportunities

Wheelchair sports incorporate a number of different sports. Wheelchair basketball is the most popular team sport. Another popular one is quad rugby (also called murderball or wheelchair rugby). This is the game that people with lesions from C6 to T1 play. The game is played with a volleyball on a basketball court with four players. The object of the game is to carry the ball over the opponents' goal line. Players can advance the ball through any combination of passing or carrying. The ball must be bounced every 10 seconds.

Besides team sports, there are a number of individual sports played, including tennis (which can be played in pairs), swimming, shooting, weightlifting, athletics (track and field), racquetball, table tennis, and archery. Advances in terms of the types of sports played and the quality of performance have been a function of a number of things; however, two of the most important are increased expectations and changing attitudes regarding the abilities of people with disabilities and enhanced technology. We have addressed this first issue extensively throughout the book. The advancement of the wheelchair technology has mirrored that of the changes in technology within society in general. The sports chair has become extremely popular not only for sports, but for everyday use. Today, the term sports chair refers to any chair that allows for maximum maneuverability. However, beyond what is now considered the typical sports chair, there are specific chairs available for racing and triathlon racing. If you would like more detailed information on wheelchairs, we refer you to the magazine *Sports 'n Spokes*.

Figure 15.1
Medical Classification System for Wheelchair Sports

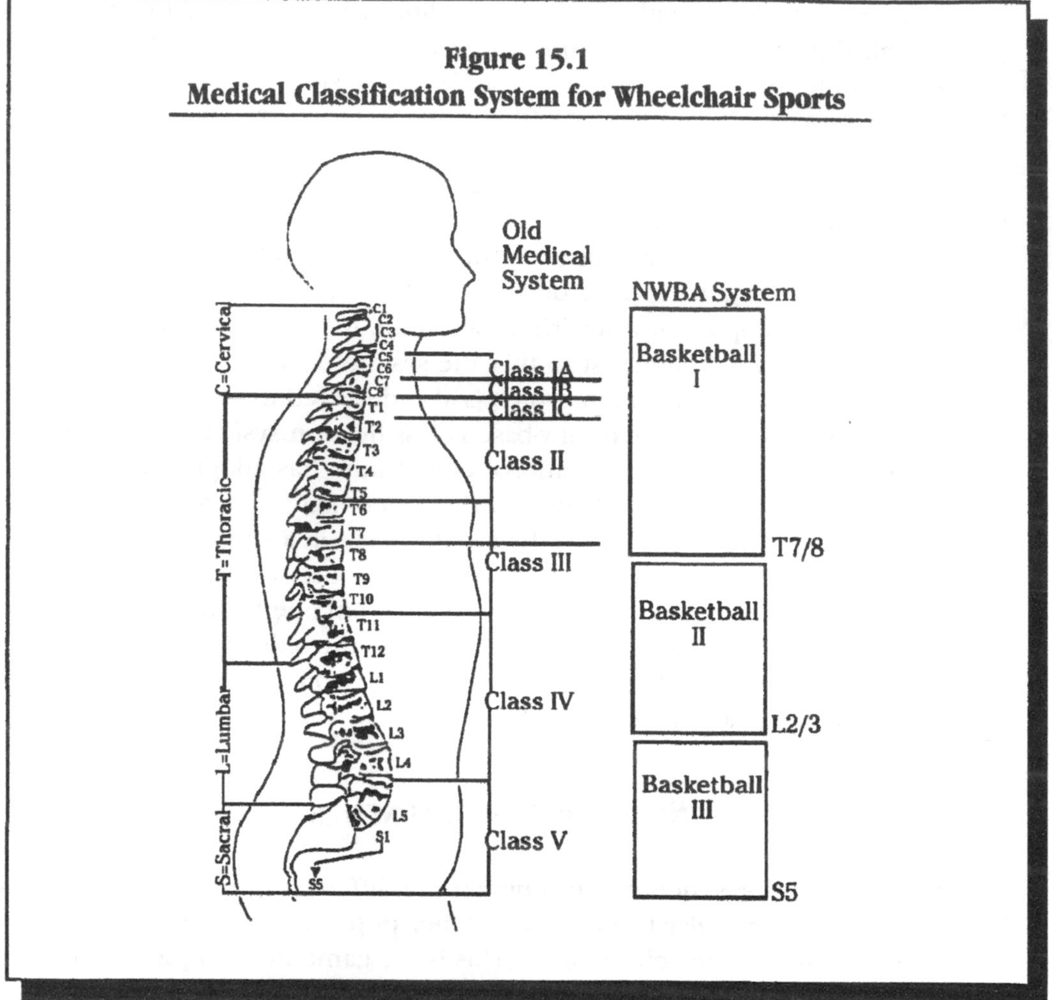

Sport Issues for People with Disabilities

Throughout this chapter we have described many of the benefits of sport participation for individuals with disabilities as well as the delivery system that has been developed during the last 40 years to facilitate such benefits. You should understand that these developments have not taken place without their share of controversy. There are varying perspectives on the most appropriate manner in which to delivered sport-related services for athletes with disabilities. We cannot highlight all of the controversial issues; however, we will touch on some of the more prominent ones.

Normalization and Integration

In the first section of this text, and throughout subsequent chapters, we discussed the significance of the principle of normalization. Clearly, we feel that this principle is foundational to the provision of recreation and sport for people with disabilities.There has been some discussion in the literature related to Special Olympics and the principle of normalization. For example, Hourcade (1989) suggested that the structure of Special Olympic competitions works in oppositions to the principle of normalization. He cited such things as huggers at the end of the finish line and the fact that Special Olympics events and programs are segregated as examples that Special Olympics does not adhere to this important principle. Others, such as Wehman and Moon (1985), have supported Hourcade's arguments.

Without a doubt, the criticisms of Special Olympics related to normalization have some foundation. However, there is evidence to suggest that Special Olympics has made significant efforts to address these issues. In fact, in a more recent article by Block and Moon (1992), this trend is recognized and applauded. In addition, recent research by Mahon (1994) indicates that strong support exists for integration within Canadian Special Olympics. In a survey of parents and coaches involved in Special Olympics. Mahon found that parents and coaches strongly supported the facilitation of training and competition opportunities in mainstream sports for athletes with mental retardation. These respondents also believed that Special Olympics should provide opportunities for athletes to become involved in community-based recreation and leisure programs. A recent initiative that has begun to address these issues is the adoption of a program/competition delivery model by Canadian Special Olympics that articulates a commitment to community integration. This model, depicted in Figure 15.2, demonstrates that CSO is committed to facilitating integrated sport and recreation opportunities for athletes with mental retardation.

Another recent example of the role that Special Olympics plays in facilitating integration is the findings of a study conducted by Studholme (1992) on integrated recreation opportunities. Studholme was commissioned by the Association for Community Living-Manitoba (formerly the Association for the Mentally Retarded-Manitoba) to conduct an investigation to determine the extent to which integrated recreation opportunities existed with the province of Manitoba. As a part of his investigation, he interviewed a large number of parents. The result that many found surprising was that Special Olympics was considered by the majority of parents to be providing the highest quality community-based recreation program.

Reverse Integration

The concept of reverse integration has been around for many years. The essence of the concept is that individuals without disabilities are asked to be a part of a traditionally segregated program as a means of facilitating interaction between people with and without disabilities. Once proposed as a method of facilitating integrated opportunities within a recreation environment, it fell out of favor because many thought it too contrived and less likely to result in less structured integrated opportunities—less likely to facilitate true social integration. Recently, reverse integration initiatives have been proposed for and in some cases used by Wheelchair Sports and Special Olympics.

In Special Olympics, the Unified Sports program has been developed. This program combines approximately equal numbers of athletes with and without

Figure 15.2
Canadian Special Olympic Program Model

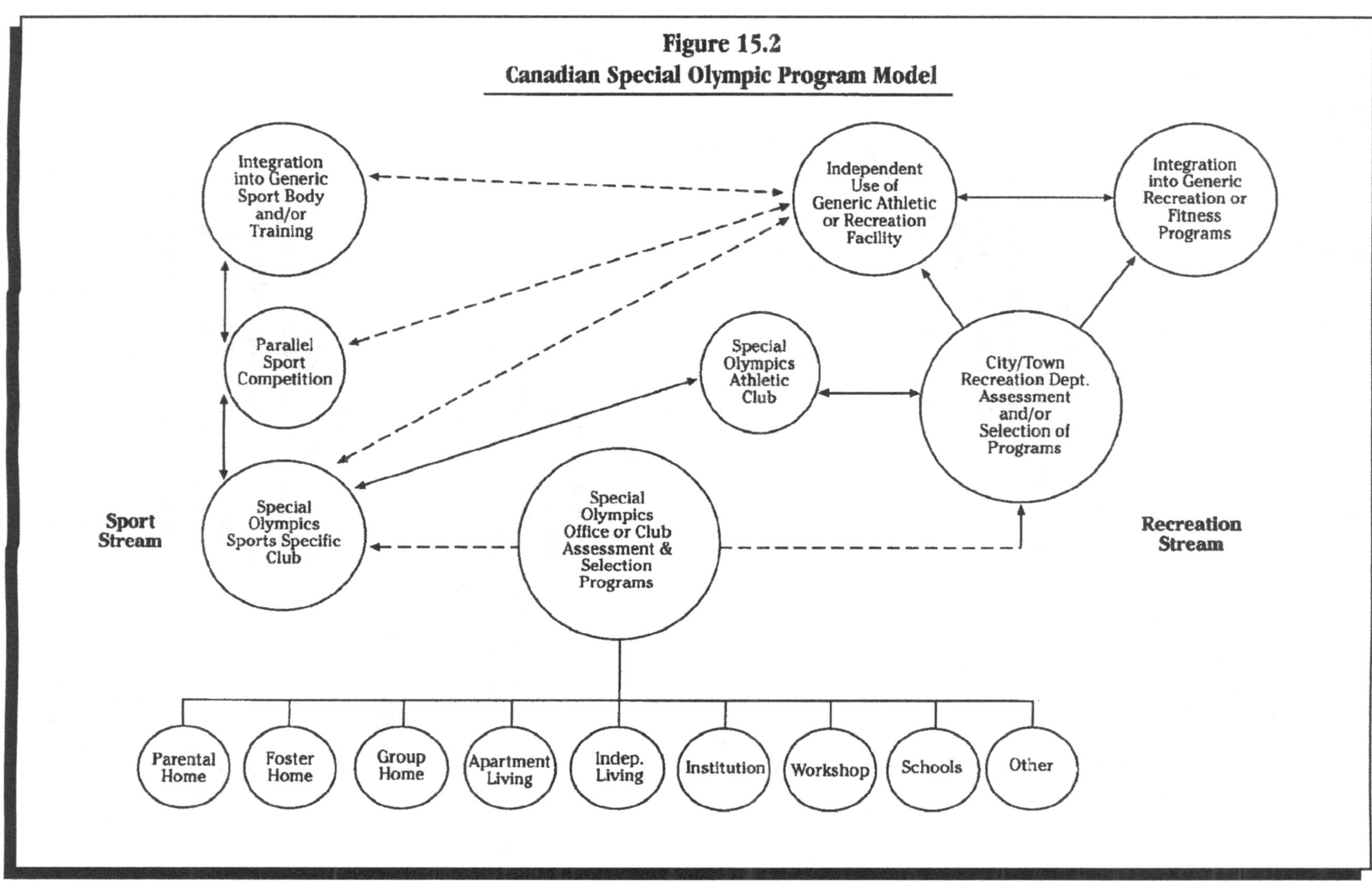

mental retardation, who are of a similar age, on teams that compete against other Unified teams.According to Special Olympics International, the Unified Sports program is unique because it provides many positive benefits:

1. It brings together athletes with and without mental retardation in a setting where everybody is challenged to improve.
2. It provides a valuable sports opportunity to individuals with mental retardation who are presently involved in Special Olympics—especially those with mild mental retardation and those in communities where there are not enough Special Olympic athletes to conduct team sports.
3. It allows athletes to develop specific sports skills and prepares them for participation in other community sports.
4. It increases public awareness of the spirit and skills of individuals with mental retardation.
5. It builds self-esteem and sports ability in all athletes by ensuring that each participant plays an important, meaningful, and valued role on the team.
6. It enables Special Olympic athletes' families to participate as team members or coaches on Unified Sports teams (Special Olympics International, 1994).

Teams that participate as a Unified team, as well as leagues themselves, can be developed by a Special Olympics group or by a community group such as a school, church, or business. The athletes with mental retardation who participate may or may not be part of a Special Olympics organization. Sports currently include basketball, bowling, distance running and walking, soccer, softball, volleyball, and cycling. Special Olympics has been commended for initiating this program, though there are those who criticize the program on the basis that it is contrived as opposed to natural integration.

Within wheelchair sports, reverse integration has been presented as an option for wheelchair basketball. Brasile (1990, p. 4) argued that the premise behind reverse integration in wheelchair athletics is:

> to promote a better comprehension of the true abilities of the disable (sic) through active participation, as well as develop an atmosphere of social integration in which all participants will be competing on an equal basis (p. 4).

Thibouot, Smith, and Labanowich (1992), in response to the Brasile article, criticize the logic of Brasile's perspective on reverse integration. They suggest that the logic behind the statement: "if integration were good, that reverse integration must also be good" is flawed. In particular, they suggest that the premise behind integration—to empower people with disabilities to be integrated into the whole of society—does not work when it is reversed; that is, that it is also useful to bring those in the mainstream (the whole) into the part (wheelchair sport). Thiboutot et al. also argue that Brasile's proposed reverse integration initiative would limit the number of opportunities wheelchair sport for athletes with disabilities.

Brasile (1992) responds to Thiboutot, et al. with the following:

> Labanowich (1978) so eloquently states "the implication for practitioners, authors, and educators in the field of recreation is that they must develop and practice a philosophy that points toward a realistic appreciation of the potential (if physically disabled individuals for normalized participation in our society)" (p. 17). Would not the acceptance of inclusion advocate a realistic appreciation of one's potential? Is not a stand against inclusion also a stand against the acceptance of wheelchair basketball as a normalized activity?

Brasile goes on to suggest:

> The inclusion of able-bodied participants cannot be reduced to a mathematical formula, as Thiboutot et al. (1992) have done. It is not an either/or situation. It is not one group versus the other group; the real fundamental issue may be related to the sociological aspects of sport participation and sport acceptance. This is an issue that goes much further than Thiboutot et al. versus Brasile. The real question is, is society ready to accept such a drastic rationale that the wheelchair takes on the aura of a piece of equipment and does not serve just as a means of confinement?

The perspective of Thiboutot el at. (1992, p. 289) would seem to have support within the National Wheelchair Basketball Association, as they indicate in their article that in 1987 the membership of the association "overwhelmingly defeated by voice vote a proposal, authored by Brasile, to admit people without disabilities as wheelchair basketball players." However, as Thiboutot et al. also point out in their article, there is support for Brasile's reverse integration initiative in Canada. Many Canadians argue that reverse integration is an important alternative for such sports as wheelchair basketball, given the population density in Canada (Personal Communication with O. Stevens, 1995, October). Even in larger urban centers it is often difficult to pull together enough athletes with disabilities to create leagues.

INAS-FMH and Special Olympics

As should be clear by now, there is no formal connection between the International Paralympic Committee, or one of its member organizations, the International Association of Sports for the Mentally Handicapped and Special Olympics. Given that both organizations claim to be international sports organizations for athletes with mental retardation, one must ask how the two coexist. First, we need to point out that INAS-FMH is a much younger organization, first established in 1986. As such, it does not, as yet, have a network that rivals SOI in size. Notwithstanding this first point, it is clear that both groups recognize each other as competition, but the same time, it appears (at least on the surface) that both groups wish to coexist and complement each other. One of the most significant differences between the two organizations relates to the form of competition each facilitates.

As was outlined earlier, SOI supports ***banded competition***, meaning that athletes participate in a similar ability grouping, or band, and each of the bands receive first-, second-, and third-place medals. In contrast, though INAS supports banded competition at lower levels, as with other Paralympic sports organizations, at international events only one winner is declared per event. In addition, only those athletes who meet a performance standard are eligible for INAS competitions.

In July of 1993, SOI and INAS-FMH met in Washington, DC. The outcome of that meeting was a memo to all chapters from Mr. Sargent Shriver, chairman and president of SOI, regarding SOI's *official* position on INAS-FMH and participation of Special Olympic athletes in non-Special Olympic events. In the memo, Mr. Shriver (1993) stated:

> I am enclosing an updated policy concerning our relationships with the International Paralympic Committee (IPC) and the International Association of Sports for the Mentally Handicapped. This follows a useful discussion on July 28th with Dr. Robert Steadward, president of IPC, and Bernard Atha, president of INAS, concerning our respective missions…SOI will not restrict or discourage any Special Olympic athlete from competing in any sporting event. At the same time, we do not permit the use of our funds, uniforms, banners, and logos in outside events. Hence, moneys raised by and for Special Olympics must be devoted only to the expansion and improvement of Special Olympics, not diverted to other athletic programs or opportunities.

What is clear from this memo is that SOI will *not* actively work against INAS-FMH, but it does not approve of Special Olympic chapters working to facilitate INAS-FMH activities. In their brochure, INAS acknowledges the position taken by SOI, but indicates that they will actively promote Special Olympic athletes participating in INAS Sponsored events. They state:

> …INAS declared its recognition of SOI as a pioneer organization which has achieved great success in its mission. It deserves and receives from INAS both respect and admiration. The philosophies of SOI and INAS differ, but they are not incompatible. SOI has a published policy which declares the right of SOI athletes to compete in any sport event of his or her choice. INAS strongly endorses this policy. INAS will work for a supportive and friendly relationship. It is not in competition with SOI. INAS hopes that SOI athletes will increasingly participate in World and Paralympic Games organized by INAS and IPC. Such athletes would remain SOI athlete before, during, and after such games, but would be part of a national team for the purpose of those games.

From the INAS brochure it is clear that INAS more actively promotes participation in paralympic competition by Special Olympic athletes than does SOI. In fact, the relationship that INAS promotes exist in at least one country. The Canadian Association for Athletes with Mental Retardation has promoted the inclusion of Special Olympic athletes in INAS competitions since its inception. Manitoba Special Olympics provided the impetus for the creation of CAAMH, which in some ways is in contravention of the policy outlined by Shiver. According to D.G. Johnson (personal communication, April 13, 1995), executive director of Manitoba Special Olympics, MSO and CAAMH (which is based in Manitoba) have a very positive relationship. MSO has contributed financially to the development of CAAMH because they believe that CAAMH and INAS-FMH provide an exciting competitive outlet for their athletes. Clearly, the goal of INAS—to have Special Olympic athletes involved in Paralympic competition—is alive and well in Canada. The relationship between SOI and INAS will continue to unfold in the coming years. As this happens, we will need to ensure that the most important issue remains front and center: the rights and choices of athletes with mental retardation.

Conclusion

In this chapter we have discussed the growth of sport for people with disabilities. The growth that has taken place regarding the participation of people with disabilities in sport in many ways mirrors the increased community-based opportunities for people with disabilities in general. These participants have more and more come to be recognized as athletes. This change in perception has resulted in increased opportunities for athletes in terms of competitions and even promotional opportunities. As with all disability-related areas, however, there is a great deal of room for growth and development. The challenge for sports organizations for people with disabilities is to attract young people with disabilities to become involved in support. In many ways, this challenge has been increased with the advent of inclusive education. Historically, young people were educated in a few settings, and as a result were more easily accessed. Today, with children attending their neighborhood schools, it is much more difficult to market opportunities to children and their families. Organizations involved in sport for people with disabilities must venture out into the mainstream to market their programs. Luckily, this challenge is balanced by the many positive images of athletes in general, and more specifically those with disabilities that exist in our culture today.

Learning Activities

1. Read the sports pages in your local newspaper. Identify a minimum of five different positive images of athletes. Are there any negative images? If so, what are they? Is there any coverage of athletes with disabilities?
2. Using the information from the conceptual cornerstones chapter, discuss the positive and negative aspects of Special Olympics and Wheelchair Sports.
3. Participate in a wheelchair basketball game or obstacle course. Discuss your feelings about the experience.

References

Alexander, M.J., (1984). Analysis of the high-jump technique of an amputee. *Palaestra, 1*, 19-23, 44-48.

Allen, A., (1981). *Sports for the handicapped.* New York: Walker and Company.

Beaver, D.P. (1998). A coming of age: Sports for athletes with disabilities and the amateur sports act. *Palaestra,* Fall, 5-6.

Block, M.E., & Moon, E.S. (1992). Orelove, Wehman, and wood revised: An evaluative review of Special Olympics ten years later. *Education and Training in Mental Retardation*, 27, 379-386.

Brasile, F.M. (1990). Performance evaluation of wheelchair athletes: More than a disability classification level issue. *Adapted Physical Activity Quarterly,* 7 (4), 289-297.

Brasile, F. (1992). Inclusion: A developmental perspective. A rejoinder to examining the concept of reverse integration. *Adapted Physical Activity Quarterly.* 9, 293-304.

Campbell, E., & Jones, G. (1994). Psychological well-being in wheelchair sport participants and nonparticipants. *Adapted Physical Activity Quarterly, 11* (4), 404-415.

Canadian Special Olympics. (1994). Canadian Special Olympics, Inc.

Coutts, K.D. (1986). Physical and physiological characteristics of elite wheelchair marathoners. In C. Sherrill (Ed.), *Sport and disabled athletes* (pp. 157-162). Champaign, IL: Human Kinetics.

Coutts, K.D. (1990). Peak oxygen uptake of elite wheelchair athletes. *Adapted Physical Activity Quarterly,* 7, 62-66.

Dahlgren, W., Boreski, S., Dowds, M., Mactavish, J., & Watkinson, E.J. (1991). The Medallion Program: Using the generic sport model to train athletes with mental disabilities. *The Journal of Physical Education, Recreation, and Dance, 62* (9), 67-73.

Davis, G.M., Tupling, S.J., & Shephard, R.J. (1986). Dynamic strength and physical activity in wheelchair users. In C. Sherrill (ed.), *Sport and disabled athletes* (pp. 169-146). Champaign, IL: Human Kinetics.

Depauw, K. (1988). Sport for individuals with disabilities: Research opportunities. *Adapted Physical Activity Quarterly, 5*, 80-89.

Fernhall, B., & Tymeson, G. (1987). Graded exercise testing of mentally retarded adults: A study of physiability. *Archives of Physical and Medical rehabilitation, 68*, 363-365.

Gibbons, S.L., & Bushakra, F.B. (1989). Effects of Special Olympics participation on the perceived competence and social acceptance of mentally retarded children. *Adapted Physical Quarterly, 6* (1), 40-51.

Gorton, B., & Gavron, S. (1987). A biomechnical analysis of the running pattern of blind athletes in the 100m dash. *Adapted Physical Activity Quarterly, 4*, 192-203.

Greenwood, C.M., Dzewaltowski, D.A., & French, R. (1990). Self-efficacy and psychological well-being of wheelchair tennis participants and wheelchair nontennis participants. *Adapted Physical Activity Quarterly,* 7 (1), 12-21.

Hedrick, B.N. (1985). The effects of wheelchair tennis participation and mainstreaming upon the perceptions of competence of physically disabled adolescents. *Therapeutic Recreation Journal, 14* (2), 34-46.

Hourcade, J.J., (1989). Special Olympics: A review and critical analysis. *Therapeutic Recreation Journal, 23* (1), 58-65.

Kennedy, D., Smith, R., & Austin, D. (1991). *Special recreation: Opportunities for persons with disabilities.* Dubuque, IA: Wm. C. Brown.

Kisabeth, K.L. & Richardson, D.B. (1985). Changing attitudes toward disabled individuals: The effect of one disabled person. *Therapeutic Recreation Journal, 19*(2), 24-33.

Labanowich, S. (1987). *The physically disabled in sports. Sports 'n Spokes, 12* (6), 33-42.

Labanowich, S. (1988). A care for the integration of the disabled into the Olympic games. *Adapted Physical Activity Quarterly, 5,* 364-372.

Mahon, M.J. (994). *A comprehensive needs assessment of the program delivery system of Manitoba Special Olympics, Inc.* Winnepeg, MD: University of Manitoba, Health, Leisure & Human Performance Research Institute.

Petetti, K., Jackson, J., Stubbs, N., Campbell, K., & Battar, S. (1989). Fitness levels of adult Special Olympic participants. *Adapted Physical Activity Quarterly, 6,* 354-370.

Pope, C., Sherrill, C., Wilkerson, J., & Pyfer, J. (1993). Biomechanics variables in spring running of athletes with cerebral palsy. *Adapted Physical Activity Quarterly, 10,* 226-254.

Reid, G. (1993). Motor behavior and individuals with disabilities. Linking research and practice. *Adapted Physical Activity Quarterly, 10,* 359-370.

Reid, G., Montgomery, D.L., & Seidl, C. (1985). Performance of mentally retarded children. *Exceptional Children, 306,* 508-519.

Sherrill, C. (1993*). Adapted physical activity, recreation and sport: Cross disciplinary and life span.* Dubuque, IA: Brown and Benchmark.

Sherill, C. (1998). *Adapted physical activity, recreation, and sport: Crossdisciplinary and life span* (5th edition). Boston, MA: WCB McGraw-Hill.

Shriver, S. (1993) *Special Olympics International executive office memo: Policy on Special Olympics athletes competing in other than Special Olympics events.* Washington, D.C.: Special Olympics, International.

Songster, T. (1986). The Special Olympics sport program: An international sport program for mentally retarded athletes. In C. Sherrill (ed.), *Sport and disabled athletes* (pp. 3-20). Champaign, IL: Human Kinetics.

Special Olympics International (1994). *Special Olympics soccer: Sport management team guide.* Washington, .C.: Special Olympics International.

Steadward, R., & Walsh, C. (1986). Training and fitness programs for disabled athletes: Past, present, and future. In C. Sherrill (ed.), *Sport and disabled athletes* (pp. 3-20). Champaign, IL: Human Kinetics.

Studholme, H. (1992). ***Manitoba report: M.I.R.L. project.*** Winnipeg, MN: The Association for Community Living—Manitoba.

Thiboutot, A., Smith, R.W., Labanowich, S. (1992). Examining the concept of reverse integration: A response to Brasile's "new perspective" on integration. ***Adapted Physical Activity Quarterly, 9 (4),*** 283-292.

Tomporowski, P., & Jameson, L. (1985). Effects of a physical training program on the exercise behavior of institutionalized retarded adults. ***Adapted Physical Activity Quarterly, 2,*** 197-205.

Walsh, C. (1986). ***The effect of pushing frequency on the kinematics of wheelchair sprinting.*** Unpublished master's thesis, University of Alberta.

Wehman, P., & Moon, M.S. (1985). Designing and implementing leisure programs for individuals with severe handicaps. In M.P. Brady & P.L. Gunter, (eds.), ***Integrating moderately and severely handicapped learners.*** Springfield, IL: Charles C. Thomas.

Williams, T. (1994). Disability sport socialization and identity construction. ***Adapted Physical Activity Quarterly, 11*** (1), 14-31.

Winnick, J. (Ed.). (1990). ***Adapted physical education and sport.*** Champaign, IL: Human Kinetics.

Related Websites

http://ed-web3.educ.msu.edu/kin866/contents.htm
(Disability Sports)

http://www.ausport.gov.au/para.html
(Australian Sports Commission — Paralympics)

http://cso.on.ca/
(Canadian Special Olympics)

http://www.specialolympics.org/
(Welcome to Special Olympics)

http://www.sni.net/nscd/
(National Sports Center for the Disabled)

http://www.dsusa.org/~dsusa/dsusa.html
(Disabled Sports USA)

http://www.eskimo.com/~jlubin/disabled/sports.htm
(Sports Training and Athletic Competition)

http://www.ausport.gov.au/partic/dislinks.html
(Australian Sports Commission Disabilities Program — Weblinks)

Chapter 16

Leisure Education

Introduction

Leisure education has become in many ways one of the cornerstones of service delivery within the recreation system. As a result, we—as professionals working in a variety of recreation settings—must develop an understanding of both the meaning of the term leisure education and some of the models and processes that have been developed. This chapter will highlight this information and provide an overview of some of the innovative leisure education programs that have been developed in both the United States and Canada during the past decade.

Definition of Leisure Education

Leisure education has become a significant component within the recreation delivery system. Yet in many ways, consensus has yet to be achieved among leisure and recreation professionals as to the definition of this term. In one of the earliest texts on leisure education, Munday and Odum (1979) described leisure education as:

> ...process rather than content. It is viewed as a total developmental process through which individuals develop an understanding of self, leisure, and the relationship of leisure to their own lifestyles and the fabric of society.

Table 16.1 highlights "What leisure education is..." according to Mundy and Odum. Remarkably, this list is still very appropriate a decade and a half later.

The Munday and Odum text on leisure education provides a very important initial framework that has served as the catalyst for the development of more recent conceptualizations of leisure education. Their conceptualization of leisure education was created within the context of the leisure service field that included the field of therapeutic recreation.

Table 16.1
What Leisure Education is...

Leisure Education is...

1. A total movement to enable individuals to enhance the quality of their lives in leisure.
2. A process to enable individuals to identify and clarify their leisure values, attitudes, and goals.
3. An approach to enable individuals to be self-determining, self-sufficient, and proactive in relation to their lives during leisure.
4. Deciding for oneself what place leisure has in one's life.
5. Coming to know oneself in relation to leisure.
6. Relating one's own needs, values, and capabilities to leisure and leisure experiences.
7. Increasing the individual's options for satisfying quality experiences in leisure.
8. A process whereby individuals determine their own leisure behavior and evaluate the long-and short-range outcomes of their behavior in relation to their goals.
9. Developing the potential of individuals to enhance the quality of their own lives in leisure.
10. A lifelong, continuous process encompassing prekindergarten to retirement years.
11. A movement in which a multiplicity of disciplines and service systems have a role and a responsibility.

(Adapted from Munday & Odum, 1979)

In addition to the early work of Munday and Odum (1979), Chinn and Joswiak (1981), in a special issue of ***Therapeutic Recreation Journal***, defined leisure education more specifically within the context of therapeutic recreation. Their article, which provides an analysis of the distinction between leisure education and leisure counseling, defines leisure education as "...the use of comprehensive models focusing on the educational process which helps to develop the leisure lifestyle of an individual, as well as any single aspect of the approach" (p. 6).

A number of similarities exist between this definition and that of Munday and Odum (1979). One significant difference in the Chinn and Joswiak (1981) definition is that any single aspect of the leisure education process can be described as leisure education. This is not necessarily a widely held belief. For many years we have thought about leisure education as a process that consists of a number of components such as leisure awareness, self-awareness, decision making, and skill development. For example, Dattilo and Murphy's (1991) text on leisure education depicts a set of stairs, with a component of leisure education on each step, ultimately leading at the top of the stairs to ***meaningful leisure experiences***. In contrast to this image, Chinn and Joswiak's definition suggests that while one individual may need all of the stairs, another may need only a step. Leisure education, as presented by these two definitions, can and should be used to describe a process that includes either a number of components or any single component. According to Chinn and Joswiak, a learn-to-paint class, a course in social skills training for people with developmental disabilities, or a one-on-one session designed to teach decision-making skills are all examples of leisure education. Each of these experiences has at least one thing in common: each is intended to enhance or contribute to the life of the person. As such, any leisure education process may be either comprehensive in nature or narrowly centered on one particular leisure goal.

Leisure education is also described by Chinn and Joswiak (1981) as helping to develop a leisure lifestyle. This, too, is significant, as it speaks to the scope of issues that leisure education can help to address. Kelly (1996, p. 33) points out that different individuals seek different styles of leisure:

> Some concentrate on one or two activities, and others do a little of 15 different things. Some do little outside the home, and others are quite involved in many kinds of community activities and organizations. Some are constantly trying to learn and develop, while others prefer to be entertained.

Kelly also indicates that the leisure lifestyle of a person relates to the combination of activity and meaning. Thus, two people may engage in the same activity but for very different reasons and, as a result, the leisure experience will hold different meanings for each. For example, some individuals may participate in competitive team sports because they love to compete, while others may do so for the socialization often inherent in team sports. Thus, according to Chinn and Joswiak (1981), leisure education is designed to facilitate the different leisure lifestyles that will be sought by various individuals.

Though there is some agreement in the field of recreation and leisure studies regarding the conceptualization of leisure lifestyle, we do not find this concept to be completely satisfactory when applied to the leisure education process. We contend that leisure education not only has an impact on the leisure lifestyles of people with disabilities, but in fact, the process can and does have an impact on their overall lifestyle. In our research we have seen many instances of a leisure education process benefiting individuals in areas outside of the domain of leisure. For example, in our study on decision making with adolescents with mental retardation (Mahon & Bullock, 1992), we found that the decision-making instruction within the leisure education program resulted in participants making more and better decisions at their jobs. Similarly, Bullock and Luken (1994) discovered that the Reintegration Through Recreation leisure education program enhanced participants' ability to manage their own money.

There are a number of other definitions of leisure education that have appeared in the literature. Each provides a unique perspective. We contend, however, that none of the present definitions is truly person-centered. None places the individual first and the process second. As a result, we propose a new definition of person-centered leisure education. It is reflective of many of the points we have addressed in this chapter. It builds on those who have defined leisure education in the past, including Mundy and Odum (1979), Chinn and Joswiak (1981), and Dattilo and Murphy (1991). This new definition is rooted in the concepts of social role valorization, integration, self-determination, and interdependence as defined in our chapter on the conceptual cornerstones of service delivery. Thus, it is particularly responsive to contemporary issues within the fields of recreation and therapeutic recreation. With that in mind, we propose that person-centered leisure education is:

> ...an individualized and contextualized educational process through which a person develops an understanding of self and leisure and identifies and learns the cluster of skills necessary to participate in freely chosen activities which lead to an optimally satisfying life.

It is useful to analyze the various components of this definition as a means of determining its implications for the fields of community recreation and therapeutic recreation. We talk about a person-centered leisure education process as being individualized and contextualized. Leisure education is designed to meet the needs of the individual. This point is crucial because it underscores the relationship between leisure education and leisure. As we have discussed in a previous chapter, leisure is a personal construct that is inextricably linked to freedom of choice and personal or intrinsic motivation. In order for leisure education to facilitate the leisure needs of a given individual, the process must encourage self-determination in leisure. Any leisure education process must therefore be closely connected and tailored to the needs of the individual, as opposed to his classification of disability. Most of us would argue that we individualize. Some of the situations in which we find ourselves, however, do not allow us to be as individualized as we would like to be. We may do an individual assessment, we may develop an individualized plan, but again, is it as individualized as we would like to be? Or as it needs to be? The leisure education process must be based on the person's needs and aspirations, as understood by that person, not as perceived by us as either the intervenor, leisure educator, or therapeutic recreation specialist.

Contextualization is a very important part of individualized services, but it is often overlooked in leisure education. The best way to explain contexualization is by using an example. Consider a person in a psychiatric hospital. Her sole reason for being there is so that she can be discharged and go back home. When you compose a contextualized program, you are creating a program with that in mind, knowing that the sole reason for a person to be in a hospital or any intervention program is for her to do something else, usually to go back where she came from—to her home, community, neighborhood, with her friends and family—i.e., her context. The contextualized process is one that takes into consideration who a person is, where she has come from, where she is returning, and what her support systems are.

Another key component of the definition of leisure education is that it is an educational process. The word education is defined in various ways:

> 1) the act of process of education or being educated; systematic instruction, 2) a particular kind or stage in education, 3) a) the development of character or mental powers, b) a stage in or aspect of this (*Webster's II*, 1984).

This definition suggests that leisure education is ongoing or continuous. The use of the term education juxtaposed with leisure suggests that the process of leisure education juxtaposed with leisure suggests that the process of leisure education results in knowledge gain and person development within the domain of leisure. It is a process that is systematic in nature and has a variety of different outcomes. In addition, according to this definition of education, leisure education can consist of one stage or any aspect of the educational process.

It is also important to understand that through leisure education a person develops an understanding of self and leisure. Leisure education helps an individual to understand what leisure means to him in the *context* of who he is right now. For example, what leisure means to you right now might be very different if you found yourself one day with a spinal cord injury. Your understanding of the concept of leisure changes over the course of your life span. As such, leisure education must be a dynamic process, not only able to meet individuals where they are but also able to change over time as individuals' perspectives grow and change.

Beyond awareness of leisure, the leisure education process can help a person to identify and to learn a cluster of skills necessary to participate in an activity. In using the term ***cluster of skills*** we are not only talking about learning how to play a game or activity, though that certainly may be part of it, we are also talking about all those things that it takes for a person to be able to do what she freely chooses to do. In the case of a person with severe mental retardation, one skill necessary to enable him to participate in something that he freely chooses might be counting money. Another skill might be riding a bus. You may be saying that these types of skills (and we use these intentionally) should be taught by an occupational therapist. At this point it becomes important to understand the notion of transdisciplinary services. A transdisciplinary service model is one that recognizes that here are many things that professionals do that overlap. Rather than trying to carve out the distinct roles of various disciplines, a transdisciplinary model encourages overlap as a means of best meeting the needs of the individual.

A cornerstone of person-center leisure education is the concept of self-determination in leisure. Earlier in the text we discussed the concept of self-determination at length. There is ample evidence in the literature that suggests that self-determination, or more specifically—perceived control, is a critical regulator of leisure. Given this, a person-centered leisure education process must ensure that the choices of individuals are front and center in the leisure education process. Emphasis must be placed on facilitating participation in ***freely chosen activities***.

The final piece that is almost self-evident is that leisure education should lead to optimal satisfaction with life. As we discussed earlier, leisure education has the potential to impact not only one's leisure lifestyle but life in general. Another way of putting this is to say that leisure education has the capacity to enhance both life and leisure satisfaction. It is important to understand that we are not downplaying the importance of leisure satisfaction. Rather, we stress the potential for leisure education to enhance a person's life that includes leisure.

Our definition of leisure education does not indicate that a leisure education process should be hierarchical or directional. Most texts and articles that present leisure education processes, however, describe a directional/hierarchical process that typically starts with self-and leisure-awareness and ends with recreation participation. In fact, some of our own work provides examples of this. The Community Reintegration Program (Bullock & Howe, 1991) that is presented in Figure 16.1 is a directional model.

Datttilo (1994, p. 157), in his text ***Inclusive Leisure Services***, presents the characteristics of a person prepared through leisure education in a figure depicting people moving up steps, with the first step titled "Aware of self in leisure" and the last labeled "Demonstrate recreation activity skills;" the term "Leisure" appears at the top of the steps. Though neither the Bullock and Howe (1991) model nor the Dattilo (1994) model specifically says that leisure education is hierarchical, the manner in which the material is presented leaves the reader with the distinct impression that leisure education is a building-block process in which a participant is expected to proceed in an orderly fashion.

Recently, we have come to believe that any leisure education process must allow the unique needs of the individual to dictate the order in which different components or elements are introduced and, indeed, whether one, some, or all of the components are necessary for the given individual. Though in many cases people will want or need to proceed through a leisure education process in an order that is quite normative, it is dangerous to assume that all individuals should or must proceed along the same path. The danger of this assumption is that an individual may not receive the type of intervention needed at a given point in time if he is bound by a prescribed process. In essence, what can happen is that the unique needs of the individual are sacrificed for the sake of maintaining a standard process.

The case of Samantha provides a useful example of the danger of adhering too closely to a hierarchical leisure education process. In Case Example 16.1, the instructor of the leisure education program was convinced that each individual must proceed through the leisure education program in a specific order to get the benefits of the program. In fact, Samantha's request called for the instructor to work with her in a few specific areas in order to get the benefits of the program. In fact, Samantha's request called for the instructor to work with her in a few specific areas in order to meet her needs. Because the instructor insisted that Samantha stick to the prescribed order, he failed in his goal of meeting the leisure needs of Samantha.

The remainder of this chapter will describe what we believe are the most significant domains and corresponding components of a leisure education process. We will also present some examples of leisure education practice models.

Figure 16.1
The Community Reintegration Program: Leisure Education Model

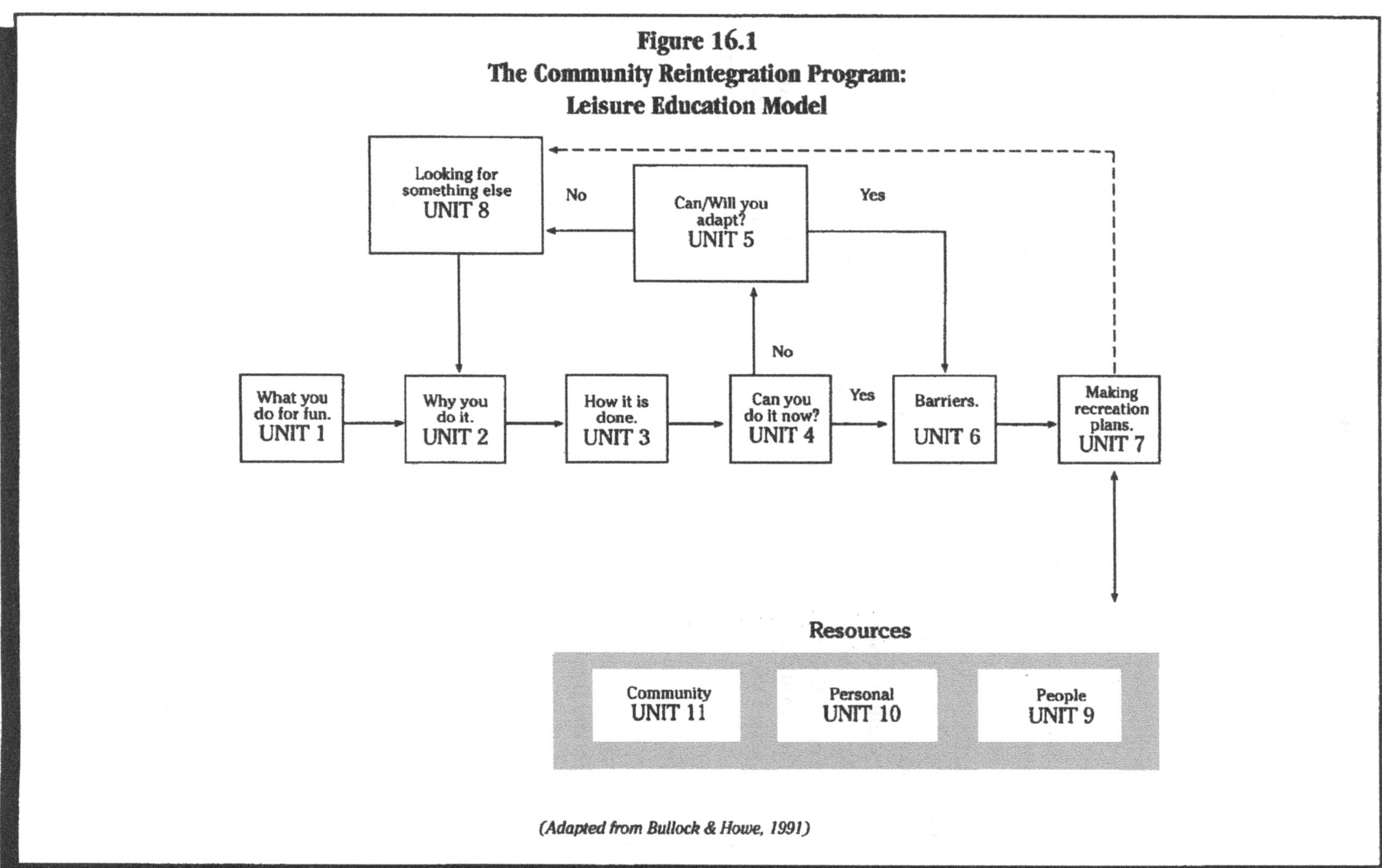

(Adapted from Bullock & Howe, 1991)

Case Example 16.1

Samantha is a 24-year-old who has cerebral palsy. She lives on her own in an apartment and works part time at a local dry cleaners. Samantha recently contacted the Independent Living Centre in her community because she wanted to become more active during her leisure time. Being quite a voracious reader, Samantha had already explored a number of activity options by taking out books from the public library on specific activities. She had read books on Tai-Chi, Pottery, Painting, and Yoga. Samantha had decided that she wanted to try out Tai-Chi. She contacted the Centre because she knew they had recreation staff who might be able to help her find a program that would be willing to include a person with a disability in their program. When she contacted the Centre and told them a little bit about what she was interested in, the recreation staff person suggested that she should enroll in a six-week leisure education program. Samantha was a little confused by this, but thought she would go to the first session and see what they had to offer. At the first session, the instructor had the eight participants spend time doing exercises that he said would help them to develop a better understanding of themselves in relation to leisure. Samantha took part in the exercises but wondered how they would help her find a Tai-Chi program. At the end of the session she approached the instructor and expressed her concern that this program did not appear to be getting her any closer to her goal of joining a Tai-Chi program. The instructor was very pleasant. He told her that it was important that she spend time developing an awareness of various leisure options first, and that by the end of the program she would have a much better sense of what she really wanted to do with her leisure time. Samantha went to one more session and then dropped out.

The Leisure Education Process

In the previous section we identified the components that Chinn and Joswiak (1981) suggest are included in most leisure education models. Since this article was published, a significant amount of research and program development has occurred in the area of leisure education. As a result of a number of years of conducting research in the area of leisure education (e.g., Bullock & Howe, 1991; Bullock & Luken, 1994; Mahon & Bullock, 1992a & b, 1993; Mahon & Searle, 1993; Mahon, Bullock, & Luken, 1993; Searle & Mahon, 1991, 1993; Searle, Mahon, Iso-Ahola, Sdrolias, & van Dyck, 1995), we have created a conceptual model for leisure education that incorporates what we believe to be the domains and corresponding components most germane to leisure education. The conceptual model is presented in Figure 16.2.

In keeping with our concern with hierarchical models of leisure education, this conceptual model is not intended to be directional in nature. The beginning, middle, and end of each process is determined by the individual in concert with the leisure education specialist. The two work in an interdependent manner to

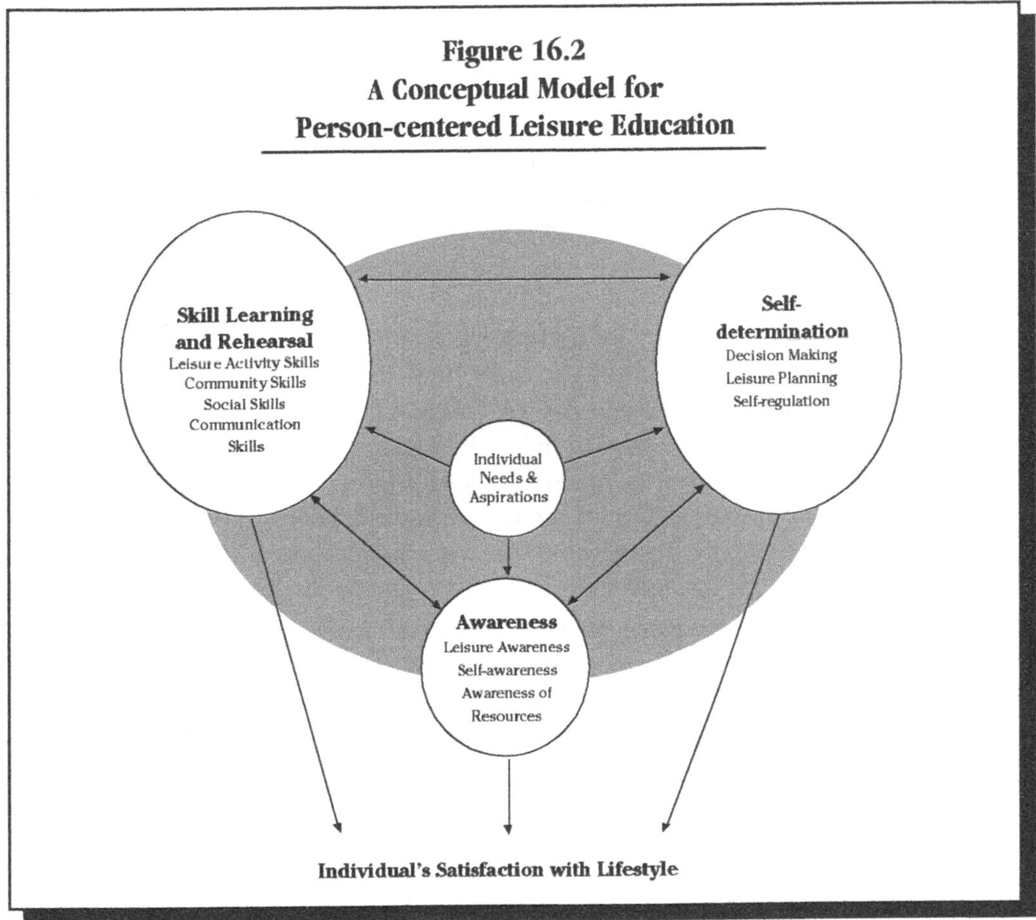

Figure 16.2
A Conceptual Model for Person-centered Leisure Education

achieve the goals identified by the individuals. So, in contrast to the scenario outlined in Case Example 16.1, if the individual expresses a very specific goal that relates to only one domain of the model, the leisure education process would only include that one domain. Thus, in center of the model, we indicate that the individual and his aspirations and needs provide unique input into the development of the individualized leisure education process. There are three domains within the leisure education conceptual model: 1) Awareness, 2) Skill Learning and Rehearsal, and 3) Self-determination. Though each are presented as separate, overlap and connection will occur. The individual and the leisure education specialist will be the ones to determine which domains and corresponding components they will access during the individualized process. As with our definition of leisure education, the ultimate goal of the leisure education process is personal satisfaction with one's lifestyle. In the following section each of the domains and corresponding components will be briefly discussed.

Domains of Leisure Education

Awareness

A cornerstone to any leisure education process is the opportunity for the individual to develop a deeper understanding of herself and her personal lifestyle within the context of leisure. This process of enhancing one's personal awareness is extremely important for achieving a satisfying leisure lifestyle. The awareness domain within our conceptual model consists of the following three components: 1) leisure awareness, 2) self-awareness, and 3) awareness of resources.

1. **Leisure awareness** centers on helping an individual to understand the concept of leisure. Depending upon the individual, this may include helping her to understand the difference between work and leisure and when and where leisure can happen. For example, often individuals with a cognitive impairment have a difficult time distinguishing between work and leisure. A leisure awareness process can help them to understand the inherent differences between the two, and why one should have the opportunity to experience both during the course of a day, week, and year. At the same time, it is also important that individuals understand that leisure can occur at various times of the day and in various locations. This is especially important for individuals with a disability whose leisure lives have often been controlled by others. Such individuals may not understand that leisure can occur at various times of their day and week and in different settings. A key aspect of the leisure awareness component is also exposing the individual to various types of leisure pursuits. These types of pursuits are often grouped under the following five headings: 1) social, 2) relaxation, 3) sports, 4) crafts, and 5) outdoors. Once again, people with disabilities and others, such as older adults and persons at risk, often have a limited understanding of the scope of leisure pursuits that are available to them. The leisure awareness of the many options that are available to them. One other important element of leisure awareness focuses on the benefits of leisure participation. For a variety of reasons—including socialization, lack of exposure, and competing commitments such as work—many individuals do not understand the many benefits of developing a satisfying leisure lifestyle. For such people, this last aspect of the leisure awareness component can be the most important. Maybe individuals are aware that options exist for them with respect to leisure but are unaware of the many inherent benefits of participating in leisure. This component is designed to enhance their awareness of the benefits.

2. **Self-awareness** is another component of the awareness building process. It helps the individual to personalize her understanding of leisure. A central goal of the self-awareness component is to help the individual become cognizant of her preferred leisure experiences. To articulate leisure preferences requires that the individual consider a number of factors. These factors are presented in the form of questions in Table 16.2.

In addition to the identification of leisure preferences, the self-awareness component is also designed to facilitate exploration of leisure attitudes, values, and motivations for participating in leisure. This requires a good deal of introspection on the part of the participant. Such introspection is easier for some than for others.

Table 16.2
Things I Can Ask Myself About Leisure

1. What are my past and present leisure pursuits?
2. Am I satisfied with what I am currently doing for leisure?
3. What benefits do I desire from leisure?
4. What new activities would I like to try?

The job of the leisure education specialist to help the participant through this process by creating an environment that is best able to facilitate the reflection necessary for the identification of attitudes, values, and motivations. This may take the form of paper and pencil exercises, open-ended discussion with the specialist, or individual reflection. For certain individuals who may have severe cognitive impairments or communication deficits, such reflection may be less feasible.

3. **Awareness of resources** is the final component of this domain. This component is intended to help focus the participant on the more pragmatic aspects of leisure participation. The resources that are addressed are both personal and community-based. Some of the issues dealt with in this component are as follows:

- home and community leisure activities,
- budgeting and money management,
- people and relationships,
- communication,
- transportation,
- leisure skills,
- personal routines.

The purpose of this component is to help the individual identify the resources that he presently has that will enable him to participate in his chosen leisure pursuits and the barriers he faces because of either a lack of personal resources within certain areas or a lack of community-based resources. Each individual is blessed with strengths within the area of resources, and most individuals who access a leisure education program are also faced with resource-based barriers. This component enables the individual and leisure education specialist to clearly articulate both strengths and barriers as a precursor to developing strategies for the utilization of identified strengths and methods of either reducing the impact on or negating barriers. The remainder of the leisure education process is designed to enable the individual to work with these strengths and barriers in order to facilitate a satisfying lifestyle.

Skill Learning and Rehearsal

An equally important domain within our leisure education conceptual model is skill learning and rehearsal.This domain consists of three components: 1) leisure activity skills, 2) community skills, and 3) social/communication skills. In one study we conducted with people with severe and persistent mental illnesses (Mahon, Bullock, Luken, & Martins, 1996), which assessed the impact of a leisure education program on the lives of a number of individuals, we asked participants what part of the leisure education process they found most valuable.The vast majority of the respondents indicated that skill learning and rehearsal was the most important domain. They felt that having increased leisure, community, and communication skills enhanced their ability to be out in the community.The other results of this study corroborated these findings. Individuals demonstrated higher levels of self-esteem and leisure satisfaction as a result of the program. Each of the areas within skill learning and rehearsal are important for facilitating the leisure goals of an individual.Whether some or all become a part of a program depends upon capacities and needs of the individual. In most cases, the areas of focus within this domain are closely associated with the barriers/areas of needs identified within the awareness section For example, if an individual decides that she is interested in trying rock climbing, it is likely that she will require some leisure activity skills instruction. Each of the three components will be briefly discussed.

1. **Leisure activity skills** form the basis for leisure participation.Any leisure activity requires some level of skill.The complexity of the skills required depends upon the activity or a few activities in which he wishes to participate, he must then determine whether he possesses the necessary skills for the activity. For example, if Bill, who has a visual impairment, decides that he wants to kayak, he must first identify whether he possesses the necessary skills. In order to help answer this question, a participant profile and an activity profile should be completed. These two procedures are discussed in depth in Chapter 13. Those individuals who do not possess the skills to participate in a chosen activity must be taught. This is a very important part of the leisure education process, as is the opportunity to practice.According to Bullock and Luken (1994, p. 224):

> The goal (of a leisure education program) is skill development and mastery. Far too often, clients are offered minimal opportunities to develop and master a selected activity skill, and thus lack the self-confidence to continue their involvement without professional assistance. Activity skill mastery requires that sufficient time be devoted to skill development, rehearsal, and application in the "real environment."

It is crucial that a lack of skill not be seen as an insurmountable barrier to a person participating in a chosen leisure pursuit. Leisure education must be seen as a mechanism for teaching new leisure activity skills or upgrading previously learned skills.

2. **Community skills** are not leisure skills, but are those collateral skills that enable a person to participate in community-based programs. Within the field of mental disabilities, these skills are often described as adaptive skills. One example of a community skill is transportation. In order to access many community-based

leisure opportunities, individuals must have access to and knowledge of how to use different types of transportation. The type of transportation an individual may use will depend on such things as her disability, whether she lives in a rural or urban setting, her financial situation, where the program is located, and what forms of transportation are readily available. For some individuals, learning how to get to a new program may be quite straightforward—as easy as knowing where the program is located so that they can choose the right bus line or the right route to drive themselves. Other individuals may need much more assistance in this area. People with visual impairments who rely on the bus for transportation will need to be guided along the new route a number of times before they can independently travel. Though transportation is not necessarily a leisure-based skill, it may be one of a cluster of skills needed to ensure success in a recreation program.

Money management is another collateral skill that may be necessary to be included in a leisure education program. Bullock and Luken (1994) found in their Reintegration Through Recreation leisure education program that for many individuals with severe and persistent mental illnesses, money management and budgeting were crucial to their successful reintegration back into community recreation programs. Once individuals with disabilities recognized the value of leisure experiences, recreation therapists and other program leaders found it necessary to convince them of the need to budget money for their leisure pursuits. As a result, the leisure education program did not pay for the individual's recreation participation.

> If the program assumes this responsibility, it lessens the likelihood that the person will be able to independently to continue participation without the TRS. It also sends a message that the person is unable to care for himself. It is important to be sensitive to real financial limitations that consumers often face, but also important to convey a belief that there are other, more empowering approaches to money management. For example, options include advocating for more reasonable fees for persons with limited incomes, while not using the disability label as a means for income assistance (Bullock & Luken, p. 228).

Thus the money management element of community skills can be a shared responsibility between the participant and the leisure education specialist. This is also true for other collateral skills.

3. **Social/Communication skills** are crucial for inclusion in community-based leisure programs. Social skills are those skills that enable an individual to interact with another individual or integrate into a social group or the larger community. A wealth of literature has identified that people with disabilities and, in particular, people with developmental disabilities often lack social skills necessary for social inclusion (Siperstein, Bak & O'Keefe, 1988; Taylor, Asher & Williams, 1987). According to Dattilo and Murphy (1991, p. 31), "Absence of social skills is particularly noticeable during leisure participation and frequently leads to isolation and inability to function successfully." In addition, other research has determined that, in general, social isolation and, as a result, more limited social networks and limited friendships, are also very common in people with disabilities (Abery, Thurlow, Johnson, & Bruininks, 1990; Bogdan & Taylor, 1987; Horner, Dunlop & Koegel, 1988).

Given this, leisure education programs must be sure to include a component focused on enhancing social skills.

A social skills component within a leisure education process can deal with a number of issues, including learning valued behaviors within different leisure setting, while in other they are completely inappropriate. The subtle difference between two spectator activities like watching a basketball game in a field house and a movie at the theater may not be understood by certain individuals. In order for the same individual to enjoy both experiences, she may need assistance in recognizing what behaviors are valued in the two different settings.

Another social skill that is strongly associated with play and leisure is cooperation. Some cooperative behavior, that are important for successful leisure participation are sharing toys and games appropriately, taking turns in structured activities, initiating an activity with a partner, and getting along with others during an activity. Bullock, Morris, Mahon, and Jones (1992) have a module in their leisure education program called Getting Along With Others. The module uses cooperative games as a means of teaching cooperative skills.

One other social skill that is so crucial that it is highlighted within the title of this component is communication. Communication is vital within games and activities that include more than one person. Communication, both verbal and nonverbal, is also strongly associated with whether people with disabilities will connect with other people within a program and develop relationships. A number of strategies for facilitating communication has been incorporated into leisure education programs (Bullock et al, 1992; Dattilo & Murphy, 1991).

Self-determination

The importance of self-determination in the lives of people with disabilities was discussed at length in Chapter 3. As was noted then, many individuals with disabilities have had little opportunity to be self-determining within the context of leisure. As a result, a focus on self-determination in any leisure education model is crucial. Our self-determination domain is divided into three areas: 1) decision making, 2) leisure planning, and 3) independent leisure initiation. This is consistent with the definitions of self-determination proposed by both Ward (1988) and Wehmeyer (1992).

1. **Decision making.** The majority of recent literature concurs that one of the most significant ways in which society can empower individuals with disabilities to become more self-determining is through enabling them to make decisions for themselves (Brown, 1988; Kennedy & Killius, 1987; Mitchell, 1988; Ward, 1988). According to Bullock (1988) and Guess and Siegel-Causey (1985), a great deal has been accomplished in teaching skills to individuals with disabilities but very little in teaching these same individuals how to make a decision or choice. Statements such as these have led to a rapidly expanding research emphasis on decision making for individuals with disabilities (Goode & Gaddy, 1976; Guess, Benson, & Siegel-Causey, 1985; Houghton, Bronicki, & Guess, 1987; Nietupski, Hamre-Nietupski, Green, Varnum-Teeter, Twedt, LePera, Scebold, & Hanrahan, 1986).

Most of the research on decision making has been related to work and daily living skills; only more recently, studies have focused their inquiry in the leisure domain (Bender & Valletutti, 1976; Duffy & Nietupski, 1985; Putnam, Werder, & Schleien, 1985; Schleien, Certo, & Muccino, 1984; Wehman & Schleien, 1981).

Mahon and colleagues have developed a process for facilitating self-determination in leisure for people with mental disabilities (Bullock, Morris, Mahon, & Jones, 1992; Mahon, 1994; Mahon & Martens, in press; Mahon & Bullock, 1992a & b, 1994). The central focus of this process is on enhancing decision making in leisure as a means of facilitating self-determined independent leisure management.

A Model for Decision Making in Leisure

The Decision Making in Leisure Model (Mahon, 1990) is based on the theoretical single-choice open model proposed by Wilson and Alexis (1962). The structure of the DML Model is adapted from Mithaug, Martin, and Agran's (1987) Adaptability Instructional Model. The leisure activity areas identified in the model are derived from Nash's (1953) original model, which was adapted by Beck-Ford and Brown (1984) for use with individuals with a mental disability. The DML Model is composed of the following four steps:

1. Identify a desired leisure experience, such as being a spectator, or involving yourself in either a social, physical, or creative/self-actualizing activity.
2. Consider alternatives that satisfy the experience desired; i.e., what specific activities within the chosen area will provide you with the leisure experience desired?
3. Describe the consequences for each alternative:
   a. the amount of enjoyment,
   b. whether a partner is required,
   c. the cost (if any) and affordability of the options,
   d. where it takes place and the available transportation, and
   e. the equipment/attire that is required.
4. Choose an alternative that satisfies the desired experience. Figure 16.3 outlines the basic steps that are followed in conducting decision-making training using the DML model.

2. **Leisure planning.** Fields and Hoffman (1991), along with Ward (1988), have suggested that independent planning and initiation are important skills related to self-determination. In addition, Wolfensberger (1972) has suggested that these are important self-determination skills in relation to the leisure domain for people with mental retardation.

The focus of planning and initiation in leisure and recreation programs for people with disabilities has tended to fall within one of two categories. The first process for facilitating planning tends to have the care-giver ***plan for*** the person with mental retardation and then facilitate initiation through such techniques as behavior modification. Once the individuals with disabilities consistently displays the behaviors on cue, the instructor then fades the behavioral intervention and

Figure 16.3
Picture Board for DML Model
(Decision Making in Leisure)

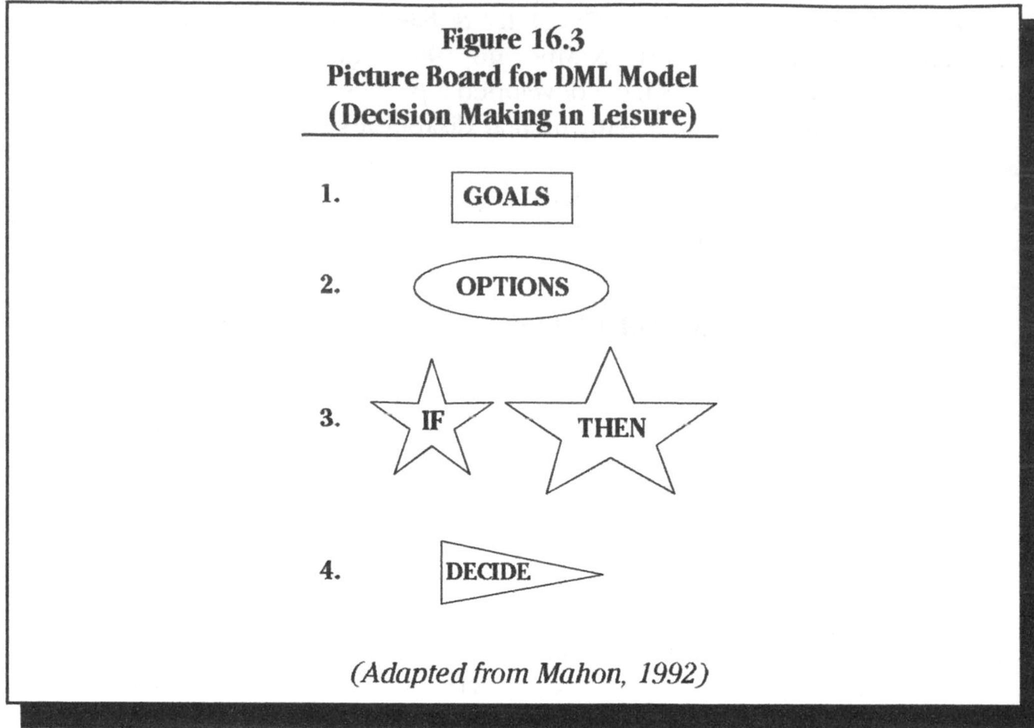

(Adapted from Mahon, 1992)

tries to facilitate generalization to independent settings. In a leisure education model proposed by Pollingue and Cobb (1986), to facilitate community integration, the instructor planned the activities to be carried out by the participant at the community-based site and facilitated the participation via the use of behavioral techniques.

The second process that has been used to facilitate independent planning and initiation encourages the individual with mental retardation to become a more active participant in planning and initiating leisure activities. Wuerch & Voeltz (1981) provided for independent leisure initiation by people with severe mental retardation by helping students to develop a "choice book" that consisted of pictures of preferred activities. Students are then trained to initiate activities during leisure time at school by selecting from their personal choice book. Other successful interventions for, in particular, facilitating independent leisure initiation, have been reported by Dattilo (1986) and Nietupski and Soboda (1982). All of the intervention strategies used within these studies utilized behavior management techniques as the primary source.

One of the few examples in the literature of a process specifically aimed at facilitating leisure planning and initiation in people with mental retardation, which did not employ behavior management techniques, is the case study data of Bullock and Copp (1991). This study, which reported on the implementation of a yearlong leisure education program incorporating weekly leisure planning, found that having students "think through" a plan had a significant impact on independent leisure planning and initiation of the students with mild and moderate mental retardation.

The self-determination training program developed by Mahon, Bullock, and colleagues also incorporates a leisure planning and initiation component based on the use of self-control techniques. As was noted earlier, Ward (1988) defines self-determination as the ability to define and carry out one's goals. Within the context of this leisure education program, this can be translated into the capacity to not only define one's own leisure goals (i.e., make a decision about what to do for leisure), but also to carry out the goal. Once participants have learned to make leisure decisions using the DML Model, they are then taught to make a leisure action plan using a leisure action plan card (see Figure 16.4). The portfolio and plan is likened to a date book used to remember appointments. Five boxes, 2" by 2", are arranged on the card, each with one of five words representing the components of the plan: what, with whom, where, stuff, and when. The reading and writing skills of the participants may preclude them from writing key words in the boxes to represent each component of the plan. Instead, participants can be taught via modeling to select sticker pictures to represent each component and place them on the leisure action plan card. An example of a participant plan follows:

1. **What?** I am going to play cards (a picture of cards is placed on the card).
2. **With Whom?** I am going to play with my brother (a picture of one male is placed on the card).
3. **Where?** At home (a picture of a house is placed on the card).
4. **Stuff?** We will need a deck of cards (a picture of cards is placed on the card).
5. **When?** After dinner (a clock with 6:30 P.M. on the face is placed on the card).

It is crucial that participants are encouraged to create their plan as independently as possible. This will enable them to eventually create leisure plans on their own. Once participants have created a leisure action plan, they are given a 6" by 9" portfolio in which to keep their plan with a brightly colored marker attached to the folder.

Figure 16.4
Leisure Action Plan Card

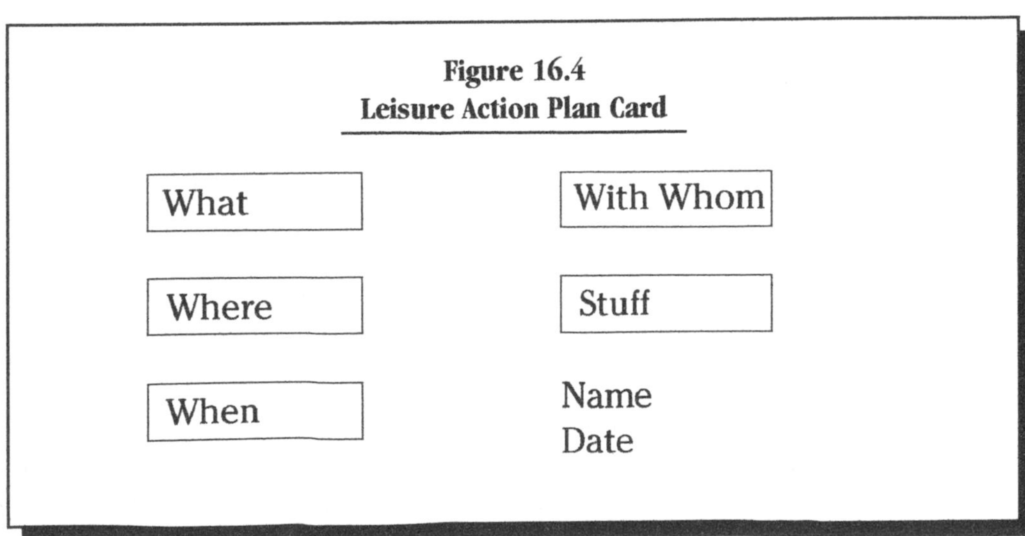

3. **Independent leisure initiation.** Independent leisure initiation is the final element within the domain of self-determination. As has been suggested by Wehmeyer (1992), self-control is an important part of self-determination. In keeping with this, Mahon (1994) has suggested that self-control strategies be used to help individuals with disabilities facilitate independent leisure initiation.

Self-regulation has been proposed as a useful community-based process for facilitating person-centered outcomes for individuals with disabilities and, particularly, people with mental retardation (Agran & Moore, 1987; Martin, Burger, Elias-Burger, & Mithaug, 1988). The use of such strategies is supported by a plethora of scholars and practitioners who concur that self-control can help individuals with disabilities control their own behaviors (Agran & Moore, 1987; Martin et al., 1988; Shapiro, 1981; Whitman, 1990). Self-regulation has been defined by Martin et al. as "the process of managing one's own behavior through self-regulation of antecedent or consequent stimuli" (p. 157). The intent of self-control training is to achieve internal control via external control procedures (Bandura, 1976).

Self-control strategies were used by Mahon (1994) to assist individuals with disabilities in independently using the Leisure Action Planning card. Once participants have made a leisure action plan, they are then taught to self-monitor using the card as means of helping them to carry out their plan.

Examples of Models

During the past decade we have initiated a number of research and demonstration projects designed to develop and test innovative approaches to leisure education. As we indicated at the beginning of this chapter, our knowledge and understanding of leisure education has grown over the years. As such, some of what we designed in our earlier work we have refined, built on, and improved. Therefore, our more recent work is most reflective of the conceptual model we have outlined in this chapter. Within this section we will describe three different models that we and our colleagues have developed. We have chosen these three because they were designed for individuals at three different points on the lifespan, and for people with quite different needs, abilities, and life situations.

The School-Community Leisure Link (SCLL)

The School-Community Leisure Link, a research and demonstration project funded by the U.S. Department of Education, is a comprehensive leisure education program within a public school system with program links to the community and student's family. The purpose of the project was to facilitate the independent leisure functioning of students with disabilities in their school and home communities. More specifically, the goal was to develop a curriculum through which students with disabilities could acquire leisure knowledge, skills, and attitudes. The underlying basis for the leisure education curriculum was the concept of self-determination (Brown, 1988; Fields & Hoffman, 1991; Ward, 1988). Implicit in the concept of self-determination, strong conceptual components were the normalization principle (Wolfensberg, 1972) and social role valorization (Woflensberger, 1983). With this conceptual base, it was clear that any curriculum would be community-based and would seek to elicit choices from students in order to empower them to take more control over all parts of their lives.

The project was designed to have a TRS function initially as a leisure education instructor within a number of classrooms. During these first two years, the TRS facilitated leisure education sessions for students with mental retardation, and at the same time she provided classroom special education teachers with a six-week course in leisure education facilitation techniques. After the two years of the project, the role of the TRS shifted to that of a consultant to classroom special education teachers who were by then trained to provide leisure education within their own classrooms. This shift in roles for the TRS allowed her to provide consultation to families and IEP teams regarding leisure-related goals for individual students, to help facilitate these goals, and to expand her role in the community to enhance opportunities in community-based recreation for children and adolescents with disabilities. The ultimate goal of the project was to investigate the impact of a school division-based TRS position on the lives of the students with disabilities in the system.

A comprehensive leisure education program, developed by Bullock et al. (1992), served as the basis for the school leisure education program. This program consisted of six units, each of which was meant to facilitate one of the goals of the overall program identified in Phase 1. The six units are as follows:

1. Leisure awareness,
2. Leisure resources,
3. Leisure communication skills,
4. Making decisions,
5. Leisure planning,
6. Activity skills instruction.

Each unit had a number of sub-objectives, each of which had corresponding exercises to be carried out in the classroom, a home-based component that parents were asked to carry out, and curriculum-based measure that were used to determine the extent to which the students had achieved the objectives of the unit. In keeping with the conceptual model outlined earlier, classroom teachers determined which components of the leisure education process were introduced, depending upon the needs and interests of the students. Research conducted by Mahon (1994) and Mahon and Bullock (1992a & b, 1993) determined that the process was successful in facilitating leisure-based decision making, planning, and initiation. In addition, teachers, parents, and students indicated that the program had a positive impact on the lives of the students with disabilities.

A five-year follow-up study is currently underway, which has broadened the original model to involve parents much more extensively in the leisure-education process. Family Link in Leisure Education has taken the original curriculum and devised a training program so that parents, siblings, teachers, and students with disabilities can share in the process of enhancing community-based recreation opportunities.

Reintegration Through Recreation (RTR)

People with severe and persistent mental illnesses may identify new interests while in the hospital, but they often encounter difficulties related to following through on their interests. After discharge, they often experience loneliness, overdependence on service providers and families, and discomfort being with others. Many also lack repertoire of individual skills that can help them to connect with people based on interests and abilities, not on disability. When back in their community, they experience fluctuating motivation and energy, limited resources, and discrimination by others (Campbell & Schrailser, 1989; Miller & Miller, 1991). Since these needs can be best addressed in the environment in which a person lives, Reintegration Through Recreation was conceptualized to be a community-based model of transitional therapeutic recreation services that is responsive to the needs of individuals.

The mission of RTR is to provide the necessary skills and supports to individuals with severe and persistent mental illnesses, so they may have satisfying and successful lives that include freely chosen and supported recreation and leisure in the settings of their choice. Overall RTR participant goals include successful community tenure that includes community membership and acceptance, improved quality of social supports, more varied leisure interest, the ability to use problem-solving skills to handle present and future concerns, improved life satisfaction, increased self-esteem, and the ability to follow through on personally chosen and planned leisure experiences.

RTR, which is a leisure education program that uses cognitive behavioral principles, is a three-phase process that facilitates the transition of skills to one's community. Phase one is conceptualization, which involves data collection, assessment, problem identification and goal setting. Phase two involves skill acquisition and rehearsal. Phase three, the most critical and often-neglected learning phase, centers on application and follow-through. It is necessary to provide gradual exposure to increasing levels of difficulty in the real environment so that maintenance and generalization of skills can occur (Meichenbaum, 1986). Also during this phase, future plans are made, with an emphasis placed on expanded circles of support, environmental resources, and the ongoing use of problem-solving skills. If skill application does not take place, rehabilitation successes likely will not last.

RTR uses a systematic leisure education program that is then individualized with each participant based on the problem identification and self-selected goals. The client is at the center of the process. The overall components of the leisure education program include an appreciation of leisure and an awareness of personal values, and understanding of self-determination and its impact on leisure choices and behaviors, the use of problem-solving skills to facilitate personal decision making, the ability to use a variety of community and personal resources, the development of social interactions kills and confidence, and the learning of specific activity skills. These leisure education topics have been translated into three core units and six resource units (see Figure 16.5) that serve as a road map for the collaboration between each participant and the TRS.

Throughout the RTR process, the TRS is careful not to overload the participant with too many techniques and procedures that may make it more difficult to succeed. The therapist's responsibility is to collaborate with the client in selecting the most useful learning strategies and individualizing a plan. The least amount of TRS time is spent on developing specific activity skills because clients can work with other community specialists for this goal (park and recreation staff, commercial recreation service providers, volunteers, etc.).

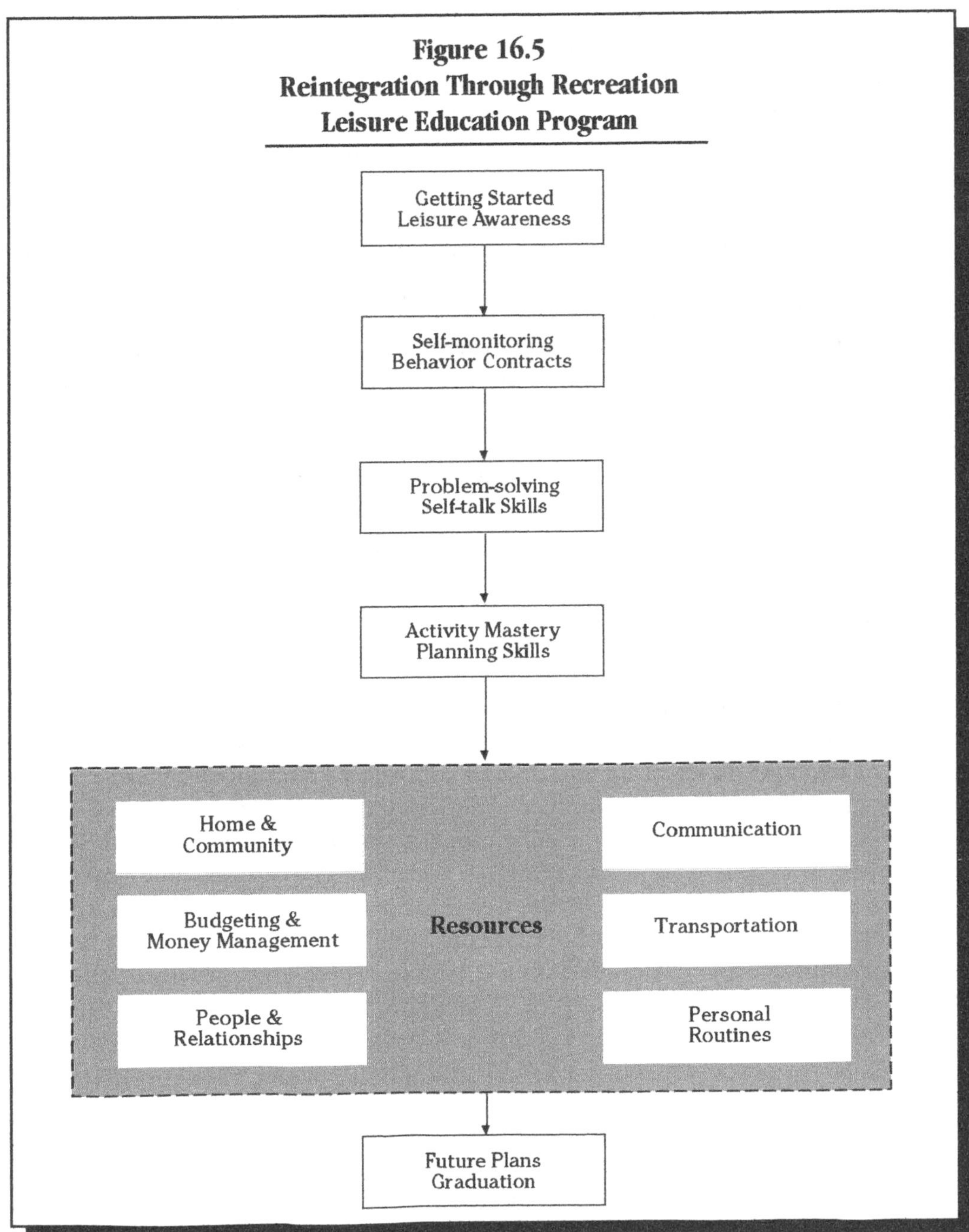

Later Life Planning Program (LLPP)

Retirement for older people with mental disabilities is a relatively new concept. Retirement age has been considered to be between 55 and 60 years of age (Stuton, Sterns, & Park, 1993). When older people with mental disabilities are faced with the option of retirement, many are not aware of the consequences of their retirement or the alternatives. Janicki (1992) reports that "older persons with mental retardation find that the loss or change of friends when moving to a new program can pose a significant barrier" and that "many seniors demur on retiring to senior programs because of fear of losing their workshop or job income and close network of friends made in the workplace" (p. 119). Pre-retirement and retirement training programs may allow older adults with mental disabilities to recognize the opportunities to develop new interests and make new friends that retirement can bring (Cotton, 1991). Structured interviews with older adults with mental disabilities revealed that views of life after retirement were initially negative due to a perceived lack of alternatives. Yet, when participants became familiar with options, attitudes were noticeably more favorable (Laughlin & Cotton, 1989).

The Later Life Planning Program was a model program developed by Mahon in conjunction with a supported employment program, Sturgeon Creek Enterprises, and the Province of Manitoba. The purpose of this research and demonstration project was to determine whether leisure education and futures planning could be used in combination to facilitate later life planning for people with mental disabilities. Individuals were elected based on their interest in retirement and the extent to which their social support networks were prepared to support a change in the individual's life. The LLPP is divided into three phases.

In phase 1, each individual begins by receiving a minimum of six leisure education sessions designed to enhance his awareness of the concepts of retirement and leisure, the resources that exist in his community to support various retirement options, and how to make decisions about what to do during retirement.

In the LLPP, individuals learned about their options by going out into the community and experiencing them. As a result, individuals took part in experiences ranging from day program for older adults without disabilities, to recreation programs at local YMCA's, volunteer experiences, and even part-time work.

Following the initial leisure education training, the subjects and their families took part in a PATH (Pearpoint, O'Brien, & Forest, 1993) planning meeting in phase 2. This is a futures planning process that has been used within a supportive employment setting to help personnel identify and facilitate the community adjustment needs of a client. Personal futures planning is a creative process "designed to help a group of people create a life of meaning and contribution for the person who is focus of the planning" (Mount & Zwernik, 1990, p. 1). It asks people involved in the process to ***dream*** about possible futures and work backwards from that perspective to very specific manageable steps that lead to the envisioned future (Pearpoint, O'Brien, & Forest, 1993). Mahon hypothesized that the PATH process would be a useful means of developing a comprehensive retirement plan operationalized in large measure by natural supports in the community.

Following the PATH meeting, in phase 3, participants were taught to engage in leisure action planning, initiation, and self-committing as a means of carrying out the action plan they identified during the PATH meeting. Each individual plan was very different, as it was based upon the needs and aspirations of the individual.

What should be evident after reviewing these three sample programs is that leisure education is a very flexible process that can be used in a variety of settings with people with quite disparate needs. The common bond between the programs described are the concepts of choice, social role valorization, community integration, and interdependence—all of which have been discussed extensively in this text. Each of the projects described also speak to the efficacy of leisure education for enhancing the quality of life of people with disabilities. So that you have further evidence of this, the final section within this chapter highlights some of the benefits of leisure education that have been described in the literature.

Benefits of Leisure Education

A long-held belief is that leisure education can provide a number of benefits to people with disabilities. This belief, often cited by educators and practitioners, was for many years unfounded. Up until very recent times, there was a dearth of research to support the many claims regarding the benefits of leisure education. During the past decade, researchers in the field of recreation and leisure studies, and in particular those interested in the efficacy of leisure education as a therapeutic recreation-based approach, have begun to explore the efficacy of leisure education through structured research studies.

People with Physical Disabilities

Zoerink (1988) and Zoerink and Lauener (1991) studies the effects of using a values-clarification approach to leisure education on young people with spina bifida and adults with head injuries. Neither group of individuals demonstrated any systematic changes in psychological well-being as a result of the leisure education program. Calwell, Adalph, and Gilbert (1989) found that their leisure education program actually resulted in increased leisure dissatisfaction in people with head injuries after they were discharged from a rehabilitation hospital. They suggested that the problem with the program is that it may have increased participants' expectations about what they could do following discharge from the hospital, while the awareness and skills developed may not have persisted following discharge.

In contrast to these three studies, Bullock and Howe (1991) found that a transitional leisure education program, the Community Reintegration Program (CRP), did facilitate successful reintegration of people with physical disabilities, including those with head injuries, back into the community. Bullock and Howe asserted that the positive changes in their participants were attributed to the fact that the CRP program took place in the community following discharge, as opposed to predischarge, as with the Calwell et al. (1989) study.

People with Mental Retardation

Research on leisure education for people with mental retardation began in the mid-1980s. One of the earliest studies, conducted by Anderson and Allen (1985), look at the impact of a leisure education program on people with mental retardation living within an institutional setting. The authors reported that the leisure education program helped to increase activity participation, but did not effect the frequency or duration of social contacts between participants. Lanagan and Dattilo (1989) conducted a community-based study of daily leisure education program in which they compared the impact of a traditional recreation participation approach to leisure education. They found leisure education to be more effective in enhancing activity involvement.

As if evident from the two aforementioned studies, early research on leisure education and people with mental retardation tended to focus on whether leisure education is effective in increasing participation in leisure activities. More recent studies with this population has focused on contemporary issues, including community integration and reintegration, self-determination, social-psychological outcomes such as perceived competence and control, and quality of life (Bedini, Bullock, & Driscoll, 1991; Williams & Dattilo, 1997; Johnson, Ashton-Shaeffer & Bullock, 1997; Mahon, 1994; Mahon & Bullock, 1992b, 1993). For example, Mahon (1994) demonstrated that a public school-based leisure education program facilitated increased decision making and independent leisure initiation in adolescents with mental disabilities. More recently, Mahon and Martens (1996) found that a similar leisure education program conducted within a supported employment program had a nearly identical impact on adults with mental disabilities.

People with Mental Illnesses

The most recent research on people with mental illnesses and leisure education is connected to the Reintegration Through Recreation Model described in an earlier section. Mahon, Bullock, Luken, and Martens (1996) reported on a study of the social validity of this leisure education program. Social validity relates to the extent to which consumers, service providers, and significant others feel that the goals, processes, and outcomes of an intervention are of value of consumers, service providers, and significant others feel that the goals, processes, and outcomes of an intervention are of value to consumers (Wolf, 1978). In addition, social validity research often looks to evaluate whether an intervention has the potential to benefit the broader community, including other consumers, family members, and service providers. In the study reported on by Mahon et al. (1996), the researchers sought to determine the social validity of the RTR Program from the perspective of consumers, service providers, and family members. All three groups were asked to evaluate the goals, processes, and outcomes of the leisure education program via three separate questionnaires. The results indicated that all three groups found the RTR program to be socially valid. Most notably, the consumers indicated that they would recommend the program to others that it had a very significant impact on their ability to become involved in recreation opportunities within their home community. It is also interesting to note that the consumers felt that the most important part of the leisure education program was skill learning and rehearsal.

Few other studies have investigated the benefits of leisure education for people with mental illnesses. Wolf and Riddick (1984) reported that a leisure education program enhanced leisure attitudes but had no impact on the self-esteem of adults who were part of an outpatient program for adults with mental illnesses. In contrast, Skalko (1990) found that a leisure education program, conducted in a group home setting with adult males with chronic mental illnesses, increased their quality of discretionary time use. The authors of all three of these studies recommended that leisure education be used as a component of community mental health services.

Older Adults

One of the first studies that documented the effects of leisure education on older adults compared leisure counseling (a component of leisure education) to traditional activity instruction, a combination of the two and no program (Backman & Mannell, 1986). This study demonstrated that the combination program had the most significant positive impacts on leisure attitudes and participation. Dunn and Wilhite (1997) found that a similar leisure education program with older women enhanced leisure participation, but did not effect psychological well-being. These results support the basic tenets of our conceptual model that indicates awareness must be combined with skill learning and rehearsal.

Following this, through a series of studies, Searle, Mahon, and their colleagues at the University of Manitoba demonstrated that leisure education can significantly impact on older adults' feelings of control and competence and is able to enhance self-esteem and reduce boredom (Mahon & Searle, 1994; Searle & Mahon, 1991, 1993; Searle, Mahon, Iso-Ahola, Sdrolias, & van Dyke, 1995). In addition, this research team also found that the effects of the leisure education program were long lasting. These studies provide quite convincing evidence that a comprehensive approach to leisure education is most effective in promoting social-psychological changes in older adults. An important side note by Searle and Mahon is that changes in leisure participation patterns are unlikely to occur unless older adults first experience enhanced feelings of control and competence. This provides clear support for a strong focus on the promotion of self-determination skills within any leisure education process.

Conclusion

Leisure education is an important therapeutic recreation-based process for enhancing life satisfaction in people with disabilities. However, as was noted in the section on benefits, there is a good deal more research needed to ensure that leisure education continues to respond to the changing needs of people with disabilities. We contend that in order for leisure education to be successful, it must be a person-centered approach that promotes collaboration between the leisure education specialist and the person with a disability. It is extremely important that recreation service providers be aware of the presence of a leisure education program in their community, that they be knowledgeable about the goals of the program, and that they support the inclusion of people with disabilities within their programs and services.

Leisure education can only be successful if people with disabilities are accepted as equal members of their community. Beyond this, there is a need for leisure education to be introduced in a variety of settings in order to ensure that the leisure needs of as many people with disabilities as possible are met. We reported on programs that have been developed in conjunction with schools, rehab program, and services for older adults. Leisure education has also been incorporated into such services as supported employment, community recreation, institutional settings, and group home settings. The challenge for the future is to increase the involvement of people with disabilities in leisure education programs in settings that are able to provide quality, person-centered opportunities.

Learning Exercises

1. Have the class discuss which components of the leisure education model are most important for them, in terms of overcoming barriers and achieving a satisfying lifestyle.
2. Organize the class into small groups. Ask each group to take one component of the person-centered leisure education model and come up with exercises that could be used with people with disabilities to deal with needs that relate to the specific component.
3. Drive or walk around your home community and determine what recreation opportunities exist. Identify which opportunities you were aware of and which you were not.

References

Abery, B.H., Thurlow, M.T., Johnson, D.R., & Bruininks, R.H. (1990, May.) ***The social networks of adults with developmental disabilities residing in community settings.*** Paper presented at the annual meeting of the American Association on Mental Retardation, Washington, D.C.

Anderson, S.C. & Allen, L.R. (1985). Effects of leisure education program on activity involvement and social interaction of mentally retarded persons. ***Adapted Physical Activity Quarterly, 2*** (2), 107-116.

Backman, S.J., & Mannell, R.C. (1986). Removing attitudinal barriers to leisure behavior and satisfaction: A field experiment among the institutionalized elderly. ***Therapeutic Recreation Journal, 20***, 3, pp. 46-53.

Beck-Ford, V., & Brown, R. (1984). ***Leisure training and rehabilitation: A program manual.*** Springfield, IL: Charles C. Thomas, Publisher.

Bedini, L., Bullock, C.C, & Driscoll, L (1991). From schools to community: Achieving independence and community integration through leisure education. ***Palaestra, 8*** (1), 38-43.

Bender, M., & Valletutti, P.J. (1976). ***Teaching the moderately and severely handicapped: Curriculum, objectives, strategies, and activities.*** Vol. 2, Baltimore, MD: University Park Press.

Bogdan, R., & Taylor, S. (1987). Toward a sociology of acceptance: The other side of the study of deviance. ***Social Policy, 18*** (2), 34-39.

Brown, P.J., (1988). ***Effects of self-advocacy training in leisure on adults with severe physical disabilities.*** Unpublished doctoral dissertation, Virginia Polytechnic Institute and State University, Blacksburg, VA.

Bullock, C. (1988). Interpretive lines of action of mentally retarded children in mainstream play settings. ***Studies in Symbolic Interaction, 9***, 145-172.

Bullock, C., & Copp, M. (1991). ***Interviewing people with mental retardation.*** Unpublished manuscript, University of North Carolina at Chapel Hill, Center for Recreation and Disability, Chapel Hill, NC.

Bullock, C., & Howe, C.Z. (1991). A model therapeutic recreation program for the reintegration of persons with disabilities into the community. ***Therapeutic Recreation Journal, 25*** (1), 7-17.

Bullock, C., & Luken K. (1994). Reintegration through recreation: A community-based rehabilitation model. In S.E. Iso-Ahola & D.M. Compton, (eds.), ***Leisure and Mental Health.***

Bullock, C., Morris, L., Mahon, M., & Jones, B. (1992). ***School-community leisure link: Leisure education program curriculum guide.*** The Center for Recreation and Disability Studies, Curriculum in Leisure Studies and Recreation Administration, University of North Carolina at Chapel Hill, Chapel Hill, NC.

Calwell, L.L., Adolph, S., & Gilbert, A. (1989). Caution! Leisure counselors at work: Long-term effects of leisure counseling. ***Therapeutic Recreation Journal, 23*** (3), 4-7.

Campbell, J., & Schrailser, R. (1989). ***Well-being project.*** Department of Mental Health, Sacramento, CA.

Chinn, K.A., & Joswiak, K.F. (1981) Leisure education and leisure counseling. ***Therapeutic Recreation Journal, 15*** (4), 4-7.

Dattilo, J. (1994). ***Inclusive leisure services: Responding to the rights of people with disabilities.*** State College, PA: Venture Publishing.

Dattilo, J., & Murphy, W. (1991). ***Leisure education program planning: A systematic approach***, State College, PA: Venture Publishing.

Duffy, A., & Nietupski, J. (1985). Acquisition and maintenance of video game initiation, sustaining and termination skills. ***Education and Training in Disabilities, 20***, 157-162.

Dunn, N. & Wilhite, B. (1997). The effects of a leisure education program on leisure participation and psychosocial well-being of older women who are home-centered. ***Therapeutic Recreation Journal,*** 31, 53-71.

Fields, S., & Hoffman, A. (1991). ***Skills for self-determination.*** Paper presented at The Project Directors' Sixth Annual Meeting, Transition Institute at Illinois, Washington, D.C.

Goode, D.A., & Gaddy, M.R. (1976). Ascertaining choice with lingual, deaf-blind, and retarded clients. *Mental Retardation, 14*, 10-12.

Guess, D., Benson, H.A., & Siegel-Causey, E. (1985). Concepts and issues related to choice making and autonomy among persons with severe disabilities. *The Journal of the Association for Persons with Severe Handicaps, 10*, 79-86.

Horner, R.H., Dunlop, G., & Koegel, R.L. (Eds.) (1988). *Generalization and maintenance: Lifestyle changes in applied settings.* Baltmore: Paul H. Brookes Publishing Co.

Houghton, J., Bronicki, G.J. & Guess, D. (1987). Opportunities to express preferences and make choices among students with severe disabilities in classroom settings. *Journal of the Association for Persons with Severe Handicaps, 12*, 18-27.

Janicki, (1992). Lifelong disability and again. In L. Rowitz (Ed.), *Mental retardation in the year 2000* (pp. 115-127). New York: Springer-Verlag.

Johnson, D., Ashton-Shaeffer, C., & Bullock, C. (1997). Families and leisure: A context for learning. *Teaching Exceptional Children*, 30, 30-34

Kelly (1996). *Leisure* (3rd ed.). Needham Heights, MA: Allyn and Bacon.

Kennedy, M., & Killius, P. (1987). Living in the community: Speaking for yourself. In S.J. Taylor, D. Biklen, & J. Knoll (eds.), *Community integration for people with severe disabilities* (pp. 202-208). New York: Teachers College Press.

Lanagan, D., & Dattilo, J. (1989). The effects of a leisure education program on individuals with mental retardation. *Therapeutic Recreation Journal, 23* (4), 62-72.

Laughlin, C., & Cotton, P.D. (1994). Efficacy of a pre-retirement planning intervention for aging individuals with mental retardation. Special Issue on Aging: Our continuing challenge. *Journal of Intellectual Disability Research, 38* (3), 317-328.

Mahon, M. (1990). *Facilitation of independent decision making in leisure with adolescents who are mentally retarded*. Unpublished manuscript, University of North Carolina at Chapel Hill, Division of Special Education, Chapel Hill, NC.

Mahon, M. (1983). *An attributional analysis of the motor performance outcomes and the development of learned helplessness in educable mentally retarded boys*. Unpublished master's thesis, University of Alberta, Edmonton, Alberta, Canada.

Mahon, M., (1994). The use of self-control techniques to facilitate self-determination skills during leisure in adolescent with mild and moderate mental retardation. *Therapeutic Recreation Journal, 28* (2), 58-72.

Mahon, M., & Bullock, C. (1992a, Fall). Decision making and leisure: Empowerment for people who are mentally retarded. *Leisure Today*.

Mahon, M., & Bullock, C. (1992b). Teaching adolescents with mild disabilities to make decisions in leisure through the use of self-control techniques. *Therapeutic Recreation Journal, 26*, 9-26.

Mahon & Bullock (1993). An investigation of the social validity of a comprehensive leisure education program. *Annual in Therapeutic Recreation.*

Mahon & Martens. (1996). Leisure education in supported employment: A process for facilitating community adjustment. *Journal of Applied Recreation Research*, 21, 283-312.

Mahon, M.J., & Searle, M.S., (1994). Leisure education: Its effects on older adults. *Journal of Physical Education, Recreation, and Dance, 65* (4), 36-41.

Mahon, M.J., Bullock, C.C., Luken, K., & Martens, C. (1996). Leisure education for people with severe and persistent mental illness: Is this a socially valid process? *Therapeutic Recreation Journal, 30*, 197-212.

Martin, J.E., Burger, D.L., Elias-Burger, S., & Mithaugh, D.E. (1988). Applications of self-control strategies to establish the independence of individuals who are mentally retarded. In N. Bray (ed.), *International review of research in mental retardation*. New York: Academic Press.

Meichenbaum, D. (1986). Metacognitive methods of instruction: Current status and future prospects. *Special Services in the Schools, Fall/Winter*, 3 (1-2), 23-32.

Meichenbaum, D., & Goodman, J. (1971). Training impulsive children to talk to themselves: A means of developing self-control. *Journal of Abnormal Psychology*, 77, 116-126.

Miller, S. Miller, R.L. (1991). An exploration of daily hassles for persons with severe psychiatric disabilities. *Psychosocial Rehabilitation Journal, 14*, 11-17.

Mitchel, B. (1988). Who chooses? *National Information Centre for Children and Youth with Handicaps, 5*, 4-5.

Mithaug, D.E., & Hanawalk, D.A. (1978). The validation of procedures to assess prevocational task preferences in retarded adults. *Journal of Applied Behavior Analysis, 13*, 177-182.

Mithaug, D., Martin, J. & Agran, M. (1987). Adaptability instruction: The goal of transitional programming. *Exceptional Children, 53* (6), 500-505.

Mount, B., & Zwernik, K. (1990). *Making futures happen: A manual for facilitators of personal futures planning*. St. Paul, MN: Metropolitan Council of the Twin Cities.

Mundy, J. & Odum, L. (1979). *Leisure education: Theory and practice*. New York: Wiley.

Nash, J. (1953). *Philosophy of recreation and leisure*. Dubuque, IA: Brown.

Nietupski, J., & Svoboda, R. (1982). Teaching a cooperative leisure skill to severely handicapped adults. *Education and Training of the Mentally Retarded, 17*, 38-43.

Nietupski, J., Hamre-Nietupski, S., Green K., Varnum-Teeter, K., Twedt, B., LePera, D., Scebold, K., & Hanrahan, M. (1986). Self-initiated and sustained leisure activity participation by students with moderate/severe handicaps. *Education and Training of the Mentally Retarded*, 259-264.

Pearpoint, J., O'Brien, J., & Forest, M. (1993). *PATH, A workbook for planning positive possible futures.* Toronto: Inclusion Press.

Pollingue, A.B., & Cobb, H.B. (1986). Leisure education: A model facilitating community integration for moderately/severely mentally retarded adults. *Therapeutic Recreation Journal, 20* (3), 54-62.

Putman, J., Werder, J., & Schleien, S. (1985). Leisure and recreation services for handicapped persons. In K. C. Lakin, & R.H. Bruininks (Eds.), *Strategies for achieving community integration of developmentally disabled citizens* (pp. 253-275). Baltimore, MD: Brooks.

Schleien, S., Certo, N.J., & Muccino, A. (1984). Acquisition of leisure skills by a severely handicapped adolescent: A data-based leisure skills instructional program. *Education and Training of the Mentally Retarded, 19* (4), 297-305.

Searle, M.S., & Mahon, M.J. (1991). Leisure education in a day hospital: The effects on selected social-psychological variables among older adults. *Canadian Journal of Community Mental Health, 10* (2), 95-109.

Searle, M.S., & Mahon, M.J.. (1993). The effects of leisure education on selected socio-psychological variables: A three-month follow-up study. *Therapeutic Recreation Journal, 27* (1), 9-21.

Searle, M.D., Mahon ,M.J., Iso-Ahola, S.E., Sdrolias, A.H., van Dykck, J. (1995). Enhancing a sense of independence and psychological well-being among the elderly: A field experiment. *Journal of Leisure Research, 27* (2), 107-124.

Shapiro, E.S. (1981). Self-control procedures with the mentally retarded. In M. Herson, R.M. Eisler, & P.M. Miller (Eds.), *Progress in behavior modification* (Vol. 12, pp. 265-297). New York: Academic Press.

Siperstein, G.N., Bak, J.J., & O'Keefe, P. (1988). Relationship between children's attitudes toward and their social acceptance of mentally retarded peers. *American Journal on Mental Retardation, 93* (1), 24-27.

Skalko, T. (1990). Discretionary time use and the chronically mentally ill. In M.E. Crawford & J.A. Card, (eds.), *Annual in therapeutic recreation: Volume 1.* Reston, VA: American Alliance for Health, Physical Education, Recreation, and Dance.

Sutton, E., Sterns, H.L., & Park, L.S. (1993) Realities of retirement and preretirement planning. In E. Sutton, A.R. Factor, B.A. Hawkins, T. Heller, & G.B. Seltzer (Eds), *Older adults with developmental disabilities: Optimizing choice and change* (pp. 95-106). Toronto: Paul H. Brooks.

Taylor, A.R., Asher, S.R., Williams, G.A. (1987). The social adaptation of mainstreamed mildly retarded children. *Child Development, 58,* 1321-1334.

Ward, M. (1988). The many facets of self-determination. *National Information Center for children and Youth with Handicaps: Transition Summary, 5*, 2-3.

Websters II: New Riverside Dictionary. (1984). New York, NY: Houghton Mifflin Co.

Wehman, P. & Schleien, S. (1981). *Leisure programs for handicapped persons*. Baltimore, MD: University Park Press.

Wehmeyer, M.L., (1992). Self-determination and the education of students with mental retardation. *Education and Training in Mental Retardation, 94*, 347-362.

Whitman, T.L. (1990). Self-regulation and mental retardation. *American Journal on Mental Retardation*, 94, 347-362.

Williams, R. & Dattilo, J. (1997). Effects of leisure education on choice making, social interaction, and positive affect of young adults with mental retardation. *Therapeutic Recreation Journal,* 31, 244-58.

Wilson, C., & Alexis, M. (1962). Basic frameworks for decisions. *J.A.M.,* 150-164.

Wolf, M.M. (1978). Social validity: The case for subjective measurement or how applied behavior analysis is finding it heart. *Journal of Applied Behavior Analysis, 11*, 203-234.

Wolfe, R.A., & Riddick, C.C., (1984). Effects of leisure counseling on adult psychiatric outpatients. *Therapeutic Recreation Journal, 18* (3), 30-37.

Wolfensberger, W. (1972). ***The principles of normalization in human services***. Toronto, Ont.: National Institute on Mental Retardation.

Wolfensberger, W. (1983). Social role valorization: a proposed new term for the principle of normalization. *Mental Retardation, 21*, 234-239.

Wuerch, B.B., & Voeltz, L.M. (1982). ***Longitudinal leisure skills for severely handicapped learners: The Ho'onanea curriculum component***. Baltimore, MD: Paul H. Brookes.

Zoerink, D. (1988). Effects of short-term leisure education program upon the leisure functioning of your people with spina bifida. *Therapeutic Recreation Journal, 22* (3), 44-52.

Zoerink, D., & Lauener, K. (1991) Effects of a leisure education program on adults with traumatic brain injury. *Therapeutic Recreation Journal, (25)*, 3, 19-28.

Related Websites

http://www6.huji.ac.il/cosell/wlra/charter.htm
(World Leisure and Recreation Association International Charter for Leisure Education)

http://www.coe.ufl.edu/special/florida/leisure.htm
(Recreation and Leisure Time as Part of the Transition Program for Individuals with Disabilities)

http://www.nau.edu/ihd/aztap/recreation.html
(Recreation and Leisure Resource List)

http://www.lin.ca/findrs.htm (type "leisure" in Keyword 1, and "education" in Keyword 2
(Leisure Information Network — Leisure Education)

Chapter 17

Issues and Conclusions

Introduction

It should be clear from the Introduction as well as chapters throughout the text that we espouse the egalitarian ideal that all people—regardless of their level of physical, mental, or social functioning; regardless of their ethnicity, income level, or values—be included as a part of the whole. We long for an environment and an accompanying social structure that are not only accepting but encouraging of *all* people. We anticipate a world in which people celebrate differences rather than denigrate others who are different from them. It is a dream that inclusive and responsive person-centered recreation services can help achieve. As we continue to stress the importance of person-centeredness, we suggest that our field move more toward a community membership paradigm (Bradley, 1994) that *presupposes* inclusion and also moves away from the current recreational paradigm that *allows* integration.

We began this text by discussing issues and concepts related to the field of disability. As we noted, it is important that you understand and embrace concepts such as self-determination, normalization, social role valorization, inclusion, and interdependence prior to any discussion of recreation programming and people with disabilities. In addition, as you will remember, we spent a good deal of time providing you with both a historical and legislative context to our future discussions on recreation and people with disabilities.

Following this, the majority of the text has centered on recreation services and people with disabilities. In this final chapter, we think it is important to return to concepts that are important for the continued development of responsive recreation services that include people with disabilities. As a result, in a final chapter we will discuss advocacy, self-advocacy, inclusive communities, technology, and then conclude with a historical and conceptual review of many of the guiding principles of this book.

Advocacy

Throughout this text we have talked all around advocacy without yet naming or defining it. *Advocacy* is a means of pleading for the cause of another. Kaufman-Broida & Wenzel (1994) described advocacy as "a process directed toward improving the quality of goods and services rendered to consumers" (p. 73). From this perspective, the purpose or basis for advocacy is first and foremost consumer-oriented. Within advocacy, we promote policies and services that will benefit our clients or consumers. We must plead for and with our clients based on their interests, not our self-interests. As a result of improved services and goods for our clients, the profession itself will benefit and advance. Shank (1995) described this concept of writing that:

> success will be measured not only by what we can accomplish for the profession directly but by what we can accomplish on behalf of the children and adults who need special assistance in accessing recreational opportunities and whose lives can be improved through recreation as clinical, rehabilitative, educational, and community service. (p. 31).

To achieve this success, two types of professional advocacy exist: political and social. Political advocacy refers to advocacy that is directed toward initiating, supporting, or changing policies regarding the delivery of services. An example is lobbying legislative and regulatory bodies. On a broader scale, social advocacy refers to marketing and public relation efforts directed toward a target group of consumers. Those consumers may consist of clients, the public, students, and related service professionals, to name a few. An example of social advocacy is the promotion of Therapeutic Recreation Week through proclamations, events, and activities.

Both political and social advocacy occur within and across many contexts. Kaufman-Broida and Wenzel (1994) proposed one model for understanding the contexts of advocacy. The authors identified six contexts of advocacy: internal, external, big stuff, small stuff, individual, and system levels of influence.

Within the field of recreation and therapeutic recreation, limited literature regarding professional advocacy exists. The writings that exist focus largely on the external, big stuff, and system contexts of professional advocacy. From this perspective, the present literature explores advocacy within the realms of the profession and public policy; thus, the examination of issues has revolved around political advocacy.

The main issue regarding professional advocacy is summarized by the simple statement that professionals must be social and political advocates on behalf of clients' interest. There are many issues that influence how the profession can efficiently and effectively advocate for and with our clients. First, therapeutic recreation has multiple organizations with varying perspectives that advocate for and with our clients. First, therapeutic recreation has multiple organizations with varying perspectives that advocate on behalf of the profession. On the national level alone, therapeutic recreation is represented by three membership organizations in the U.S.—the American Therapeutic Recreation Association (ATRA), National Therapeutic Recreation Society (NTRS), the National Consortium on Physical Education and Recreation for Individuals with Disabilities (NCPERID)—and one in Canada—the Canadian Therapeutic Recreation Association—as well as a nonpartisan certification body—the National Council on Therapeutic Recreation Certification (NCTRC). Second, the organizations that represent therapeutic recreation have limited human and financial resources to dedicate to promoting the field. Therapeutic recreation advocacy efforts must rely upon the commitment and resources of volunteers. Third, the therapeutic recreation profession often relies on the use of passionate appeals rather than research-based facts to support its advocacy arguments (Shank, 1995, p. 29). A final issue is the lack of involvement on the part of individual professionals to take on advocacy roles.

Training for advocacy roles does not have to emphasize participation on the national level. Shank (1995) suggested that "state level action may be more critical than action at the federal level," as most legislation affecting educational, rehabilitative, and developmental disability services is implemented through state agencies (p. 28). Each state determines its priorities for developmental disabilities services and vocational rehabilitation services; thus, therapeutic recreational professionals must advocate at the state level to promote the needs of its consumers (Shank). The state of Colorado has moved forward in this area by designing a model to train therapeutic recreation professionals in developing advocacy skills (Shank).

According to Shank (1995), advocacy "is a genuine reflection of our values, beliefs, and ethics" (p. 25). Kaufman-Broida and Wenzel (1994, p. 75) suggest that "Therapeutic recreation professionals are responsible for advocating for/with individuals with disabilities and for the profession." By the virtue of being a member of the therapeutic recreation profession, a professional must be a constant advocate for therapeutic recreation and its services to clients. During each interaction that a professional has regarding recreation and therapeutic recreation, he is delivering a message to an audience. Every time a person speaks as a recreation or a therapeutic recreation professional, he is in essence acting as an advocate. Who is better prepared to advocate regarding the benefits of recreation and therapeutic recreation than those who are intimately involved in the delivery of the service?

Unfortunately, the membership numbers of therapeutic recreation organizations at national and state levels indicate the existence of a lack of involvement and commitment by individuals to the profession. Some professionals might argue that with the demands of jobs and life, they do not have the time or resources to involve themselves in advocacy. Some professionals would suggest that they lack the knowledge or qualifications necessary to be professional advocates. These "barriers" to participation in advocacy imply a focus on self-interests, rather than a focus on benefits for clients.

Fortunately, Kaufman-Broida and Wenzel (1994) have suggested practical ways to break these barriers to fulfill our ***individual responsibility to advocacy***. The authors' six-point guideline to becoming involved include the following:

1. Acknowledge your limitations and establish your goals within these parameters.

2. Take advantage of information provided within conferences, workshops, and professional journals to learn skills for effective advocacy.
3. Choose an issue or task with which you are comfortable. Being involved in advocacy does not mean you have to lobby on Capitol Hill. Advocacy can occur within your own environment.
4. Do not do it all yourself. Support your efforts by collaborating with colleagues as well as with resource materials from professional associations.
5. Establish time lines and target dates for the completion of tasks.
6. Adjust your advocacy plans and efforts as necessary.

Schroder (1993c) provides a personal perspective on being an advocate for a recreational cause. He suggested numerous factors that contribute to the success of advocacy participation. Six of those suggestions are summarized here:

1. Recognize and acknowledge your individual motivation for becoming in volved in the issue.
2. Recognize and utilize your individual strengths, skills, and talents.
3. Develop support through collaborating with others.
4. Establish goals and specific objectives to guide your efforts.
5. Be prepared and specific objectives to guide your efforts.
6. Learn the system within which you will advocate; i.e., the political system, the community system, or the hospital system.

We challenge you to ***accept individual responsibility*** for advocacy. Several learning experiences have been suggested at the end of this chapter. Learning experiences occur within every context of our professional and personal lives; thus, the suggestions we offer are meant to challenge you to find a comfortable starting point.

As you embrace the challenge, keep in mind that our guiding force as a human services professional is the person who is involved in recreation or therapeutic recreation services. Without this important group or group of people, there would be no need for us or our services. To move our profession forward, recreation and therapeutic recreation must maintain this most central focus. As Shank (1995) has said, "Our success as a profession will be measured by what we accomplish for those we serve." In a more global way, Sylvester (1995) has said that we must "seek the good of the profession in the good of the public" (p. 102).

Self-Advocacy

Only a page ago we asked the question, "Who is better prepared to advocate regarding the benefits of recreation and therapeutic recreation than those who are intimately involved in the delivery of the service?" Professionals, those who are intimately involved in the delivery of the service, are indeed well prepared and in fact, have a responsibility to advocate.

But the question may be answered differently by different publics. Who *is* better prepared to advocate regarding the benefits of recreation and therapeutic recreation? Many would say that the people themselves who are the recipients or potential recipients of services are better qualified to advocate regarding the benefits of recreation and therapeutic recreation that they have or may receive. This type of advocacy is called self-advocacy.

Self-advocacy refers to an individual or an independent group of people with disabilities working together by helping each other take charge of their live and to fight discrimination. It teaches individuals how to make decisions and choices that affect their lives so that they can be more independent. It also teaches about rights; but along with that. It teaches about responsibility. In the end, self-advocacy is about giving people with disabilities the confidence to speak for themselves (Adapted from the definition of self-advocacy approved at the 2nd Annual People First Conference, 1991, September) (Nelis, 1994).

Hutchison and McGill (1992, p. 58) suggest that there are some limitations to individual self-advocacy:

> In very complex situations, many people who have been devalued do not have the confidence, skills, and political know how to make changes on their own. In addition to this, making changes to massive power structures is not possible without large numbers of people...As a result of these limitations, many people who experience similar barriers come together to form self-advocacy organizations to take collective action.

One of the best examples of a group of people who have come together as self-advocates is People First. It is now an international network of self-advocates with mental retardation that began as a small group of people interested in furthering their rights a citizens of a democratic society. As suggested by Hutchison and McGill (1992), groups such as People First have become organized and continue to grow, in part due to external support. Chaikin (1994) proves guidelines for people wishing to provide support to self-advocates. Although specific to people with developmental disabilities, this information is generalizable to any person or group of people with any type of disability. Chaikin's guidelines are presented in Table 17.1.

It is important for people within the field of recreation to understand that they can contribute as both an advocate for people with disabilities and as a supporter of self-advocates. In fact, in order to create an interdependent environment within a recreation or therapeutic recreation setting, both roles have to be encouraged and nurtured. In moving from the role of advocate to that of a supporter of

Table 17.1
Guidelines for Providing Information to Self-Advocates

1. Always work from that premise that people with developmental disabilities can understand. I can't count the number of times I have given presentations to professionals who immediately decide that the people they serve are simply not capable of speaking out for themselves or making chooses in their lives. We, as professionals must be open-minded and work from the assumptions that people with developmental disabilities want information, are capable of understanding information, and that it is our job to ensure their comprehension.
2. Include people with disabilities in developing the information that will be disseminated. If I am going to develop anything for people with disabilities, then I have to do it with the expertise of people with disabilities.
3. Communicate like a "real" person. Forget the professional jargon and big words. Sometimes I say that I have a dual personality. When in the professional arena I communicate accordingly, and when working with people with developmental disabilities it is also necessary that I make a shift in the way I speak and/or write.
4. Provide information in a variety of formats, including written and audio. Because of the diversity of people with developmental disabilities there is no set format for presenting information. Even if something is written in a very simple manner, this does not ensure that everyone will understand. When I prepare information I write simply and concretely. I also incorporate clip art or icons that are associated with the words. If needed, I provide the material on audio tape. When presenting information, be flexible.
5. No matter what format you use, support must be available to assist in "processing" the information. As previously stated, there is no way to present information that will be accessible to all people. There must be personal contact to explain, to problem solve, and to answer questions.

(Adapted from Chaikin, 1994, p. 12)

self-advocates, the recreation or therapeutic recreation professional demonstrates a commitment to the reciprocal relationship necessary within an interdependent environment.

Inclusive Communities

The goal of advocacy and self-advocacy is to ensure that undeserved or underrepresented persons or groups (in our case people with disabilities) receive fair, equitable, and appropriate treatment and services. As we have said and implied so many times throughout this book, people with disabilities have the same needs, hopes, desires, and feelings common to all people. They are entitled to the full benefits of citizenship, including all of its rights, privileges, opportunities, and responsibilities. People with disabilities must be able to live, learn, work, play, and retire in environments of their choice. They must be encouraged and supported to achieve their full potential, yet be afforded the dignity of risk. People with disabilities must be primary participants in all aspects of the planning, implementation, monitoring, and evaluation of services and supports. In addition, service and support systems for persons with disabilities and their families must do the following:

- provide safeguards to ensure freedom from harm, discrimination, and stigma;
- to be developed around the individual's and the family's strengths, capabilities, and choices and rely, whenever possible, on informal or natural supports;
- be provided in as normal an environment as possible;
- employ or develop specialized services only when those used by the general public cannot reasonably accommodate the needs and choices of the individual;
- be coordinated, enabling, affordable, efficient, accountable, fully accessible, and culturally sensitive and empower consumers and families as the primary decision makers; and
- be directed by and toward the enhancement of quality of life and the achievement of independence, contribution, and inclusion into the community.

Many people feel a deep commitment to creating inclusive communities that support the membership, both active and valued participation, and the learning of each child and adult within the community. Realizing this vision of inclusive community can be very hard work and can often involve significant conflict.

The words ***community***, ***conflict***, and ***inclusion*** would most likely be seen on a list of frequently used words in the current literature on change. Although some view these as simply buzz words reflecting fads that are not here to stay, we believe the meaning behind these words is substantial and the ideas are here to stay. So, what is this thing called community? Does the adjective ***inclusive*** add anything to the meaning of community or is it redundant? What is the relationship between conflict and community?

What is Community?

Some refer to any group of people in lose physical proximity as a community. However, living together in the same apartment building does not necessarily mean that sense of community exists. A place where people live or go to school can be a community, but it does not necessarily become one. So, what makes a group a true community of people?

Defining community is somewhat like defining friendships; it is easy to experience and feel yet difficult to truly capture the concept. Sheldon Berman (1990) offers the following definition:

> A *community* is a group of people who acknowledge their common purpose, respect their differences, share in group decision making as well as in responsibility for the actions of the group, and support each other's growth.

Drawing from Berman's definition, we see a number of basic elements in an effective community. The people comprising a community do the following:

1. **Acknowledge their connection and commonalties.** In a community there is recognition of individuals' relatedness and interdependence with one another. A sense of community includes a sense of *we* and a feeling of cooperation brought to life by the expressions "we sink or swim together," "together we are better," and "it takes everyone in the village to educate a child."
2. **Experience belonging.** Belonging is not *earned* but rather unconditionally given to anyone who wants to commit to being a part of that community. A sense of belonging is just as important as the tasks the community accomplishes.
3. **Respect differences.** Differences are valued and viewed as strengthening the community. Healthy communities strive to build upon people's differences instead of hiding or downplaying them.
4. **Develop relationships.** Members have personal connections and get to know one another as *people.* The heart of community is relationships! A sense of community cannot exist without people interacting and experiencing each other on a personal level. Take away the personal contact and you do not have a community but rather a group of people swimming laps together in a pool—physically close but not connecting anymore deeply.
5. **Share the responsibility for decision making.** Communities have norms and procedures for making decisions, handling conflicts, etc., whether implicitly or explicitly stated. There are shared responsibilities helping children and adults grow in a community, for decision making, for taking action, and for living with the process and outcomes of decisions.
6. **Have a common purpose or shared vision.** All these elements are necessary, but not sufficient, if the goal is to have a healthy, effective community that sustains and stays "alive" over time. With a shared vision, members perceive a common reason for being together, which strengthens the senses of we and commitment to the relationships and decisions within a community. With a shared vision may come increased group ownership for both celebrations and crises. The group acknowledges and celebrates individual and collective contributions and accomplishments. The group also works together to solve issues and concerns that confront the community.

In reviewing the characteristics of an effective community, it appears that communities as we have defined them are inclusive. The concept of an ***inclusive*** community has placed emphasis on the element of belonging. That is, children or adults whose needs are different in any way (e.g., different abilities, ethnic backgrounds, or social-economic status) should be supported as a valued member, active participant, and learner in typical environments or activities rather than viewed as different and needing to be served separately in specialized programs that only perpetuate differentness. In addition, people's differences should be respected and valued for the potential contributions to the entire community. Yet, contributions would not be realized or would simply go unnoticed if the person whose needs are different and the people who support them were served as if two communities existed in one. This type of service delivery would also have a negative impact and would discourage the other elements of an effective community, which include the following: 1) an acknowledgment of connections and commonalties; 2) the development of relationships; 3) shared decision making; and 4) a common purpose or goal. In other words, dissonance and conflict would be around the development and maintenance of inclusive communities.

Connections Between Community and Conflict

A conflict is a disagreement. There are a variety of responses that an individual or group chooses once a conflict occurs. An effective community certainly influences how conflict is viewed and handled. This can be true of conflicts within an individual, with another person, as well as within and between groups. The following section identifies specific ways that an effective (inclusive) community deals with conflict and leads to the resolution of challenging issues:

1. **Trust** is more likely to develop within a safe, supportive community. Trust leads to risk taking in conflicts. Efforts to build trust between and within groups will potentially have a positive impact on the community's ability to effectively resolve conflict.
2. **Acceptance and belonging** within a community means a person experiences belonging even when in conflict with other members of the community. Acceptance does not need to be earned based upon the outcomes of a conflict. In an inclusive community, there is more contributing to resolving conflict.
3. **Strong, valuing relationships** exist in a caring community and may often be helpful in resolving conflict. Increased commitment may result in helping to reach a satisfactory outcome for everyone (i.e., "win-win") and not just oneself (i.e., "I win—you lose") due to the importance placed upon maintaining valuing relationships.
4. **Communities built upon diversity** can create more opportunities for conflict since differences of opinion are more likely. Also, adding multiple perspectives, abilities, cultures, personalities, and ways to approach things can make the conflict more complex. However, what may have increased the likelihood for conflict also may improve the community's ability to resolve and creatively solve the conflict: diversity!
5. **A community's response to crisis** depends upon the strength of the community (as well as other variables such as the nature or frequency of conflict). Conflict can pull an already-fragile community completely apart. If conflict occurs in a

situation where people are already disconnected, conflict can be the catalyst that pushes people totally away or even at each other. People may "remove themselves" mentally, physically, or emotionally from the problems, having little commitment to resolution. Another response may be to point fingers of blame or lash out. If there is little or no community, conflicts are likely to escalate. However, crisis can bring a community together. People's growth, commitment, and sense of membership can be strengthened when they "rally together" to address a crisis.

6. **New growth and commitment** to the community can occur within conflicts. Through effectively resolving conflict, people can grow individually and in relationships with others. In dealing with conflict, new perspectives and feelings can be discovered.

Belonging appears to be an essential part of any discussion on creating caring, inclusive communities. Being in a community with others and experiencing belonging is the base from which a person can grow and thrive in a community; getting conflict out in the open and working together for solutions also appear to be important in healthy communities.

One of the best ways to help people with disabilities, especially severe disabilities to live life to the fullest and to fit into their communities,is through a process called "futures planning." Personal Futures Planning is a creative process designed to help people create a life of meaning and contribution (Mount & Zwernik, 1990). It asks people involved in the process to dream about possible futures and work backwards from that perspective to very specific manageable steps that lead to the envisioned future (Pearpoint, O'Brien & Forest, 1993). The process is not so future oriented that it forgets the here and now. The objective of planning is that people have good day-to-day experiences in the present. This type of planning also focuses on the capacities and gifts of individuals with disabilities rather than the more traditional planning process which often focuses on deficits. Traditional planning tends to restrict individuals to the goals of specific programs or the values and decisions of the professionals with whom they are involved. The personal futures planning process places the individual with the disability in the position to direct the action in his/her own life (Mount & Zwernik). In this way planning is closely linked to self-determination. Self-determination refers to the importance of people taking control of their lives and making the decisions that affect them. Both self-determination and personal futures planning support the value of individuals with disabilities making the decisions that affect their lives. Personal futures planning can help to build healthy individuals who are a part of caring inclusive communities.

Assistive Technology

Earlier in this book, we talked about the Tech Act and how technology assists people with disabilities in becoming more involved in the communities in which they live.

In addition to assistive technology, an enormous amount of information is already available as a result of advances in technology. In the future there will be increasing amounts of information available about various types of disability, advocacy, and services.

Many people with disabilities have functional limitations that heretofore made living in the community nearly impossible. This was a significant problem in the past but is less of one today. With the passage and subsequent reauthorization of the Technology Related Assistance Act (Tech Act) discussed in Chapter 4, each state has a Tech Act-funded project that is designed to build a national capacity to provide appropriate technology-related assistance—including devices, services, information, and expertise—to all people with disabilities.

Most simply stated, assistive technology increases independence and enables people with disabilities to enjoy learning, living, working, and playing more fully. Assistive technology is any device or piece of equipment that can be used by a person with a disability to become less dependent. Examples of assistive technology include the following:

- computers,
- seating systems,
- manual and power wheelchairs,
- communications devices,
- magnifiers,
- closed-circuit television,
- assistive listening devices,
- sit ski,
- beep balls,
- outrigger skis, and
- many, many more.

As you can see, assistive technology does not mean high cost, complex, technology items. Rather, assistive technology can include low technology and even homemade devices. What is important to remember is that many things are available or can be made to enhance the lives of people with disabilities. It is incumbent on you as a professional in recreation or therapeutic recreation to be aware of assistive technology. In many cases, what a person needs may not even exist, while in other cases it is readily available. As we have said so many times in this text, the person with a disability is probably the best person to determine the most appropriate assistive technology for himself. As a professional you must be aware of what is available or possible.

But how can you know? The Tech Act was passed to help you obtain this information. No one knows all there is to know about assistive technology. The Tech Act, however, supports a staff that is available to help answer questions about specific devices, programs, funding, advocacy, and the laws themselves that are in place regarding assistive technology.

Each state's assistive technology project has increased the following:

1. Awareness of the needs of individuals with disabilities for assistive technology devices and services;
2. Awareness of policies, practices, and procedures that facilitate or impede availability or provision of assistive technology services;
3. The availability of and funding for the provision of assistive technology devices and assistive technology services for people with disabilities;
4. Awareness and knowledge of the efficacy of assistive technology devices and assistive technology services among individual with disabilities, the families or representative of individuals with disabilities, individuals who work for public agencies and private entities that have contact with individuals with disabilities (including insurers), employers, and other appropriate individuals;
5. The capacity of public and private entities to provide technology-related assistance, particularly assistive technology devices and assistive technology services, and to pay for the provision of assistive technology devices and assistive technology services;
6. Coordination among state agencies and public and private entities that provide technology-related assistance, particularly assistive technology-related assistance, particularly assistive technology devices and assistive technology services; and
7. The probability that individuals of all ages with disabilities will, to the extent appropriate, be able to secure and maintain possession of assistive technology devices as such individuals make the transition between services offered by human service agencies or between settings of daily living (Curtin & Hayward, 1992).

States have considerable flexibility in determining how best to pursue the legislated objectives of the program. Some states may emphasize an explicit ***systems change*** approach that places a priority on removing policy and financial barriers and improving coordination among consumers, providers, and government agencies. Other states may opt for a service delivery approach, with the bulk of project resources used to purchase devices, to provide assessments, or otherwise to attempt to address immediate consumer needs for technology assistance, with the view that changes in the system will follow increased service capacity. Still other states may implement a project that incorporates both systems change and indrect service components (Curtin & Hayward, 1992).

Technology can help to empower people with disabilities. It can help many people to participate in recreation activities at levels that are more normative and less special and segregated. But, there is no device or piece of equipment that is good for every person who is deaf or for all people with mental retardation. Almost certainly, however, some technology can assist an individual whatever the disability.

The Past to the Present

In the past two decades, participation by individuals with disabilities in the activities of our nation has greatly enriched society as a whole. Yet, people with disability as a group still occupy an inferior status in our society, are severely disadvantaged socially, educationally, vocationally, and economically and are segregated and relegated to lesser services, programs, activities, benefits, and jobs.

The continuing existence of discrimination, attitudinal barriers, and prejudice has been shown to be directly related to the segregation and exclusion of individuals with disabilities from participation in activities in which individuals without disabilities typically engage.

Full inclusion of individuals with disabilities into all aspects of life and areas of society can only occur when supports, accommodations, and modifications necessary for such individuals are provided. As we conclude, let us take a look at where we have been in relation to services and programs for people with disabilities and where we need to head in order to implement and sustain person-centered, responsive services.

In the past, people with disabilities were seen as burdens to family, friends, and community and, therefore, were separated from them by institutionalization, supposedly for the families' sake and for their own. At that time, institutions, foster care, specialized adoption, and even family support (by special subsidies to the family) were seen as necessary and appropriate. Currently, a person with a disability is entitled to live with her family because the family is a better place for growth. Thus, the perspective moves from institutionalization to a recognition of the importance of family and natural supports.

In the past, people with disabilities were thought to be unable to learn or to earn. Currently, people with disabilities, while not always able to be economically productive, make contributions. The perspective has moved from people who are unable, to those who can be productive, to those who can contribute.

In the past, people with disabilities were seen as a group who would always be dependent on others and be segregated because the differences were so great; they were kept separate and apart. Then over time, they were seen as people who need not be segregated necessarily, but whose full integration or full inclusion was not warranted. Currently, people with disabilities are seen as people who can, with accommodations, be integrated and included in the lives and life activities of people without disabilities. Thus, the perspective moved from segregation, to integration, to inclusion.

In the past, people with disabilities were seen as people who necessarily were second-class citizens because of their disabilities and, therefore, were without status, rights, and roles similar to those without disabilities. Then over time, people with disabilities were viewed as people who have limited roles, such as living outside of institutions but in group homes or other protected and separate settings, or such as working in a sheltered workshop or playing in a specialized recreation program. Currently, people with disabilities are seen as people who can, with support, be employed in competitive settings and involved in regular recreation settings. Thus, the perspective moves from those who had second-class status to those of a somewhat less than second-class status but not yet full.

As a society we have wrestled with issues of dignity, rights, responsibility, and the like; we have begun to understand the deeply philosophical implications of the change of our language—from ***the disabled*** to "people first" terms, from a concept of ***independence*** to ***interdependence***, from ***productivity*** to ***contributions***, from ***integration*** to ***inclusion***. Are these changes in terminology our way of saying that there is something more to life than competing, that in fact cooperating, being ***of*** not just ***in*** the community, is itself a greater good?

Have we begun to justify integration and inclusion in schools and residential neighborhoods not only on the grounds that segregation is wrong but also on the ground that integration and inclusion themselves have values to people without disabilities, allowing them to display their concern, responsibility, and care for others, and to people with disabilities, allowing them to enrich the lives of other people?

Have we belatedly begun to think about the role of choices, consent, preferences, and self-determination because we ourselves know how important it is to our own self-fulfillment and self-esteem to be able to choose what we do, with whom, and when?

Almost any professional working in a service or helping profession would insist that the ultimate goal of his service/program is to encourage the persons with whom he is involved to become more independent and self-determining. The reality is, however, that far too often it is the recreation leader or the recreation therapist who is "in charge" and the participant/client who is being "helped" and controlled.

Conclusion

It is the proper goal of the nation to ensure inclusion of individuals with disabilities into all aspects of life and areas of civic responsibility.

Despite legislative action and advocacy supporting inclusion of individuals with disabilities, a number of factors continue to ***inhibit*** the full inclusion of individuals with disabilities:

1. The lack of universal access to assistive technology services and devices that can liberate individuals with disabilities from barrier encountered in everyday life and can enable them to move from spectator to participant in the home, the school, the workforce, and the community.
2. The lack of access to augmentative communication technology and other emerging telecommunication services and products that can significantly enhance the ability of all individuals to experience increased choice, communication, and control in there lives; to participate fully in their civic responsibilities; and to otherwise exercise their right to free expression.
3. Architectural and transportation barriers.
4. The lack of accessible housing and Community Supported Living Arrangements to insure that individuals with disabilities are able to live in and participate fully within the community.

5. The lack of personal assistance services as well as family support services.

We have come a long way, but as you can see from the list, many factors still inhibit the full inclusion of individuals with disabilities into the community in which they increasingly live. In closing, we want to share with you portions of a policy on full inclusion adopted on May 1, 1993, by the United Cerebral Palsy Association. If you and the agencies in which you work and the communities in which you live were to adopt policies similar to these, there would be no need for a textbook such as this that espoused person-centered, responsive recreation and therapeutic recreation services.

> United Cerebral Palsy Associations, Inc. and its affiliate organizations support the goal of full inclusion of individuals with disabilities into every aspect of life and area of society, including the home, the school, the workforce, and the community, regardless of severity of disability, as enumerated in the Americans with Disabilities Act. United Cerebral Palsy Associations, Inc. and its affiliate organizations pledge to invest our collective time and resources for a more inclusive society that recognizes and embraces the talents of all...(UCP, 1993).

Our challenge to you is to become advocates on behalf of people with disabilities in your work and your personal lives. The future of recreation and therapeutic services is in your hands. It is up to you to take what we have presented as a starting point as you help develop inclusive communities that promote person-centered, responsive recreation, and therapeutic services. We wish you the best in this endeavor!

Learning Activities

1. Identify advocacy and professional organizations at the local, state/provincial, and national levels that share similar interests with recreation and therapeutic recreation. Do not forget to include self-advocacy and disability support groups/organizations. Review their materials and/or attend a meeting to discover possible shared purposes and avenues for collaboration.
2. Devise a personal advocacy action plan. Select an issue that is of importance to you. Establish your goals, your plan of action, and your timeline for completion. Most importantly, follow through with your plan.
3. Think of the town in which you grew up. Based on our discussion of inclusive communities, would you describe your town (or even parts of your town) as an inclusive community? What made it an inclusive community or what would have make it a more inclusive community?
4. In the technology section we discussed technology, especially electronic communication. Dream a little; let the sky be the limit. As you look into the future of technology, what technological advances or implications do you see that will have an impact on the lives of people with disabilities?

References

Berman, S. (1990). Editing for social responsibility. *Educational Leadership, 48*, 3, pp. 75-80.

Bradley, V.J., Ashbaugh, J.W., & Blaney, B.C. (Eds.). (1994). *Creating individual supports for people with disabilities. A mandate for change at many levels.* Baltimore, MD: Paul H. Brooks, Publishing Co.

Chaikin, M. (1994). Guidelines for providing information to self-advocates. *Impact,* 7 (1), 12.

Charlton, J. I. (1998). *Nothing about us without us.* Berekely, CA: University of California Press.

Condeluci, (1991). *Interdependence:The road to community.*Winter Park, FL: GR Press, Inc.

Curtin, T.R., & Hayward, B.J., (1992). *National evaluation of state grants for technology-related assistance for individuals with disabilities programs: Final report.* Research Triangle Park, NC: Research Triangle Institute.

Curtis, E., (1998). It's my life: Reference-based planning for self-directed goals. In M. L. Wehmeyer and Deanna J. Sands, *Making it Happen: Student involvement in education planning, decision making, and instruction.* Baltimore, MD: Paul H. Brooks Publishing Company, Inc.

Ebel, M.L. (1994).The barriers I face in my environment. *Impact,* 7 (1), 5.

Hayden, M.F. (1994). When the student is ready, the teacher enters, *Impact* 7 (1), 10.

Hutchison, P., & McGill, J. (1992). *Leisure, integration, and community.* Concord, Ontario: Leisureability Publications, Inc.

Kaufman-Broida, J., & Wenzel, K. (1994). Shaping our future through advocacy. *Parks and Recreation,* 29 (4), 72-77.

Martin, J. E., (1998). Choice Maker: Choosing, planning, and taking action. In M. L. Wehmeyer and Deanna J. Sands, *Making it Happen: Student involvement in education planning, decision making, and instruction.* Baltimore, MD: Paul H, Brooks Publishing Company, Inc.

Mount, B., & Zwernik, K. (1990). *Making futures happen. A manual for facilitators of personal futures planning.* St. Paul, MN: Metropolitan Council.

Nelis, T. (1994). Self-advocacy: Realizing a dream. *Impact,* 7 (1), 1.

Pearpoint, J., O'Brien, J., & Forest, M. (1993). *Planning alternative tomorrows with hope: A workbook for planning better futures.* Chicago: Inclusion Press.

Roberts-DeGennaro, M. (196). Building coalitions for politically advocacy. *Social Work,* July-August, 308-311.

Rupp, W. (1994). Citizens in action: Self-advocacy and systems change. *Impact* 7 (1), 4.

Schroeder, T. (1993). Confessions of an advocate. *Parks and Recreation,* 28 (10), 69-73.

Shank, J.W. (1997). Engaging the legislative process: Legislative and regulatory imperatives for therapeutic recreation. In D.M. Compton (Ed.), *Issues in therapeutic recreation*:Toward the new millennium (pp. 77-102). Champaign, IL: Sagamore Publishing.

Shapiro, J.P. (1993). *No Pity: People with disabilities forging a new civil rights movement*. New York, NY: Times Books

Sylvester, C. (1995). Critical theory, therapeutic recreation, and health care reform: An interactive example of critical thinking. *Annual in Therapeutic Recreation*, 5, 94-109.

The ARC Today. (1995, Spring). Vol. 44, No. 1, p. 12.

Van Reussen, A. K., (1998). Self-advocacy strategy instruction: Enhancing student motivation, self-determination, and responsibiity in the learning process.. In M. L. Wehmeyer and Deanna J. Sands, *Making it Happen: Student involvement in education planning, decision making, and instruction*. Baltimore, MD: Paul H, Brooks Publishing Company, Inc.

Ward, N. A., & Keith K. D. (1996). Self-advocacy: Foundations for quality of life. In R.I. Schalock (ed.), *Quality of Life: Volume 1.* Washington D. C.: American Association on Mental Retardation

Wehmeyer, M. L. , (1998). Whose future is it anyway? A student directed transition planning program. In M. L. Wehmeyer and Deanna J. Sands, *Making it Happen: Student involvement in education planning, decision-making, and instruction.* Baltimore, MD: Paul H, Brooks Publishing Company, Inc.

Wehmeyer, M. L., Agran, M. & Hughes, C., (1998). *Teaching self-determination to students with disabilities: Basic skills for successful transition.* Baltimore, MD: Paul H, Brooks Publishing Company, Inc

Yom, S. (1998). Disabilities: Looking back and looking ahead. *JAMA, The Journal of the American Medical Association*, Vol. 279, No. 1, p. 78.

Related Websites

http://www.esmerel.org/adapt/
(Esmerel's List of Adaptive Technology Resources)

http://www.mdri.org/
(Mental Disability Rights International)

http://www.osalink.com/freepress/research/selfadvo.htm
(Introduction to Self-Advocacy)

http://www.advocacyinc.org/arweb.htm
(Annual Report 1997— Advocacy Incorporated's Web Site)

http://www.c-c-d.org/
(Consortium for Citizens with Disabilities Home Page)

http://www.protectionandadvocacy.com/
(Protection and Advocacy)

http://www.teleport.com/~abarhydt/
(The Disability Rights Activist)

http://inclusion.org/
(The Inclustion Network)

Appendix A

The Americans With Disabilities Act Checklist For Readily Achievable Barrier Removal

Checklist for Existing Facilities

Title III of the Americans with Disabilities Act requires public accommodations to provide goods and services to people with disabilities on an equal basis with the rest of the general public. The goals are to afford every individual the opportunity to benefit from our country's businesses and services and to afford our businesses and services the opportunity to benefit from the patronage of all Americans.

By January 26, 1992, architectural and communication barriers must be removed in public areas of existing facilities when their removal is readily achievable—in other words, easily accomplished and able to be carried out without much difficulty or expense. Public accommodations that must meet the barrier removal requirement include a broad range of establishments (both for-profit and nonprofit)—such as hotels, restaurants, theaters, museums, retail stores, private schools, banks, doctors' offices, and other places that serve the public. People who own, lease, lease out, or operate places of public accommodation in existing buildings are responsible for complying with the barrier removal requirement.

The removal of barriers can often be achieved by making simple changes to the physical environment. However, the regulations do not define exactly how much effort and expense are required for a facility to meet its obligation. This judgment must be made on a case-by-case basis, taking into consideration such factors as the size, type, and overall financial resources of the facility and the nature and cost of the access improvements needed. These factors are described in more detail in the ADA regulations issued by the Department of Justice.

The process of determining what changes are readily achievable is not a one-time effort; access should be reevaluated annually. Barrier removal that might be difficult to carry out now may be readily achievable later. Tax incentives are available to help absorb costs over several years.

Purpose of this Checklist

This checklist will help you to identify accessibility problems and solutions in existing facilities in order to meet your obligations under the ADA.

The goal of the survey process is to plan how to make an existing facility more usable for people with disabilities. The Department of Justice recommends the development of an Implementation Plan, specifying what improvements you will make to remove barriers an when each solution will be carried out: "...Such a plan...could serve as evidence of a good faith effort to comply..."

Technical Requirements

The checklist details some of the requirements found in the ADA Accessibility Guidelines (ADAAG). However, keep in mind that full compliance with ADAAG is required only for new construction and alterations. The requirements presented here are to serve as a guide to help you to determine what may be readily achievable barrier removal for existing facilities. Wherever possible, the ADAAG should be used in making readily achievable modifications. If complying with ADAAG is not readily achievable, you may undertake a modification that does not fully comply with ADAAG using less stringent standards, as long as it poses no health or safety risk.

Each state has its own regulations regarding accessibility. To ensure compliance with all codes, know your state and local codes and use the more stringent technical requirement for every modification you make; that is, the requirement that provides greater access for individuals with disabilities. The barrier removal requirement for existing facilities is new under the ADA and supersedes less stringent local or state codes.

What this Checklist is Not

This checklist does not cover all of ADAAG's requirements; therefore it is not for facilities undergoing new construction or alterations. In addition, it does not attempt to illustrate all possible barriers or propose all possible barrier removal solutions. ADAAG should be consulted for guidance in situations not covered here.

The checklist does not cover Title III's requirements for nondiscriminatory policies and practices and for the provision of auxiliary communication aids and services. The communication features covered are those that are structural in nature.

Priorities

This checklist is based on the four priorities recommended by the Title III regulations for planning readily achievable barrier removal projects.

Priority 1: Accessible entrance into the facility.
Priority 2: Access to goods and services.
Priority 3: Access to rest rooms.
Priority 4: Any other measures necessary.

How to Use this Checklist

√ **Get Organized:** Establish a time frame for completing the survey. Determine how many copies of the checklist you will need to survey the whole facility. Decide who will conduct the survey. It is strongly recommended that you invite two or three additional people, including people with various disabilities and accessibility expertise, to assist in identifying barriers, developing solutions for removing these barriers, and setting priorities for implementing improvements.

√ **Obtain Floor Plans**: It is very helpful to have the building floor plans with you while you survey. If plans are not available, use graph paper to sketch the layout of all interior and exterior spaces used by your organization. Make notes on the sketch or plan while you are surveying.

√ **Conduct the Survey**: Bring copies of this checklist, a clipboard, a pencil or pen, and a flexible steel tape measure. With three people surveying, one person numbers key items on the floor plan to match with the field notes, taken by a second person, while the third takes measurements. Think about each space from the perspective of people with physical, hearing, visual, and cognitive disabilities, noting areas that need improvement.

√ **Summarize Barriers and Solutions**: List barriers found and ideas for their removal. Consider the solutions listed beside each question and add your own ideas. Consult with building contractors and equipment suppliers to estimate the costs for making the proposed modifications.

√ **Make Decisions and Set Priorities**: Review the summary with decision makers and advisors. Decide which solutions will best eliminate barriers at a reasonable cost. Prioritize the items you decide upon and make a timeline for carrying them out. Where the removal of barriers is not readily achievable, you must consider whether alternative methods exist for providing access that is readily achievable.

√ **Maintain Documentation**: Keep your survey, notes, summary, record of work completed, and plans for alternative methods on file.

√ **Make Changes**: Implement changes as planned. Always refer directly to ADAAG and your state and local codes for complete technical requirements before making an access improvement. References to the applicable sections of ADAAG are listed at the beginning of each group of questions. If you need help understanding the federal, state, or local requirements, contact your Disability and Business Technical Assistance Center.

√ **Follow Up**: Review your Implementation Plan each year to reevaluate whether more improvements have become readily achievable.

> To obtain a copy of the ADAAG or other information from the U.S. Department of Justice, call (202) 514-0301 Voice, (202) 514-0381 TDD, (202) 514-0383 TDD. For technical questions, contact the Architectural and Transportation Barriers Compliance Board at (800) USA-ABLE.

Priority 1: Accessible Entrance

People with disabilities should be able to arrive on the site, approach the building, and enter the building as freely as everyone else. At least one path of travel should be safe and accessible for everyone, including people with disabilities.

Path of Travel
(ADAAG 4.3, 4.4, 4.5, 4.7)

Question

Is there a path of travel that does not require the use of stairs?

☐ Yes ☐ No

Possible solutions

☐ Add a ramp if the path of travel is interrupted by stairs.
☐ Add an alternative pathway on level ground.

Question

Is the path of travel stable, firm, and slip-resistant?

☐ Yes ☐ No

Possible solutions

☐ Repair uneven paving.
☐ Fill small bumps and breaks with beveled patches.
☐ Replace gravel with hard top.

Question

Is the path at least 36-inches wide?

☐ Yes ☐ No

Possible solutions

☐ Change or move landscaping, furnishings, or other features that narrow the path of travel.
☐ Widen pathway.

Question

Can all objects protruding into the path be detected by a person with a visual disability using a cane?

In order to be detected using a cane, an object must be within 27 inches of the ground. Objects hanging or mounted overhead must be higher than 80 inches to provide clear headroom. It is not necessary to remove objects that protrude less than 4 inches from the wall.

☐ Yes ☐ No

Possible Solutions

☐ Move or remove protruding objects.
☐ Add a cane-detected base that extends to the ground.
☐ Place a cane-detected object on the ground underneath as a warning barrier.

Question

Do curbs on the pathway have curb cuts drives, parking, and drop-offs?

☐ Yes ☐ No

Possible Solutions

☐ Install curb out.
☐ Add a small ramp up to curb.

Ramps
(ADAAG 4.8)

Question

Are the slopes of ramps no greater than 1:12?

Slope is given as a ratio of the height to the length. 1:12 means for every 12 inches along the base of the ramp, the height increase one inch. For a 1:12 maximum slope, at least one foot of ramp length is need for each inch of height.

☐ Yes ☐ No

Possible Solutions

☐ Lengthen ramp to decrease slope.
☐ Relocate ramp.
☐ If available space is limited, reconfigure ramp to include switch backs.

Question

Do all ramps longer than 6 feet have railings on both sides?

☐ Yes ☐ No

Possible solution

☐ Add railings

Question

Are railings sturdy and between 34 -and 38-inches high?

☐ Yes ☐ No

Possible Solutions

☐ Adjust height of railings

☐ Secure handrails.

Question

Is the width between railings at least 36 inches?

☐ Yes ☐ No

Possible Solutions

☐ Relocate with railings.

☐ Widen the ramp.

Question

Are ramps nonslip?

☐ Yes ☐ No

Possible Solution

☐ Add nonslip surface material.

Question

Is there a 5-foot long level landing at every 30-foot horizontal length of ramp, at the top and bottom of ramps, and at switchbacks?

The ramp should rise no more than 30 inches between landings.

☐ Yes ☐ No

Possible Solution

☐ Remodel or relocate ramp.

Parking and Drop-off Areas (ADAAG 4.6)

Question

Are an adequate number of accessible parking spaces available (8-feet wide for car plus 5-foot striped access aisle)? For guidance in determining the appropriate number to designate, the table below gives the ADAAG requirements for new construction and alterations (for lots with more than 100 spaces, refer to ADAAG):

Total Spaces	Accessible
1 to 25	1 space
26-50	2 spaces
51-75	3 spaces
76-100	4 spaces

☐ Yes ☐ No

Possible Solution

☐ Reconfigure a reasonable number of spaces by repainting stripes.

Question

Are 16-foot wide spaces, with 98 inches of vertical clearance, available for lift-equipped vans?

At least one of every 8 accessible spaces must be van-accessible spaces.

☐ Yes ☐ No

Possible Solution

☐ Reconfigure to provide a reasonable number of van-accessible spaces.

Question

Are the accessible spaces closest to the accessible entrance?

☐ Yes ☐ No

Possible Solution

☐ Reconfigure spaces.

Question

Are accessible spaces marked with the International Symbol of Accessibility?

Are there signs reading "VanAccessible" at van spaces?

International Symbol of Accessibility: ♿

☐ Yes ☐ No

Possible Solution

☐ Add signs, placed so that they are not obstructed by cars.

Question

Is there an enforcement procedure to ensure that accessible parking is used only by those who need it?

☐ Yes ☐ No

Possible Solution

☐ Implement a policy to check periodically for violators and report them to them proper authorities.

Entrance (ADAAG 4.13, 4.14)

Question

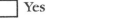

If there are stairs at the main entrance, is there also a ramp or lift, or is there an alternative accessible entrance? Do not use a service entrance as the accessible entrance unless there is no other option.

☐ Yes ☐ No

Possible Solutions

☐ If it is not possible to make the main entrance accessible, create a dignified alternate accessible entrance. Make sure there is accessible parking near accessible entrances.

Question

Do all inaccessible entrances have signs indicating the location of the nearest accessible entrance?

☐ Yes ☐ No

Possible Solution

☐ Install signs at or before inaccessible entrances.

Question

Can the alternate accessible entrance be used independently?

☐ Yes ☐ No

Possible Solution

☐ Eliminate as much as possible the need for assistance—to answer a doorbell, to operate a lift, or to put down a temporary ramp, for example.

Question

Does the entrance door have at least 32 inches clear opening (for a double door, at least one 32-inch leaf)?

☐ Yes ☐ No

Possible Solutions

☐ Widen the door.

☐ Install offset (swing-clear) hinges.

Question

Is there at least 18 inches of clear wall space on the pull side of the door, next to the handle?

A person using a wheelchair needs this space to get close enough to open the door.

☐ Yes ☐ No

Possible Solutions

☐ Remove or relocate furnishings, partitions, and obstructions.

☐ Move door.

☐ Add power-assisted door opener.

Question

Is the threshold level (less than 1/4 inch) or beveled, up to 1/2 inch high?

☐ Yes ☐ No

Possible Solutions

☐ If there is a single step with a rise of 6 inches or less, add a short ramp.

☐ If there is a high threshold, remove it or add a bevel.

Question

Are doormats 1/2 inch-high or less and secured to the floor at all edges?

☐ Yes ☐ No

Possible Solutions

☐ Replace or remove mats.
☐ Secure mats at edges.

Question

Is the door handle no higher than 48 inches and operatable with a closed fist?

The "closed fist" tests for handles and controls; try opening the door or operating the control using only one hand, held in a fist. If you can do it, so can a person who has limited use of his or her hands.

☐ Yes ☐ No

Possible Solutions

☐ Replace inaccessible knob with a lever or loop handle.
☐ Retrofit with an add-on lever extension.

Question

Can doors be opened without too much force (maximum of 5 dbf)? You can use a fish scale to measure the force required to open a door. Attach the hook of the scale to the doorknob or handle. Pull on the ring end of the scale until the door opens and read off the amount of force required. If you do not have a fish scale, you will need to judge subjectively whether the door is easy enough to open.

☐ Yes ☐ No

Possible Solutions

☐ Adjust the door closers and oil the hinges.
☐ Install power-asserted door openers.
☐ Install lighter doors.

Question

If the door has a closer, does it take at least 3 seconds to close?

☐ Yes ☐ No

Possible Solution

☐ Adjust the door closer.

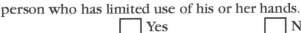

Emergency Egress
(ADAAG 4.13, [14], 4.28)

Question

Do all alarms have both flashing lights and audible signals?

☐ Yes ☐ No

Possible Solution

☐ Install visible and audible alarms.

Question

Is there sufficient lighting in egress pathways such as stairs, corridors, and exits?

☐ Yes ☐ No

Possible Solution

☐ Upgrade, add, or clean bulbs or fixtures.

Priority 2: Access to Goods and Services

Ideally, the layout of the building should allow people with disabilities to obtain goods or services without special assistance. Where it is not possible to provide full accessibility, assistance or alternative services should be available upon request.

Horizontal Circulation (ADAAG 4.3)

Question

Does the accessible entrance provide direct access to the main floor, lobby, or elevator?

☐ Yes ☐ No

Possible Solution

☐ Add ramps or lifts.
☐ Make another entrance accessible.

Question

Are all public spaces on an accessible path of travel?

☐ Yes ☐ No

Possible Solution

☐ Provide access to all public spaces along an accessible path of travel.

Question

Is the accessible route to all public spaces at least 36-inches wide?

☐ Yes ☐ No

Possible Solution

☐ Move furnishings such as tables, chairs, display racks, vending machines, and counters to make more room.

Question

Is there a 5-foot circle or a T-shaped space for a person using a wheelchair to reverse direction?

☐ Yes ☐ No

Possible Solution

☐ Rearrange furnishings, displays, and equipment.

Doors
(ADAAG 4.13)

Question

Do doors into public spaces have at least a 32-inch clear opening?

☐ Yes ☐ No

Possible Solutions

☐ Install offset (swing-clear hinges).

☐ Widen doors.

Question

On the pull side of doors, next to the handle, is there at least 18 inches of clear wall space so that a person using a wheelchair can get near to open the door?

☐ Yes ☐ No

Possible Solutions

☐ Reverse the door swing if it is safe to do so.

☐ Move or remove obstructing partitions.

Question

Can doors be opened without too much force (5 dbf maximum)?

☐ Yes ☐ No

Possible Solutions

☐ Adjust or replace closers.

☐ Install lighter doors.

☐ Install power-assisted door openers.

Question

Are door handles 48 inches high or less and operable with a closed fist?

☐ Yes ☐ No

Possible Solutions

☐ Lower handles.
☐ Replace inaccessible knobs or latches with lever or loop handles.
☐ Retrofit with add-on lever extensions.
☐ Install power-assisted door openers.

Question

Are all thresholds level (less than 1/4 inch), or beveled, up to 1/2 inch high?

☐ Yes ☐ No

Possible Solutions

☐ Remove thresholds.
☐ Add bevels to both sides.

Rooms and Spaces (ADAAG 4.2, 4.4, 4.5, 4.30)

Question

Are all aisles and pathways to all goods and services at least 36-inches wide?

☐ Yes ☐ No

Possible Solution

☐ Rearrange furnishings and fixtures to clear aisles.

Question

Is there a 5-foot circle or T-shaped space for turning a wheelchair completely?

☐ Yes ☐ No

Possible Solution

☐ Rearrange furnishings to clear more room.

Question

Is carpeting low-pile, tightly woven, and securely attached along edges?

☐ Yes ☐ No

Possible Solutions

☐ Secure edges on all sides.
☐ Replace carpeting.

Question

In routes through public areas, are all obstacles cane-detectable (located within 27 inches of the door or protruding less than 4 inches from the wall), or are they higher than 80 inches?

☐ Yes ☐ No

Possible Solutions

☐ Remove obstacles.
☐ Install furnishings, planters, or other cane-detectable barriers underneath the obstacle.

Question

Do signs designating permanent room and spaces, such as rest room signs, exit signs, and room numbers, comply with the appropriate requirements for accessible signage?

☐ Yes ☐ No

Possible Solution

☐ Provide signage that has raised and Brailled letters, complies with finish and contrast standards, and is mounted at the correct height and location.

Controls
(ADDAAG 4.27)

Question

Are all controls that are available for use by the public (including electrical, mechanical, window, cabinet, game, and self-service controls) located at an accessible height?

Reach ranges: The maximum height for a side reach is 54 inches; for a forward reach, 48 inches. The minimum reachable height is 15 inches.

☐ Yes ☐ No

Possible Solution

☐ Relocate controls.

Question

Are they operable with a closed fist?

☐ Yes ☐ No

Possible Solution

☐ Relocate controls.

Seats, Tables, and Counters
(ADAAG 4.2, 4.32)

Question

Are the aisles between chairs or tables at least 36-inches wide?

☐ Yes ☐ No

Possible Solution

☐ Rearrange chairs or tables to provide 36-inch aisles.

Question

Are the spaces for wheelchair seating distributed throughout?

☐ Yes ☐ No

Possible Solutions

☐ Rearrange tables to allow room for wheelchairs in seating areas throughout the area.

☐ Remove some fixed seating.

Question

Are the tops of tables or counters between 28- and 34-inches high?

☐ Yes ☐ No

Possible Solution

☐ Lower at least a section of high tables and counters.

Question

Are knee spaces at accessible tables at least 27-inches high, 30-inches wide, and 19-inches deep?

☐ Yes ☐ No

Possible Solution

☐ Replace or raise tables.

Vertical Circulation (ADAAG 4.3)

Question

Are there ramps or elevators to all levels?

☐ Yes ☐ No

Possible Solutions

☐ Install ramp or lifts.
☐ Modify a service elevator.
☐ Relocate goods or services to an accessible area.

Question

On each level, if there are stairs between the entrance and/or elevator and essential public areas, is there an accessible alternate route?

☐ Yes ☐ No

Possible Solution

☐ Post clear signs directing people along an accessible route to ramps, lifts, or elevators.

Stairs (ADAAG 4.9)

Question

Do treads have a nonslip surface?

☐ Yes ☐ No

Possible Solution

☐ Add nonslip surface to treads.

Question

Do stairs have continuous rails on both sides, with extensions beyond the top and bottom stairs?

☐ Yes ☐ No

Possible Solution

☐ Add or replace handrails.

Elevators
(ADAAG 4.10)

Question

Are there both visible and verbal or audible door opening/closing and floor indicators (one tone = up, two tones = down)?

☐ Yes ☐ No

Possible Solution

☐ Install visible and verbal or audible signals.

Question

Are the call buttons in the hallway no higher than 42 inches?

☐ Yes ☐ No

Possible Solutions

☐ Lower call buttons.
☐ Provide a permanently attached reach stick.

Question

Do the controls outside and inside the cab have raised and Braille lettering?

☐ Yes ☐ No

Possible Solution

☐ Install raised lettering and Braille next to the buttons.

Question

Is there a sign on the jamb at each floor identifying the floor in raised and Braille letters?

☐ Yes ☐ No

Possible Solution

☐ Install tactile signs to identify floor numbers, at a height of 60 inches from the door.

Question

Is the emergency intercom usable without voice communication?

☐ Yes ☐ No

Possible Solution

☐ Replace communication system.

Question

Are there Braille and raised-letter instructions for the communication system?

☐ Yes ☐ No

Possible Solution

☐ Add simple tactile instructions.

Lifts
(ADAAG 4.2, 4.11)

Question

Can the lift be used without assistance? If not, is a call button provided?

☐ Yes ☐ No

Possible Solutions

☐ At each stopping level, post clear instructions for use of the lift.

☐ Provide a call button.

Question

Is there at least 30 by 48 inches of clear space for a person using a wheelchair to approach to reach the controls and use the lift?

☐ Yes ☐ No

Possible Solution

☐ Rearrange furnishings and equipment to clear more space.

Question

Are controls between 15- and 48-inches high (up to 54 inches if a side approach is possible)?

☐ Yes ☐ No

Possible Solution

☐ Move controls.

Priority 3:
Usability of Rest Rooms

When rest rooms are open to the public, they should be accessible to people with disabilities. Closing a rest room that is currently open to the public is not an allowable option.

Getting to the Rest Rooms
(ADAAG 4.1)

Question

If rest rooms are available to the public, is at least one rest room (either one for each sex or unisex) fully accessible?

☐ Yes ☐ No

Possible Solution

☐ Reconfigure rest room.
☐ Combine rest room to create one unisex accessible rest room.

Question

Are there signs at inaccessible rest rooms that give directions to accessible ones?

☐ Yes ☐ No

Possible Solution

☐ Install accessible signs.

Doorways and Passages
(ADAAG 4.2, 4.13)

Question

Is there tactile signage identifying rest rooms?

Mount signs on the wall, on the latch side of the door.Avoid using ambiguous symbols in place of text to identify rest rooms.

☐ Yes ☐ No

Possible Solutions

☐ Add accessible signage,placed to the side of the door (not on the door itself).
☐ If symbols are used, add supplementary verbal signage.

Question

Is the doorway at least 32-inches clear?

☐ Yes ☐ No

Possible Solutions

☐ Install offset (swing-clear) hinges.
☐ Widen the doorway.

Question

Are doors equipped with accessible handles (operable with a closed fist), 48 inches-high or less?

☐ Yes ☐ No

Possible Solutions

☐ Lower handles.
☐ Replace inaccessible knobs or latches with lever or loop handles.
☐ Retrofit with add-on lever extensions.
☐ Install power-assisted door openers.

Question

Can doors be opened easily (5 lbf maximum force)?

☐ Yes ☐ No

Possible Solutions

☐ Adjust or replace closers.
☐ Install lighter doors.
☐ Install power-assisted door openers.

Question

Does the entry configuration provide adequate maneuvering space for a person using a wheelchair?

A person using a wheelchair needs 36 inches of clear width for forward movement and a 5-foot diameter clear space or a T-shaped space to make turns. A minimum distance of 48 inches, clear of the door swing, is needed between the two doors of an entry vestibule.

☐ Yes ☐ No

Possible Solution

☐ Rearrange furnishings such as chairs and trash cans.
☐ Remove inner door if there is a vestibule with two doors.
☐ Move or remove obstructing partitions.

Question

Is there a 36-inch wide path to all fixtures?

☐ Yes ☐ No

Possible Solutions

☐ Remove obstructions.

Stalls
(ADAAG 4.17)

Question

Is the stall door operable with a closed fist, inside and out?

☐ Yes ☐ No

Possible Solutions

☐ Replace inaccessible knobs or labels with lever or loop handles.
☐ Retrofit with add-on lever extensions.

Question

Is there a wheelchair-accessible stall that has an area of at least 5 feet by 5 feet, clear of the door swing, OR is there a stall that is less accessible but that provides greater access than a typical stall (either 36 by 69 inches or 48 by 69 inches)?

☐ Yes ☐ No

Possible Solutions

☐ Move or remove partitions.
☐ Reverse the door swing if it is safe to do so.

Question

In the accessible stall, are there grab bars behind and on the side wall nearest to the toilet?

☐ Yes ☐ No

Possible Solutions

☐ Add grab bars.

Question

Is the toilet seat 17 to 19 inches high?

☐ Yes ☐ No

Possible Solution

☐ Add raised seat.

Lavatories
(ADAAG 4.19, 4.24)

Question

Does one lavatory have a 36-inch wide by 48-inch deep clear space in front? A maximum of 19 inches of the required depth may be under the lavatory.

☐ Yes ☐ No

Possible Solutions

☐ Rearrange furnishings.
☐ Replace lavatory.
☐ Remove or alter cabinetry to provide space underneath. Make sure hot pipes are insulated.
☐ Move a partition or wall.

Question

Is the lavatory rim no higher than 34 inches?

☐ Yes ☐ No

Possible Solution

☐ Adjust or replace lavatory.

Question

Are there at least 29 inches from the floor to the bottom of the lavatory apron (excluding pipes)?

☐ Yes ☐ No

Possible Solution

☐ Adjust or replace lavatory.

Question

Can the faucet be operated with one closed fist?

☐ Yes ☐ No

Possible Solution

☐ Replace faucet handles with paddle type.

Question

Are soap and other dispensers and hand dryers 48-inches high or less and usable with one closed fist?

☐ Yes ☐ No

Possible Solutions

☐ Lower dispensers.

☐ Replace with or provide additional accessible dispensers.

Question

Is the mirror mounted on the bottom edge of the reflecting surface 40-inches high or lower?

☐ Yes ☐ No

Possible Solutions

☐ Lower or tilt down mirror.

☐ Replace with larger mirror.

Priority 4: Additional Access

When amenities such as public telephones and drinking fountains are provided to the general public, they should also be accessible to people with disabilities.

Drinking Fountains
(ADAAG 4.15)

Question

Is there at least one fountain with clear floor space of at least 30 by 48 inches in front?

☐ Yes ☐ No

Possible Solution

☐ Clear more room by rearranging or removing furnishings.

Question

Is there one fountain with its spout no higher than 36 inches from the ground, and another with a standard height spout (or a single "hi-lo" fountain)?

☐ Yes ☐ No

Possible Solutions

☐ Provide cup dispensers for fountains with spouts that are too high.

☐ Provide an accessible water cooler.

Question

Are controls mounted on the front or on side near the front edge and operable with one closed fist?

☐ Yes ☐ No

Possible Solution

☐ Replace the controls.

Question

Does the fountain protrude no more than 4 inches into the circulation space?

☐ Yes ☐ No

Possible Solution

☐ Place a planter or other cane-detectable barrier on each side at floor level.

Telephones
(ADAAG 4.30, 4.31)

Question

If pay or public use phones are provided, is there clear floor space of at least 30 by 48 inches in front of at least one?

☐ Yes ☐ No

Possible Solutions

☐ Move furnishings.

☐ Replace booth in open station.

Question

Is the highest operable part of the phone no higher than 48 inches (up to 54 inches if a side approach is possible)?

☐ Yes ☐ No

Possible Solution

☐ Lower the telephone.

Question

Does the phone protrude no more than 4 inches into the circulation space?

☐ Yes ☐ No

Possible Solution

☐ Place a cane-detectable barrier on each side at floor level.

Question

Does the phone have push-button controls?

☐ Yes ☐ No

Possible Solution

☐ Contact phone company to install push-buttons.

Question

Is the phone hearing aid compatible?

☐ Yes ☐ No

Possible Solution

☐ Contact phone company to add an induction coil (T-switch).

Question

Is the phone adapted with volume control?

☐ Yes ☐ No

Possible Solution

☐ Contact phone company to add volume control.

Question

Is the phone with volume control identified with appropriate signage?

☐ Yes ☐ No

Possible Solution

☐ Add signage.

Question

Is one of the phones equipped with a text telephone (TT or TDD)?

☐ Yes ☐ No

Possible Solutions

☐ Install a text telephone.

☐ Have a portable text telephone available.

Question

Is the location of the text telephone identified by accessible signage bearing the International TDD Symbol?

International TDD Symbol:

☐ Yes ☐ No

Possible Solution

☐ Add signage.

Additional Information

To obtain additional copies of this checklist for existing facilities, contact our Disability and Business Technical Assistance Center. To find out the name and number of your regional center, call 1-800-949-4ADA or refer to Fact Sheet 6. This checklist may be copied as many times as desired by the Disability and Business Technical Assistance Centers for distribution to small businesses but may not be reproduced in whole or in part and sold by any other entity without written permission of the authors.

Barrier Free Environments, Inc. and Adaptive Environments Center, Inc. are authorized by the National Institute on Disability and Rehabilitation Research (NIDRR) to develop information and materials on the Americans with Disabilities Act (ADA). However, you should be aware that NIDRR is not responsible for enforcement of the ADA. The information presented here is intended solely as informal guidance and is neither a determination of your legal rights or responsibilities under the act nor binding on any agency with enforcement responsibility under the ADA.

Americans with Disabilities Act: A Selected Bibliography

The materials listed below may be borrowed from the Library at the Institute for the Study of Developmental Disabilities, 2853 E. Tenth St., Bloomington, IN 47405, (Voice) (812) 855-9396. The library has additional ADA resources available upon your request.

The ADA maze: What YOU can do. (videorecording). (1991). West Des Moines, IA: American Media, Inc.

Allen, J.G. (1993). *Complying with the ADA: A small business guide to hiring and employing the disabled.* New York: John Wiley.

The Americans with Disabilities Act. [videorecording]. (1991). Oak Forest, IL: Foundation for Exceptional Children.

The Americans with Disabilities Act. [videorecording]. (1992). Urbana, IL: Reed Martin.

The Americans with Disabilities Act: An overview. (1992). Indianapolis: Very Special Arts Indiana.

Americans with Disabilities Act handbook. (1991). Washington, D.C.: Equal Employment Opportunities Commission.

The ADA: Questions and answers.

Americans with Disabilities Act: Reed Martin. Legal Challenges in Special Education series [videorecording]. (1992) Urbana, IL: Carle Media.

Americans with Disabilities Act: transportation for individuals with disabilities—Department of Transportation final regulations (1992?). Indianapolis: Governor's Planning Council for People with Disabilities.

...And justice for all: A celebration of the Americans with Disabilities Act. [videorecording]. (1991). Dunbar, WV: West Virginia Research and Training Center.

The basics of the Americans with Disabilities Act. [videorecording]. (1992). Colorado Springs, CO: Franklin Video Seminars.

Caring for children with special needs: The Americans with Disabilities Act and child care. (1993). San Francisco, CA: Child Care Law Center.

Cochrane, C., & Woods, W. (Eds.) (1992). *Desk reference on the Americans with Disabilities Act.* Richmond, VA: The Association for Persons in Supported Employment.

Compliance guide to the Americans with Disabilities Act. (1990). Washington, D.C.: Small Business Legislative Council.

Doggett, L., & George, J. (1993). *All kids count: Child care and the Americans with Disabilities Act.* Richmond, VA: The Association for Persons in Supported Employment.

Ellexson, M.T., Kornblau, B.L. (1993). *Functional job analysis and pre-placement screening.* [videorecording]. (1990). Cleveland, OH: Classic Video.

Every page spelled liberty. [videorecording]. (1990). Cleveland, OH: Classic Video.

Fasman, Z.D. (1992). *What businesses must know about the ADA: 1992 compliance guide.* Washington, D.C.: U.S. Chamber of Commerce.

Foos, D.O., & Peck, N.C. (1992). *How libraries must comply with the Americans with Disabilities Act (ADA).* Phoenix, AZ: Oryx.

Gostin, L.O., & Beyer, H.A. (1993). *Implementing the Americans with Disabilities Act: Rights and responsibilities of all Americans.* Baltimore, MD: Paul H. Brookes.

Jarrow, J.E. (1992). *Title by title: The ADA's impact on post-secondary education.* Columbus, OH: Association on Higher Education and Disability.

Kailes, J.I., & Jones, D. (1993). *A guide to planning accessible meetings.* Houston, TX: ILRU Program.

The National Senior Citizens Law Center. (1992). ***Implementation of the Americans with Disabilities Act.*** Washington, D.C.: American Association of Retired Persons.

Parry, J. (Ed.) (1992). ***The Americans With Disabilities Act manual: State and local public accommodations.*** Washington, D.C: American Bar Association.

Providing public transportation to everyone [videorecording]. (1992). Chicago, IL: National Easter Seal Society.

Scott, K.M. (1988). ***The Americans with Disabilities Act: What will it mean to you?*** Silver Spring, MD: Governor's Planning Council on Developmental Disabilities.

Wehman, P. (1993). ***The ADA mandate for social change.*** Baltimore, MD: Paul H. Brookes.

West, Jane (Ed.). (1991). ***The Americans with Disabilities Act from policy to practice.*** New York, NY: Milbank Memorial Fund.

Work in progress. [videorecording]. (1993). Raleigh, NC: Barrier Free Environments.

Zuckerman, D., Debenham, K., & Moore, K. (1993). ***The ADA and people with mental illness: A resource manual for employees.*** Washington, D.C.: American Bar Association.

Appendix B

An Example of A Disabilities Awareness Event

Legislative Forum

A good way to increase public awareness about disability issues is to host a legislative forum in your community. The forum has two purposes: 1) it educates people about disability issues by facilitating a lively discussion; and 2) it gives state and federal legislators an opportunity to discuss disability legislation that is underway as well as listen to constituents' concerns.

Planning the Event

Before inviting legislators, make sure a location is available to hold the event. Generally, when legislators make a local appearance, especially to discuss issues, there is a large crowd. Choose a location with a large stage area for the legislators to sit or a podium where they can easily be seen. There should be plenty of seating for the audience.

You should also make sure the location is accessible for wheelchair users and provide an interpreter for people who are deaf. The Governor's Planning Council has resource material on how to plan an accessible meeting. For more information, call the Council at (Voice) (317) 232-7770 or (317) 232-7771.

Free and ample parking is another consideration when choosing a location.

It is important to schedule legislators weeks or even months in advance. Their availability depends on the schedule of the legislative session. If you know when legislators will be on recess, try to schedule the legislative forum during that time. Hopefully, you will be able to have the forum in March to coincide with Disabilities Awareness Month. If not, it is still an excellent event to improve community awareness. And, a well-organized legislative forum can be just as beneficial to legislators as it is to your community.

Call the offices of your local and federal representatives. Explain that your group is organizing a legislative forum and would like the senator or representatives to participate. Provide the details of the forum, including topic of discussion, date, time , place (if known), and other invited participants. You can describe the topic of discussion as local disability issues and concerns and request a progress report on new or pending disability legislation.

The legislative assistant will probably ask you to send a formal request in writing (see same on page 406). If so, mail it right away and then follow-up a few days later to make sure the letter was received. Since it may take awhile to get a response, the sooner you make the initial contact with the representatives' offices, the better. Once all the invited legislators have responded, sent a confirmation letter to those who will be attending the forum (see sample on page 409). One week prior, to the event, contact the legislators' offices to reconfirm.

Room Setup

Coordinate with the building manager or your contact about how you want the stage and audience areas setup. This includes seating, sound, and lighting. If legislators will be sitting panel style, have a microphone for each of them. Or, if you are using a podium, have a microphone attached to the podium. Arrange for two or three standing microphones to be placed around the room so audience members can ask questions.

Ask someone from your group to be Hospitality Chairperson. That person will be responsible for making name cards to sit in front of each legislator, if applicable, or name tags. A pitcher of water and glasses should be available for the legislators. The Hospitality Chairperson should also greet legislators and media representatives at the event.

One week prior to the event, reconfirm the room reservation and all equipment and setup requests.

Forum Procedure

Ask someone from your community or group who is an active disability advocate and understands local issues to serve as moderator of the forum. Several weeks before the forum, your group should meet with the moderator to determine what issues to discuss and what specific questions to ask the legislators. Once the questions are decided, mail copies to all the legislators that are attending so they can prepare.

It will be the moderator's job to keep the discussion on track. He or she will present an issue and pose a question. The moderator should also make sure that each legislator gets a chance to respond. Since the discussion might lead to other issues, it is important that the moderator has a solid understanding of disability issues so he can ad lib other questions. This part of the forum should last about on hour and then discussion should be opened to the audience. Have a set time for the question and answer session. Limit each audience member to one question and two minutes at the microphone. Try to keep the forum no longer than two hours since the legislators have other obligations.

Media Relations

Approximately three weeks before the event, send a calendar release to local newspaper editors (see sample on a page 494) and a public service announcement to radio public service directors (see sample on page 495). Call a few days later to make sure the release or PSA was received and ask for the newspaper or station's help in publicizing the event.

One week before the event, fax a media advisory (see sample on page 496) to print and broadcast media outlets. For print publications, attention the advisory to either government reporters, disability reporters, city editors, or photo editors. For broadcast outlets, attention the advisory to government reporters or news directors. Again, follow-up by phone and try to get a confirmation from each media outlet.

At the forum, be sure to take black and white photos to mail to newspapers that did not send a photographer but do accept photos. Also prepare a release about the forum (see sample on page 497), describing the issues and legislation that were discussed. Mail the release to any media outlet that did not send a reporter.

After the event, mail thank you notes to all media outlets that provided coverage before or after the event (see samples on pages 498 & 499). Let the reporter/editor know that the Anytown Planning Council for People with Disabilities appreciated the coverage of the forum since it will help educate people about disability issues in Anytown.

Another way to promote the event is to send notices to community groups and ask them to announce the forum at their meetings.

The Day of the Event

Arrive at the site about an hour early to make sure the room is properly arranged. Check the seating, sound system, and lighting, if necessary, of both the stage and audience areas. Also, check the accessibility of the room for wheelchair users. The Hospitality Chairperson should have the name cards and water pitchers and be ready to meet and greet legislators and media representatives.

Have an information table by the door staffed with representatives from your organization. The person can answer questions, distribute materials about your group or Awareness Month, and serve as a check-in point for legislators and the media. The staff member should remain there throughout the forum in case there are media representatives who show up late.

The moderator will give a brief introduction about Disabilities Awareness Month and your organization and discuss the format of the forum. He or she can then introduce the legislators and begin with the first issue and round of questions. It is the moderator's duty to keep track of time. Remember, try to keep the forum at or under two hours.

Assign someone to take black and white pictures. The pictures should be good quality since you are sending them to newspapers.

During the audience's question and answer session, you and the Hospitality Chairperson can select audience members who have questions. Have one person at each microphone at all times and have the moderator call on audience members in a continuous order. This will keep the questions moving at a steady pace. Each audience member should only ask one question at a time.

After the question and answer session, the moderator should end the forum by thanking the legislators and reminding the audience to celebrate Disabilities Awareness Month. If your group has other events planned, the moderator can discuss those as well.

After the Event

Mail a news release and photo(s) to any print publications that did not attend. Identify everyone in the photo(s) by typing their names on an adhesive label and attaching it to the back of each photo.

The final step is thanking everyone who was involved in the forum. Send thank you letters to the legislative representatives, media representatives, building manager/contact, or anyone else who volunteered their time or resources (again, see samples on pages 412 & 414).

Note: For more information about lobbying or contacting your legislators, the Governor's Planning Council offers a brochure entitled "The Legislative Process." To order a brochure free of charge, please call the Council at (Voice) (317) 232-7770 or (TDD) (317) 232-7771.

Sample Invite Letter for Legislators

Date

Representative Joe Smith
c/o Ann Jones, Legislative Assistant
Indiana General Assembly
Address
City, State Zip

Dear Representative Smith:

In celebration of Disabilities Awareness Month, the Anytown Planning Council for People with Disabilities is hosting a legislative forum to discuss disability issues. We invite you to be part of our legislative panel to discuss the progress of disability legislation and to listen to the concerns of constituents with and without disabilities.

The forum will take place Tuesday, March 3 at 7 P.M. in the Anytown High School Auditorium. Our group will provide you with a list of issues and questions to be discussed. There will also be an audience question and answer session. The forum should last no longer than two hours.

We hope this forum will serve as an educational tool for you and people in our community and will demonstrate that people with disabilities are vital, contributing members of the community. Our goal is to raise awareness of disability issues and disability-related legislation.

We appreciate your support of people with disabilities and hope to see you at the forum. I'll be contacting your legislative assistant, Ann Jones, to confirm your attendance.

Sincerely,

John Doe
President
Anytown Planning Council for People with Disabilities

Sample Confirmation Letter for Legislators

Date

Representative Joe Smith
c/o Ann Jones, Legislative Assistant
Indiana General Assembly
Address
City, State Zip

Dear Representative Smith:

The Anytown Planning Council for People with Disabilities is pleased that you will be participating in our Disabilities Awareness Month Legislative Forum.

The Forum will take place Tuesday, Mach 3, at 7 p.m. at the Anytown High School Auditorium. Please plan on arriving at the school approximately 15 minutes early. The forum should last no longer than two hours.

Enclosed are disability issues that will be addressed at the forum as well as a list of questions. We would also like for you to give the audience an update on recent or pending disability legislation.

Please call me at (555) 123-4567 if you have any questions. I look forward to seeing you in March.

Sincerely,

John Doe
President
Anytown Planning Council for People with Disabilities

enclosure

Sample Calendar Release

For Immediate Release
Date

Contact:
Your name
Your phone

CALENDAR RELEASE

The Anytown Planning Council for People with Disabilities is hosting a Legislative Forum in celebration of Disabilities Awareness Month on Tuesday, March 3 at 7 p.m. at the Anytown High School Auditorium. (List participating legislators) will discuss local and national disability issues and recent or pending legislation. There will be an open question and answer session at the end. The forum is open to the public and admission is free. For more information, contact John Doe at 123-4567.

Sample Radio PSA

Your Name
Your Phone

Start: February __, 19__
Stop: March __, 19__

Time: 15 seconds

Legislative Forum

ANNOUNCER: IN CELEBRATION OF DISABILITIES AWARENESS MONTH, THE ANYTOWN PLANNING COUNCIL FOR PEOPLE WITH DISABILITIES IS HOSTING A LEGISLATIVE FORUM, TUESDAY MARCH 3 AT 7 P.M. AT THE ANYTOWN HIGH SCHOOL AUDITORIUM. STATE AND FEDERAL LEGISLATORS WILL DISCUSS DISABILITY ISSUES AND RELATED LEGISLATION AND ANSWER AUDIENCE QUESTIONS. THE EVENT IS FREE AND OPEN TO THE PUBLIC.

Sample Media Advisory

For Immediate Release
Date

Contact:
Your Name
Your Phone

MEDIA ADVISORY

What Disabilities Awareness Month Legislative Forum

State and federal legislative representative will discuss disability issues on the local and national levels and report on recent or pending legislation. Audience members will be able to ask questions at the end of the program.

Who List participating legislators and titles

When Tuesday, March 3, 7-9 p.m.

Where Anytown High School Auditorium

Why March is Disabilities Awareness Month. The Anytown Planning Council for People with Disabilities is sponsoring the forum to increase public under standing about disability issues.

Note The forum is open to the public. Admission is free.

Sample News Release

For Immediate Release	Contact:
Date	Your Name
	Your Phone

Legislators Discuss Disability Issues at Public Forum

Anytown, Ind.—(List legislators and titles) attended a legislative forum hosted by the Anytown Planning Council for People with Disabilities last night at Anytown High School. Local and federal disability issues were discussed as well as recent and pending disability legislation such as (specify legislation).

"The legislative forum was a good way to raise awareness about The abilities of people with disabilities as well as the disability issues facing our community," said John Doe, president of the Anytown Planning Council for People with Disabilities, which hosted the event.

Representative Joe Smith reported on disability legislation in the Indiana General Assembly. (Give details...)

The legislators answered questions posed by Moderator Sue Johnson, title, for about one hour, followed by questions from the audience. Approximately (give no.) people attended the forum, which was one of several Disabilities Awareness Month activities planned throughout the month.

Sample Thank You Letter for Legislators

Date

Representative Joe Smith
c/o Ann Jones, Legislative Assistant

Indiana General Assembly
Address
City, State Zip

Dear Representative Smith:

On behalf of the Anytown Planning Council for People with Disabilities, thank you for participating in the Disabilities Awareness Month Legislative Forum.

The forum provided our residents with important information about disability issues and hopefully increased awareness and understanding. We hope that you gained some insight about concerns facing our community. We're pleased to have legislators such as you that are truly interested in listening to the concerns of people with disabilities, their families, and friends.

Sincerely,

John Does
President
Anytown Planning Council for People with Disabilities

Sample Thank You Letter for Media

Date

Ms. Jane Doe
City Editor
The Anytown Courier
Address
City, State Zip

Dear Ms. Doe:

On behalf of the Anytown Planning Council for People with Disabilities, thank you for providing pre- and post-event coverage of the Disabilities Awareness Month Legislative Forum.

The forum provided Anytown residents with important information about disability issues as well as an opportunity to express their concerns with legislators. We hope our community will continue to study the issues and work toward improving opportunities for people with disabilities.

We appreciate your interest in increasing disability awareness.

Sincerely,

John Doe
President
Anytown Planning Council for People with Disabilities

Legislative Forum Timeline Checklist

**This timeline checklist should b adjusted accordingly to your specific planning time frame.

Three months before the forum:

_____ Check the availability of locations that are suited for the forum.

_____ Based on location availability, select a date for the forum.

_____ Contact your legislators' offices and invite them to participate in the forum.

_____ Mail a written request to legislators after the initial phone call.

Two months before the forum:

_____ Confirm the legislators' participation.

_____ Confer with the building manager/contact about the room arrangement, sound and lighting, and accessibility.

_____ Appoint a Hospitality Chairperson and assign him or her duties.

_____ Assign duties to other members of your organization.

_____ Send flyers/notices to other members of your organization.

One month before the forum:

_____ Ask a community representative who is an active disability advocate to serve as moderator of the forum.

Three weeks before the forum:

_____ Mail the calendar release to newspaper editors and the PSA to radio public service directors.

Two weeks before the event:

_____ Meet with volunteers to discuss last minute details and their duties the day of the event.

One week before the event:

_____ Reconfirm with legislators.

_____ Reconfirm location reservation, equipment needs, and room arrangement with building manager/contact.

_____ Mail the media advisory.

The material located in Appendix B was provided by The Indiana Governor's Planning Council for People with Disabilities, (5-LF-95).

Index

AUTHORS' PAGE

Charles C. (Charlie) Bullock became professor and chair of the Department of Health Ecology at the University of Nevada, Reno, on July 1, 1996. Prior to that, Dr. Bullock was on the faculty of the Curriculum in Leisure Studies and Recreation Administration at the University of North Carolina at Chapel Hill for 17 years. While at the UNC at Chapel Hill, he was chair of the curriculum from 1995-96. He was also founder and director of the Center for Recreation and Disability Studies, which brought together creative, innovative, and forward-thinking professionals to conceive and conduct exemplary training, research, and demonstration projects in the area of recreation and disability. He is past president of the National Consortium of Physical Education and Recreation of Persons with Disabilities. During his professional career, Charlie has written, presented, and consulted extensively in the areas of special recreation, therapeutic recreation, integration, reintegration, transition, and leisure education.

Michael J. (Mike) Mahon is professor, Associate Dean, and Director of the Health, Leisure, and Human Performance Research Institute in the faculty of Physical Education and Recreation Studies at the University of Manitoba, Canada. Dr. Mahon has been actively involved in the disability field as both a practitioner and researcher for over 15 years. He first worked as program director of Manitoba and Canadian Special Olympics before joining the faculty of Physical Education and Recreation Studies at the University of Manitoba in 1989. During a leave from the faculty to complete his Ph.D., he was a research associate at the Center for Recreation and Disability Studies, Curriculum in Leisure Studies and Recreation Administration, University of North Carolina at Chapel Hill. His current research, which focuses in the area in the area of disability and aging, includes numerous presentations, articles, and book chapters on decision making, leisure education, efficacy research, and social integration over the life span and later life planning for persons with mental disabilities. He is a past coeditor of the Therapeutic Recreation Journal and past chair of the Research Committee for the Canadian Centre for Disability Studies.